MORE THAN ONE WAY

Day Hiking
the Appalachian Trail

Dennis Heller

©2014 More than One Way, LLC

ISBN: 978-0-578-13648-6

More than One Way, LLC
PMB #281
3140 Tilghman Street
Allentown, PA 18104

www.more-than-one-way.com

Printed in the United States of America

Contents

Foreword

I was driving home to Pennsylvania from southwest Virginia after hiking four days on the Appalachian Trail (AT). I had stayed at Woods Hole, enjoying the hospitality of Michael and Neville. It was early May of 2011, and I was beginning my tenth year of AT section hiking. I had met many hikers at Woods Hole this trip, all with a story of some sort. I decided that I have a story about my adventures on the trail as well. Writing would be a stretch for me though. Accountants are notoriously horrible at writing. My adventures would undoubtedly include the stories of the people I had met. Did I have enough, or too much to say? Do I have the skill? None of that really matters much. This book was rattling around in my head, and it had to come out. I will tell the story, and maybe some others will read it. I believe it will bring some fond memories to those who have hiked all or parts of the trail.

I had few notes from the last ten years, but lots of pictures to trigger my memory. The names had faded. I sometimes changed or invented names or trail names to protect anonymity, or if I could not remember the real names. There are no composite characters. I had a rudimentary log of the date of each day's hike. I mean *day's hike,* because I truly am a day hiker. To this point I have not slept on the ground once, even though I have hiked over half of the trail (the middle half). Instead, I meet a shuttle each morning, leave my car at my end point, get shuttled to my start point, and hike back to my car. I almost always hike alone. I stay mostly in inexpensive motels, and eat in sports bars each night. A cold beer and a shower after a hike can be the best part of the day. Actually, for the first five years, I did not even stay in motels or drink the beer. I was just driving a lot. I'd get up early, drive to my starting point, meet my shuttle, hike, and then drive home. Eventually I got too far from Pennsylvania to do that anymore. I began to stay over in an area and hike three, and then more, days at a time. I have still put almost 100,000 miles on my car in the last three years, and countless miles on my feet.

Who am I? When I started hiking the AT in 2002, I was 54 years old. I'd been married to Virginia since 1970, and we had two great kids who had recently both graduated from college. Virginia and I met at Penn State, where we both graduated in 1969, she with high distinction in elementary education. I was in the top five fifths of my class in the business school. We settled in Allentown, Pennsylvania. It was the big city for me, growing up in Boyertown, Pennsylvania, twenty miles down the road. Virginia was from Westfield, New Jersey. She went to Gettysburg College for a year before transferring to Penn State. Virginia taught first grade for seven years before we had Ben and Bethany. I went to work for a local CPA firm in 1969. I was a much better accountant than I was a student. I passed the CPA exam in 1972 on my first try, and became a partner in the firm in 1975. In many ways, I was in the right place at the right time. I have had only that one job. For over thirty years, building my career and family was my main focus. I worked hard and put in long hours. Long hours were an expected part of the profession at the time.

Benjamin was born in 1978, and Virginia has been raising the family ever since. She is the glue and support system for all of us. Ben was always a special kid. He's spoken like an adult since he was three. He was always good in school. He played some soccer and was on the high school tennis team. I coached his youth baseball team when he was 8 to 10 years old. He took piano lessons for four years, and then switched to the French horn. He was an all-state band French horn player. Ben scored 1560 on his SATs (800 in math) and was accepted to the Penn State honor's college on a full tuition scholarship. When he finished in December of 2000, he was the student marshal of the business school, graduating with the highest GPA of the thousand or so students. He went to work for a boutique consulting firm in New York City. After about five years, he gave up the road warrior life for a job in sourcing with a large national industrial gas company. He and his wife Michelle gave us our first grandchild, John, in October of 2011.

Our daughter Bethany was born in 1980, and always had her dad wrapped around her little finger. She would dispute that. She was quiet, since Ben was more verbal and tended to dominate family dinner. That changed later. Bethany started piano lessons about a year after Ben, and took off to be a star pianist in the area. She accompanied the elementary, junior high and high school chorus' and won the area "Friends of Music" competition. She won another competition, with the prize being organ lessons, and during her high school years she was an organist at a small local church. I was her softball coach in local youth leagues for nine years, from ages 9 to 17. I coached one more year without her, but coaching was not the same after she gave up the sport. Bethany got some scholarships to go to Indiana University in Bloomington Indiana as a piano performance major. She graduated in just three years, in 2001. She had strong communication and interpersonal skills, and to combine those with her love of music, she got a job in sales with Steinway and Sons in the New York City area. She paid her dues in a retail showroom and visiting churches, but in four years became the institutional sales manager for the New York metro area. Juilliard and Yale became her customers. She married her best friend from college, Kevin, in 2005.

But that's enough about me and my family. Why did I start to hike the trail? I was a Boy Scout until I was sixteen. I never made Eagle, but was the last step (Life) before it. I was also "Order of the Arrow", but remembered little of that. When I was about 14, in the summer of 1962, I did go to the National Boy Scout Camp, Philmont, in New Mexico. We were out on the trail for about ten days, with a four day bus ride each way. Since high school, I really had not camped or hiked at all. Virginia and the kids never showed any interest, nor did I. We had traveled some, and did Yosemite and maybe a few other parks, but that was it. I was not necessarily looking for something, or felt like something was missing. Even though Ben and Bethany were out on their own and had good jobs with their own health insurance, I felt like I had plenty to do with working, and a full client load. I had grass to cut and golf on weekends. Then, two events may be what set things in motion.

First, my Kiwanis club in Emmaus, Pennsylvania had an AT thru-hiker as a speaker sometime over the winter of 2001-2002. He was an early 20-something and had the usual slide show. I don't remember his talk being particularly inspiring. It was probably not his fault, since his audience were a bunch of ROMEOs (Really Old Men Eating Out). But somehow, the idea of hiking part of the AT was intriguing. It kind of stuck that, if I would hike, it would be with a point of working toward some kind of goal. I would have no interest in hiking just a random trail and coming home and saying that was nice. But, hiking some part of the AT, say, all of Northern Pennsylvania, from the Susquehanna to the Delaware, had an appeal to me. It may have stopped there, but then...

The second event was in May of 2002. I had always loved pictures of Banff in the Canadian Rockies, so Virginia and I took a trip up there. We bought hiking shoes before we went, but really did not need them for the things we did. It seemed like there was a lot of hiking going on, but Virginia clearly was not interested in hiking. Although she would have been happy to let me go off on my own for a day, it did not seem like the Canadian Rockies was a place to learn to hike. We took the gondola up to the top of the mountain near Banff, and I was amazed that people actually hiked up or down the mountain instead of taking the gondola. This almost seemed like suicide. It seemed steep and difficult, and like it would take forever. I think it was a few miles long, and up a few thousand feet.

We drove the Icefields Parkway up to Jasper National Park and stayed there a few days before driving back to Banff. The mountains and lakes were all gorgeous throughout the entire area. We toured around in the rented Jeep. We stopped off at many vistas, but never really had to walk very far. We saw a lot of wildlife. Elk roamed the streets of Banff, and deer were all over Jasper. We walked around the Jasper resort lake during elk rutting season, which horrified Virginia to no end. Female elk are particularly ornery during rutting season. From the dining room, we saw a bear dive into the lake. We even spotted a moose and a wolf on our drive back from Jasper. I think I was becoming hooked on the outdoors.

We came home from Banff, and I joined the Appalachian Trail Conference (as it was called at the time). I bought the book and map set for the AT in Pennsylvania. The ATC publishes very complete book and map sets for each state or pair of states. They can be found through the ATC website or in many bookstores. I loved looking at the maps. After reading the do's and don'ts of hiking, and studying the maps endlessly, I scheduled my first day.

2002 – Starting Out

The closest AT trailhead to our home in Allentown was up at Blue Mountain Summit, on Route 309, on the way up to Tamaqua. For my first day I decided to go easy, and planned a 4.9-mile section from there to the Bake Oven Knob. I just wanted to see what it was like. How hard could it be? Just follow the white blazes. It was Saturday, June 22. Virginia agreed to follow me up to the Bake Oven Knob parking lot. I would leave my car, and then she would drop me off at Route 309. She was on her way to a bridal shower at Lake Hauto. The road up to the Bake Oven Knob parking lot was washed out quite a bit. Virginia was horrified, but we made it. I had an old backpack from one of the kids' high school days. I had plenty of water and other items from the AT book checklist. At this point in my life, I was generally overweight (not sure, but maybe over 225 pounds at 6 feet) and out of shape. I'm not sure I realized it at the time.

The first two miles were easy, along an old woods road. Then the trail became very rocky, hardly seeming like a trail at all. About a mile later I was on all fours, scrambling across The Cliffs, a knife edge that you can see from the valley below. It was not terribly difficult, but was a little more than I expected. The view from The Cliffs was great, despite the somewhat hazy day. The valley floor went on for miles, it seemed. In another half-mile I came to Bear Rocks. I could hear voices, and there were four packs at the intersection of the blue-blazed trail to the top, where there were 360 degree views. Somewhat intimidated by the rock pile, I just continued on to the parking lot. To my amazement, my car was there. That is the beauty of maps. Out of the woods at the far end of the parking lot was a mountain of a southbound thru-hiker. He had a large pack and a long beard. He did not stop, and disappeared into the woods.

At the office the next week, people asked how my hike went. I said I enjoyed it, but it was a little harder than I'd expected. The trail over the last few miles was very rocky. There was little climbing, as most of the trail in this part of Pennsylvania runs across the top of the ridge of the mountains.

Almost a year later, on Father's day of 2003, Bethany and I hiked the section again. I was much more "experienced" then. We both scrambled across The Cliffs, and we both climbed Bear Rocks. It was a very nice day. There were some clouds, but it was not as hazy as the year before, so all the views were great.

My second day on the trail was a week after my first, on June 29. Ben came with me. Ben was working in New York City for a consulting firm, but came home on weekends to see his girlfriend (and us). I was in my still-new hiking shoes that I had bought for our trip to Banff. Ben was in sneakers and gym shorts. Off we drove in our two cars to Lehigh Gap, to leave a car on the south side of the river. Then we headed back to Bake Oven Knob, and up the washed-out dirt road. I did not really have a plan about where to hike next, but this just seemed logical. We started our hike, and soon arrived at Bake Oven Knob. The area around it was disappointing, as this was obviously a gathering point for area teens to have beer parties. Trash and beer cans were strewn all over. We did not stick around, as we had a full 8.4 miles to hike to get to the car. During the day, we came to very open areas along the top of the ridge that had great views, especially to the northwest. You could see the Pennsylvania Turnpike; actually, in this section we hiked *over* the turnpike tunnel, which burrows through the mountain far below.

After lunch, we arrived at the junction of the North Trail, off of which there was a side trail leading down to Devil's Pulpit. The side trail was extremely steep, and it seemed like we were bushwhacking down the side of the mountain; but there were blue blazes marking this "trail". I led the way down. The view from Devil's Pulpit was fantastic. I had driven through Lehigh Gap for years. This area around Palmerton, Pennsylvania was just beginning to recover. Years of zinc mining had decimated the vegetation. The steep mountains on either side of the river made a dramatic scene. I barely made it back up the quarter-mile trail. I had to stop and catch my breath multiple times. Ben was waiting for me at the top.

The 2-mile hike down the mountain seemed steep and annoying. There were rocks, and what seemed like an uncomfortable grade. About halfway down we stopped at the Outerbridge Shelter for a snack. This was actually the first shelter that I saw on the trail. Shelters are mostly three-sided structures, with an overhanging roof and a wood floor. They hold anywhere from 6 to 20 people. This particular shelter apparently does not get much use, since it is a short two miles into town from Lehigh Gap. Long-distance hikers need the stop in Palmerton to resupply, and often stay in the jail (with permission). I was tired from the side trip to Devil's Pulpit, and was glad when we got to Ben's car.

My third Saturday (July 6) in a row, I was up in Lehigh Gap again, starting my next section. I left my car in Delps (where?) at a parking lot about a mile down a side trail from the AT. It seemed logical, since it was halfway through the 20 miles of Section 2 (Lehigh Gap to Wind Gap). Delps and the parking lot seemed hard to find, but after asking three different neighbors, Virginia and I got there. It might have been smarter to leave my car at Smith Gap Road, but that would have meant a lot more driving around the north side of the mountain. The trail down from the AT to the Delps parking lot was very steep, but was mitigated somewhat by wonderful rock steps that someone had built many years before.

Virginia dropped me off on the southwest side of the bridge, where I immediately met Tin Man and Godiva. They were married thru-hikers who had stayed alone at the George W. Outerbridge Shelter the night before. They had enough supplies, so did not plan to go into Palmerton. They had been hiking since April, and explained to me that they were maybe the tail end of the thru-hikers for the season, since most thru-hikers who reached Katahdin, Maine (the northern terminus of the AT) before it closes for the winter were through Pennsylvania by the Fourth of July. They were hopeful to make it to Katahdin. I wonder if they did.

I went ahead, across the bridge over the Lehigh River, up the road, through the parking lot and started the climb up out of Lehigh Gap. Wow. Since I had studied the maps and elevation endlessly, I knew the climb was about 1,000 up in about a mile. I did not know what that meant, exactly. It was tough, and I had to stop multiple times to catch my breath. At one point I did not think I could pull myself up, and almost quit. I couldn't quit. My car was 10 miles ahead. Tin Man blew by with his huge pack, followed shortly by Godiva. I was nervous, but I made it up the steepest part; but it kept going up. I was scrambling up through the rocky hillside. The views of Lehigh Gap were again spectacular. I could identify Devil's Pulpit across the way. It was a beautiful day, but hot, and I was sweating like a pig. At the top, the trail leveled off, and soon entered the woods. There were still plenty of rocks on the trail, but I made good time, and was cruising as I was approaching Little Gap. I met Tin Man and Godiva again, who were taking a break. Just before crossing the road, I noticed multiple crates with gallon jugs of water. It was a dry year, and trail angels were leaving water and some snacks for thru-hikers. Several years later, I recall reading in the newspaper that there were fires up on this mountain during the hiking season. The local trail angels posted themselves at times to shuttle the hikers around the fire, since the trail was closed.

I crossed the road and started up a steep 400 foot climb. I was soon breathing hard again. Tin Man and Godiva passed me like I was standing still. The rest of the hike did not seem too difficult. I was a little worried that I might not find the junction with the Delps Trail, but right on cue, Tin Man and Godiva were there, resting. I offered that my car was at the bottom of the hill if they needed anything or needed to resupply, but they were only 10 miles from Wind Gap, and were fine. They had made it 1,300 miles without me, I guess, so I did not persist. I was encouraged that I was able to keep pace (more or less) with thru-hikers. They did have the handicap of 30 pounds on their backs. I headed down the Delps Trail and reached my car, tired but happy. I have heard people say that sometimes the best part of a hiking day is getting back to your car. The tough climbs out of Lehigh and Little Gaps gave me a lot of satisfaction and feeling of accomplishment. I had hiked over 11 miles, including the hike down. My feet were killing me, but somehow I felt good.

I actually let two weeks go by until Saturday, July 20. Virginia and I found Delps again, and she dropped me at the top of the borough of Wind

Gap. After getting lost in a mobile home park, I realized that the trail followed the road, crossing under Route 33, followed by a left turn and up a 500-foot climb via switchbacks up out of Wind Gap. The climb included some scrambling up some rock piles on hillsides. It surprised me that there would not have been an easier way, but I have learned that trail builders are not trying to make it easier, but more interesting. Once on top of the ridge, I was cruising for the rest of the day. There were some good views along the way, both north and south. I passed the shelter and Smith Gap Road, then down the Delps Trail to my car. During my first few days, I saw only a limited number of people; and other than Tin Man and Godiva, did not really talk to people that much. Most were local people. All the thru-hikers had been through. Between being stiff and having sore feet, the drives home were not always that pleasant.

On Sunday, August 4, I left my car in Wind Gap, and Virginia took me up to the Route 191 trailhead at Fox Gap, 8.6 miles from my car. Sarbanes Oxley was signed into law that week, reflecting the accountancy scandals such as Enron and WorldCom. These scandals had a large effect on my profession, although not necessarily my practice.

Since the trail intersected Route 191 right at the top of the mountain, there was virtually no climbing that day. The trail could not have been more level. During the day, I met a retired couple from New York State. They were section-hiking from Delaware Water Gap to Lehigh Gap on this trip. They had two cars. They were camping some and staying in inexpensive motels some. He had jury-rigged a white handkerchief under his hat to keep the bugs away. There was an easy descent down into Wind Gap. I was looking forward to my next day, since I would then have completed Pennsylvania sections 1, 2 and 3, from Delaware Water Gap to Blue Mountain Summit. I felt like I was making some progress. I started to think in terms of making it to the Susquehanna River that year, and therefore finishing half of Pennsylvania. It seemed like a doable goal.

On Sunday, August 10, Bethany offered to join me on the hike from Delaware Water Gap to Route 191. Bethany finished college in three years and had been working for a year for Steinway and Sons. She shared an apartment in Hoboken, New Jersey with a nurse who was also just out of school.

Bethany was paying her dues and learning in her sales job with Steinway, but it was great, since it kept her in the music industry that she loved. It would ultimately be a great fit for her. She became the institutional sales manager for them. She has wonderful interpersonal skills, and was becoming quite an outstanding young woman. She did seem to honestly want to hike with her dad. How great was that?

The hike southbound out of Delaware Water Gap was spectacular. Although it was up 1,000 feet over two miles to the top of Mount Minsi, it did not seem that difficult. There were lots of places to view the Delaware River and the I-80 corridor on the way up, so Dad could rest often. The last five miles were partially open along some old roads, and then some very rocky sections through the woods. The rocks were a little problematic for Bethany, since she was in sneakers. We stopped at the Kirkridge Shelter. Two guys were there just chillin'. I think they were section-hiking. Bethany got their attention, so we moved on.

We met a couple from Philadelphia who liked to hike the AT. They were doing in and outs and seemed envious that we had two cars and did not have to retrace our steps. We drove back to Delaware Water Gap to get my car, had lunch in a nice restaurant, and then Bethany was on her way back to Hoboken, New Jersey.

It was less than a year since 9/11. Since Ben and Bethany both lived in the New York City area at the time, they were greatly affected, as we all were. Ben was sharing an apartment in Brooklyn, but was in London on the day of the attacks. He actually phoned Bethany in Hoboken to alert her of what was going on. Bethany and her roommate went down to the water in Hoboken (just across the Hudson from Manhattan) just after the Towers came down. When Ben got back to New York City, he took a week's vacation to volunteer with the Red Cross.

I drove back to Allentown with my sore feet. I did not know how I could ever hike more than one day at a time.

I was encouraged that I had hiked 50 contiguous miles. It seemed like some sort of milestone. I was becoming pleased with myself, and began talking about it.

For my next time out, I planned the hike from Hawk Mountain Road back to Route 309 at Blue Mountain Summit. A semi-retired partner at the firm who lived in that area near Kempton said that he'd hiked in that area as a Boy Scout a lot, and to watch out for the rattlesnakes. I never saw any. It was August 16, a Friday, and I did not see a soul on the trail that day. Other days so far it might be 4-8 people, mostly locals or section-hikers. Shortly after Virginia dropped me off, I got bitten by a large horsefly. I bled all over my cotton shirt. I still had not graduated to synthetic shirts, and was usually soaked at the end of each day. It was the normal hot and humid summer in Pennsylvania, and a very dry year. Many of the springs that the long-distance hikers relied on were dry. Trail angels seemed to be helping out by leaving jugs of water near the trailheads. I never had to worry about it, since I always carried the water I needed for the day.

About a mile from Hawk Mountain Road, the trail started to climb. The trail was good, but fairly steep. It was 1,000 feet up to Dan's Pulpit, over two miles. Dan conducted Sunday services there back in the day. I took the little side trip to Tri-County Corner, atop a pile of rocks with some good views of Berks, Lehigh and Schuylkill counties. There was a mixture of easy old woods road-type of trail, and some extremely rocky sections that were starting to become a pain. Someone explained the difference between a walk and going for a hike was that on a hike, you have to stop to look around and enjoy the scenery. True. I took a break at the Allentown Shelter. It seemed new, and had its own outhouse. The hike out to the road was on easier trail, almost a passable road, and it seemed to me that the Allentown Shelter could be accessed by Jeep or pickup. I logged 11 miles that day.

On Monday, August 26, I took another day's vacation to do my longest section to date, over 14 miles from Port Clinton to Route 183. This was a stretch. There were some side trails to break up the section, but I passed on those. I had to wait for a train to pass before crossing the tracks to start the climb out of Port Clinton. The trains out of Port Clinton are mostly fall foliage tours. We were getting close to that time of year. Actually, many leaves were already down with the drought, which I really noticed this day. It was very steep coming up out of Port Clinton, and I was soaked with sweat after the first mile, 1,000 feet up. This is the Northern Pennsylvania theme. You climb up out of the trailhead gaps, but then it's hiking across the top of a flat ridge. There were rocks galore on the trail for much of this day. I could begin to see why many people quit in Pennsylvania. If you were hiking day after day in these rocky sections, it could get to you. There were times it was just not fun. Hikers who reside in Pennsylvania respond that, "Yes, we grow rocks," or "Yes, we sharpen the rocks," when outsiders complain about the rocky trail in Pennsylvania.

It was a clear day, and there was a great view at Auburn Lookout. I did run into an older couple just out for the day. They were hiking some sort of loop on those side trails. They were amazed that I would be hiking the full 14-mile section. The trail got better around the Eagles Nest Shelter. I went to the shelter even though it was a third of a mile off the trail. There was a small ravine that you had to navigate. I'm not sure why the shelter needed to be this far from the trail. It was probably because of the spring a little bit further on the way to the Eagles Nest Lookout. The trail seemed to be going through a wooded area where there were mostly saplings. It was like walking through a forest of sticks. There were multiple crossings with forest service roads in this area. Some had quite wide right of ways, maybe because of fire breaks. By the time I got to the parking lot at Route 183 I was exhausted and sore (feet and pack straps). Driving the 40 miles home was tough.

The next Saturday, I decided on a short section. I would hike six miles in the morning, and be home in time for the Penn State football game. We dropped my car at the Hamburg Reservoir near the Windsor Furnace Shelter, and Virginia drove me back over to the Port Clinton train station. I crossed over, and then went down along the Schuylkill River. It was early, and cooler than I had been used to. I went under Route 61 and then up, fairly steep at first, then not so bad. On the way up there we some views through the trees back down into the Schuylkill River Valley. Since it was a Saturday, there was some activity in this area, including some on horse-back, which was permitted in the area. The parking lot was full, and I could barely get my car out. This lot is used heavily on weekends for outings up to the Pinnacle. I think I beat Virginia home (she ran some errands) which annoyed her. She likes the days of solitude when I'm out hiking.

I was getting into this hiking business, and was out the next Saturday on September 7, my tenth day out. Virginia drove me back to the Hamburg reservoir, and then off we went to Hawk Mountain Road. It was a long and steady climb up to the ridge. I passed a troop of Boy Scouts who were out for an overnight. The leaders were bringing up the rear, some gasping for air with the heavy packs. Then came a heavy kid or two. The rabbits were out in front. They were strung out over a mile or so. I don't believe they were going far. I was always surprised about the relatively few miles that scout or college groups that I met on the trail, had planned. I guess when you have a diverse group, you have to tone down the mileage to suit those of lesser ability. It only makes sense. I still thought they were wimps. I was now a tough, experienced hiker.

Once on top of the ridge, I could cruise on easy trail on to the Pinnacle. The Pinnacle is considered the best view on the AT in Pennsylvania. It was busy. People were sunning themselves. There was the token 20-something yuppie with his dog with doggie backpacks. I stopped to have lunch and enjoy the view. I think I could pick out Little Round Top, which the semi-retired partner from the firm talked about. I got sweaty palms when people would get close to the edge.

The trail down to Windsor Furnace was much more rocky and difficult than the way up. There were some short-but-steep descents. Overall it was flat to Pulpit Rock (not to be confused with Dan's Pulpit), where there was another good view. I must have passed 100 people of all shapes and sizes on their way up to the Pinnacle. This was no easy hike, I thought. Would they all make it without getting hurt? Maybe *I* am the wimp. The view at Pulpit Rock was similar to the Pinnacle, so I did not dillydally, and was soon on my way down to my car. The parking lot was a zoo. I made a note to myself; if I ever take the family up to the Pinnacle, don't go on a fall weekend.

I had now hiked 90 contiguous miles for the year. It might have been a stopping point, but I was up for more.

The next Saturday, September 14, Virginia followed me out to the trailhead at Route 501 off of I-78. We then proceeded to Swatara Gap, two miles north of Lickdale. She took some pictures at the historic Waterville Bridge. The pictures are not kind to me. I looked very overweight. I'm not sure this hiking is helping the weight problem. Over the years since, I have learned that exercise alone does not do it for me. I really had to change the way I ate.

At the office, I was king of the donuts. Since I worked all the time during tax season, I would finish all of Saturday's leftover donuts on Sunday (and be proud of it). Oh well, it took me a while longer to get that to sink in. The exercise could not hurt.

I would return to Swatara Gap a few years later to reciprocate for a shuttle driver who helped me immensely in Connecticut. Greg, who was retired military and a retired prison guard and now driving a school bus, had hiked a lot of the trail in New England, and was working on Pennsylvania. Greg knew a lot about the trail and talked a lot about the Green Mountains, the "Whites", and the "Mahoosucs." I was not always sure what he was referring to, since those areas were not on my radar yet. He had a passion for the trail, and it was infectious.

I picked Greg up at Port Clinton one weekday morning and took him out to Swatara Gap. It was VERY hot. I was sweating in my shirt and tie as I took a few pictures for him, even though it was only about 8:00 A.M. I worked that day, and then later visited my parents. I only used my cell phone in the car, and it was off most of the time at that point. When I left my parents, I had a voicemail from Greg. With the hot and humid day, he was in trouble. He had run out of water, and was suffering from dehydration. He had called about 2:00 P.M. and it was now 6:00 P.M. I felt terrible. I called him back right away. With great difficulty, he'd made it to the Route 501 shelter, was able to get some water, and was starting to recover. I said I would be right up to get him, but he had already made arrangements with a Trail Angel that was close by and had a sign at the Route 501 shelter. The Angel would pick him up and take him back to his car shortly. Greg told me later that he collapsed in a motel room at the Route 61/I-78 intersection near Cabela's, and when he woke the next morning, realized he had left the door to his room open all night. It took him a week to recover fully.

Getting back to my day's hike; over the Waterville Bridge I went, onto an old macadam road and under I-81. It would be the first of four times I would cross I-81. Crossing an interstate highway was always a milestone to me. As usual, there was the initial climb out of Swatara Gap. As usual, it was a total of 1,000 feet; steep at first, and then very gradual. My hiking pace seemed very fixed. I would cover an average of two miles an hour, including breaks. If I hiked 10 miles, I would be at my car in 5 hours. I could almost set my watch by it. I did not hurry or lag, either. I stopped at the viewpoints, and sometimes the shelters. The viewpoints were truly the rewards of hiking. I also just liked the idea of working toward a goal of the AT. I had no delusions and did not admit that I was trying to hike the whole trail. Right now, I was just thinking of getting to the Susquehanna River at Duncannon this year.

Before I knew it, I was at the William Penn Shelter. I did not actually see the new shelter, since there was an older, smaller one that held four people right on the trail. As I approached Route 501, I came to Kimmel's Lookout. There were two unattended hang gliders there. It looked like a good spot for it. Years later, Ben, Bethany, Kevin and I would try hang gliding. I'll leave that story for another time. The miracle of the map worked again, and I came out right at my car.

The following Thursday, I filled in the section between Route 183 and Route 501. Virginia dropped me at Route 183 after leaving my car at Route 501. I'm not sure why I did it in this direction, since it added driving. Both the Route 183 and Route 501 trailheads are at the top of the ridge of the Blue Ridge Mountains, so there would be little climbing this day.

Soon after the start, there was a historical marker showing the site of an old fort, Dietrich Snyder, that was used by the local militia in the French and Indian War. I snapped a picture and was off. I arrived in Shubert's Gap, a pretty area in a low on the ridge. I took the blue-blazed side trail down to a nearby pond and dam. The water was very green with algae, and still. The dam was out of place in the middle of nowhere. It was hard to figure its origin, and there did not seem to be any nearby roads, either visually or on the map. I stayed in Shubert's Gap for lunch. While there, a man appeared. He seemed about my age, with a big pack. He was from New Jersey, and after I told him I was from Pennsylvania, he said, "I hate Pennsylvania." He had been section-hiking the trail over the years, and was backpacking a large part of Pennsylvania this time, starting in Delaware Water Gap. He did not seem to be having fun, and was cranky. After about two weeks out, the rocks on the trail were getting to him.

I hiked out of Shubert's Gap and on to my car. I stopped at the Route

501 Shelter, which was more of a large cabin. It had electricity, tables and chairs. It had an outdoor cold-water shower. There was a caretaker of sorts who lived in a nearby house, who sold sodas and snacks. It was the nicest shelter that I have seen on the trail to the point that I am writing this.

I was now at 111 miles on the trail in 12 days of hiking.

A few weeks went by, but I had the itch, so I took another day off from work on Wednesday, October 2. I had planned a few previous days, but rain or threat of rain delayed me. I was definitely a fair-weather hiker. I joked that if there was greater than a thirty percent chance of showers, I would not go out. I had met enough long-distance hikers by now who had slogged through a rainy couple of days. They did not have fun.

Hiking the section near Indiantown Gap Military Reservation seemed difficult logistically. It was 17 miles, with no road breaks. I studied the map and book endlessly, and figured out that I could go through the base and use the Cold Spring Trail for access to the AT. I was stretching Virginia's limits. This day did not help. We dropped my car at Swatara Gap, and then proceeded to the base. I was somewhat familiar with the base, since I had been in the Pennsylvania National Guard. I spent a few summer camps there. It was an "open base," though after 9/11 I thought there might be some additional security. I did call the base, and they said it was no problem to go on the base to access the trail. We proceeded up Cold Spring Road, and the big red "Caution: Watch for Tanks and Track Vehicles" sign was intimidating to Virginia. She hung tough and took me all the way into the state game lands parking lot. The road after leaving the base was horrible, but it was only a mile or so. It was important that Virginia had her small SUV (RAV4). A car would not have made it. There were a few trucks at the parking lot, hunters scouting, I thought. She dropped me off and headed out.

It was a 1-mile hike up the Cold Spring Trail to the AT junction. The hike into Rausch Gap was easy and interesting. Back in the 1800s, there had been coal mining activity here. It seemed remote. Rausch Gap was interesting as well. It was a pleasant area. An old railroad bed had been transformed into a nice rail trail. Some bikers were taking advantage of the nice day. A sign indicated the Village of Rausch Gap had as many as 1,000 people living there, and I enjoyed looking around what little was left of tiny houses and buildings (just rudimentary foundations) and an old well. I wandered down into the creek to take a picture of an old railroad bridge, and slipped and fell on a mossy rock and got very wet.

The hike out to Swatara Gap was a mixture of open areas on easy, old roads and some rocky trails. I met a local woman who hiked this area almost every day. She seemed interested in "my story" of having hiked over 100 miles of the AT this year. It took a while, but I eventually spied my car parked along Route 72.

The next Sunday, October 6, we were off again. The drives were getting longer as we had to go out past Harrisburg and up along the Susquehanna River to Dauphin. The trailhead was at the top of the ridge at Route 225. The trail crossing at Route 225 was considered dangerous, since it was at the top of the hill, and somewhat blind in either direction. A few years later, I read in *A. T. Journeys* that the ATC built a hiker bridge across the road. On my way to a Penn State football game a year or so after that, I stopped to look at it. It was beautiful, and must have cost a fortune. Being an accountant, I wondered about the cost benefit; but I guess it was a big safety thing. I had not heard if anyone had actually been hurt, or of any close calls at the crossing.

It seemed like a long drive out Route 325 to the trailhead. From there it was 9.4 miles to my car. It was an immediate strong climb (800 feet) up out of Clark's Valley. The trail on most of this section before the shelter was very rocky, a prelude of things to come for the northbound thru-hiker. There was a gorgeous view down into the valley. The hawks were flying in full force. I reached the Peter's Mountain Shelter. I almost missed it, since the tiny (sleeps four) old shelter was still there. The new shelter was gorgeous. It was a 2-story design with a loft for sleeping and room for tables. For maybe the first time, I read the hiker's journal in the shelter. The theme for southbound hikers was "they could hardly wait to get to Duncannon (10 miles south) to get some pizza." I enjoyed the peace over lunch. On my way out, I got a picture of Table Rock, the first of many table rocks along the trail. About a mile from my car, I met Dave from Baltimore. He was about my age, and backpacking about 60 miles on the AT this trip. He was on his way to the shelter. He asked about water there, and I said that there was a sign there that the nearby spring was dry. That was problematic for him, but I gave him all my remaining water since I was only a mile from my car. He seemed to be a great guy, and loved being out. He would be able to get water at the creek in Clark's Valley. Water is always a big issue for the long-distance hiker. I never had to worry about it.

A few Sundays later, on October 20, Bethany and her boyfriend Kevin wanted to go out with me, so we decided to hike the New Jersey side of the Delaware Water Gap. After dropping a car at Camp Road about eight miles up the trail, we started at the parking lot, a beautiful area about a mile in from the I-80 bridge. This meant I had a gap of a few "road walk" miles across the I-80 Bridge, since Bethany and I had started in a parking lot in Delaware Water Gap a few months before. I thought I would come back sometime to hike that gap over the bridge. I have not yet as I am writing this, but I will. There is a pledge that some thru-hikers make about passing every white blaze. I personally don't get too excited about not doing a road walk, but I have and will go out of my way to make up for a missed section on actual trail. To each, his own.

The hike up to Sunfish Pond was a steady climb, not too taxing. There were a lot of people out, as it was a beautiful day. It was about 1,000 feet, but over 2 ½ miles. I had a bright-orange T-shirt on, which Virginia insisted I wear because of hunting season. We passed some hikers who had been out for the weekend who wanted to know about the Penn State game when they saw my hat. We had lunch when we got to Sunfish Pond.

I was at Sunfish Pond about five years later. My baby sister (by 14 months) and two high school friends who were hikers, and with whom she had stayed in touch, wanted to go out. We chose this area, but came up a side trail off of River Road. We got caught in a massive, frightening thunderstorm at Sunfish Pond. It was quite a day. Although we had intended to hike around the pond, we headed down, and had lunch soaking wet in the park below.

The hike on the AT along Sunfish Pond was extremely rocky and actually a little difficult, especially for Bethany, who was in sneakers. The rocky shoreline of the pond had many rock cairns, or sculptures, that creative types had built. I have wondered how these withstand the test of time, but they always seem to. I believe it is a real talent and actually, the advice I have heard is "don't try to build these unless you know what you are doing."

The hike along the ridge had many great views, both east and west down to the Delaware River. I have a lot of great pictures. I took a lot with the disposable cameras I was still buying. There must have been 50 people at the last wonderful, unnamed viewpoint. I'm not sure where they all hiked up from. The hike down to Camp Road was not that long or steep, but seemed uncomfortable. I took a picture of Bethany and Kevin at the bridge over the creek at Camp Road. I have a similar one of Ben a few years later. We had some pizza on the way back to the Gap, and Bethany and Kevin were off to Hoboken.

In was Saturday, November 9. The Angels had beaten the Giants in the World Series. It would be my last day out for the year, so I decided I would like to make the 7-mile hike out to the Susquehanna River from Route 225. I would not quite make my goal of doing everything north of the Susquehanna, since I still had the other half of the section through Indiantown Gap. I dropped my car at the north side of the bridge at Clark's Ferry. Virginia dropped me back at the top of the ridge, and off she went. I snapped a cute picture of her RAV4 headed down the hill. She had a 2-hour drive home. The hike along the ridgeline was rocky, but no climbing. At the shelter there were two guys from Maryland. They had left work on Friday evening in Washington DC and were just out for the weekend. They got to Clark's Ferry after dark and hiked in with their headlamps. I did not even own one, which I promptly went out to get the next week. It was a cold night and even though it was around 11:00AM, they were just getting moving for the day. I think they were headed up to Peters Mountain shelter and then back to Maryland. The hike down from the shelter was great. The path got better, and there were many great views of the Susquehanna. Then finally, the Route 322 bridge came into view between the trees. I felt like I had accomplished something.

I was new to it, but I had hiked 145 miles on 16 different days of the year. I reflected on the drive home (sore feet and all) about my new hobby.

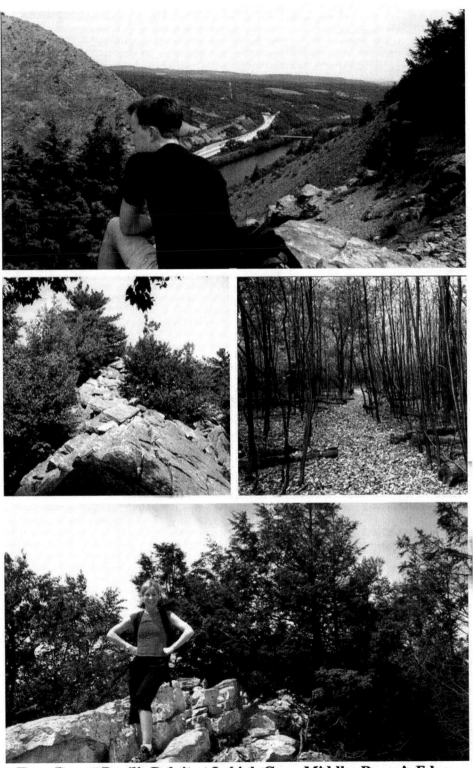

Top: Ben at Devil's Pulpit at Lehigh Gap. Middle: Razor's Edge; Forest of Sticks. Bottom: Bethany at Bear Rocks.

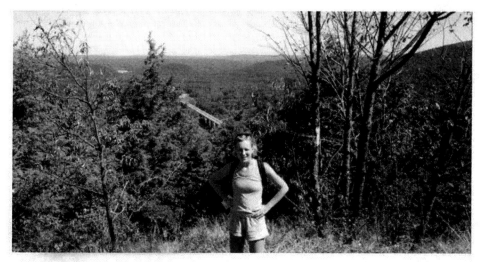

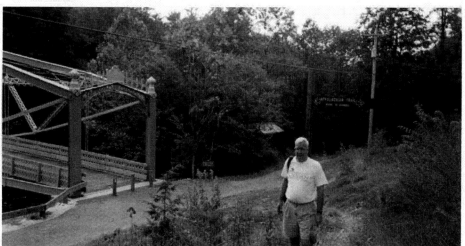

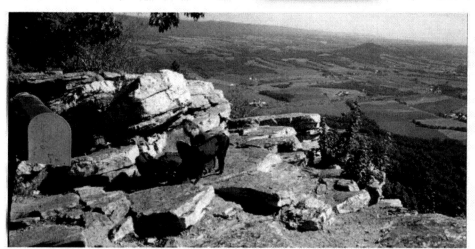

**Top: Bethany at Delaware Water Gap. Middle: Waterville Bridge
Bottom: The Pinnacle.**

2003 – Penn's Woods

The fall/winter of 2002-2003 was eventful. Ben and Michelle got engaged on November 23, and planned to get married in August of 2003. Ben proposed after the final home game at Penn State, on the field. Michelle was in the Blue Band. Ben and Michelle were in the Blue Band seven straight years, but never together. Ben had graduated in December of 2000, as did Michelle, and was working in New York City. Michelle stayed at Penn State and was working on her PhD in bio-mechanical engineering. They were both in the Honors College. You could add their GPAs together and divide by four, and I would have barely been above them.

The US had launched a war against Iraq, and the Columbia space shuttle exploded. The Tampa Bay Buccaneers won the Super Bowl.

My first day out hiking was unfinished business. It was that 8.7-mile section from Clark's Valley into Indiantown Gap. I'm not sure why I did not get out until Tuesday, June 10. Tax seasons were running longer. Virginia followed me up the tank road, but we decided that the road down to the Cold Springs trailhead would not suit my sedan, so I parked at the top of the hill. Off we went to Clark's Valley. It was a nice day, but it had rained the day before, and the trail was very wet. In fact, running water was pouring down the trail from Stony Mountain. The trail was wet, steep and rocky all the way up. I reached the junction of the Horseshoe Trail which goes all the way to Valley Forge, 137 miles away.

Past Stony Mountain, the section was dark woods all the way to Yellow Springs Village, an abandoned coal mining community. Unlike Rausch Gap Village 10 miles to the north, there was little that remained. I might have missed the village altogether except for a mailbox with hand-painted letters on its side. There was a trail journal in the mailbox.

Down the Cold Spring trail I went, and started the climb up the road; but a hunter who was scouting the state game lands picked me up and took me to my car. I drove around the military base a little before heading home. Soon after I had bought some new hiking shoes, I discovered that the ones I had been wearing for a year were 1 ½ sizes too small. Dumb me. I won't be whining about my feet anymore!

The next Sunday was Father's Day, and Bethany and I hiked out to Bake Oven Knob. For Father's Day, Bethany bought me a new day pack, so I did not have to use the old one from her high school days.

On Friday, June 27, I left my car at Route 850, an open area next to farmer's fields. Virginia drove me back to Clark's Ferry. This would be Virginia's last day of shuttling me for now. It was only fair. The drives were getting long, and Virginia was always worried about getting lost in some of the more remote areas. It was just not her thing. She drove four hours this day, as did I.

When she dropped me at the Clark's Ferry Bridge, several thru-hikers were starting their ascent up Peter's Mountain. I noticed that one was not wearing hiking boots, but a pair of some sort of hiking sandals with his wool socks. Footwear on the trail is varied, to say the least. I crossed the bridge and started the street walk through Duncannon. I did not stop, not even at the infamous hotel (The Doyle) where thru-hikers often stay. Many thru-hikers do not have much good to say about The Doyle, with its hot upstairs rooms and windows that do not open. Duncannon is a popular trail town, with pizza shops and plenty of beer. On the other side of town, the trail turns, and heads straight up Cove Mountain. After crossing a rock slide, I almost stepped on a box turtle. There were several great, sweaty-palm views from Cove Mountain down into the Susquehanna Valley. It was a nice, clear day, and you could see miles of farmlands to the north.

I encountered a set of thru-hikers about my age or older, two men and a woman. They had large packs, and were lunching on cans of tuna. They seemed weary, especially the woman, who seemed envious that I was day-hiking. I did not have a sense of how far they would make it. Thousands start at Springer Mountain in Georgia each year, and only a few hundred actually make it to Katahdin, Maine in the same year. Some never finish.

When I reached my car, there was a woman sitting on a lawn chair next to her car, with a cooler next to her. She was a Trail Angel, just waiting for hikers to come by so she could offer them a soda. I don't think business was that brisk this day. After a brief chat, I was off to Allentown.

Back home, I began my search for shuttle drivers. Fortunately, the ATC website has a shuttle list of those willing to assist hikers. I hit the jackpot when I called Bob Freeman. Bob was a little older than I, and lived near the trail between Pine Grove Furnace and New Caledonia State Parks. He had thru-hiked the trail. We decided to meet in Boiling Springs at the ATC Regional Office. Bob was very knowledgeable about the trail, and the whole hiking community. Many times he spoke as if I knew what he was referring too, but I was still a greenhorn in most all respects. He, like Greg from Connecticut, clearly had a passion for the trail. He had built a bunkhouse for thru-hikers on his property, and was willing to help them in most any way he could. I'm not sure how many took advantage of his hospitality. During some time in his life he did trail support for some people of means, dropping them off each morning, and then meeting them at the end of their hike and taking them to town, or cooking an evening meal for them. I came to learn the term *slack packer*. They are ones who have full-time trail support, usually family, whom they meet up with each evening. I guess I was one, except I was not doing it day after day. Bob supported one crazy woman who made several failed attempts to thru-hike the AT. He told stories of her leaving her pack halfway through her hike because she was tired, and Bob would hike in to retrieve it.

Bob would shuttle me every day I hiked for the rest of the year. He spoiled me. I tried to be generous with what I paid him, but I'm not sure that is why he continued to help me. He just loved being involved, even with a rookie.

I left my car at Boiling Springs, and Bob took me 8.8 trail miles south to Route 94. It was Tuesday, July 8. Many of my hikes were now on weekdays. I had the vacation time and was not that busy at work in the summer. From Route 94, the trail made a short climb to Rocky Ridge. Trail builders, or the local hiking club, had a sense of humor, as the trail wove through a maze of unusual rock formations when it could have just as easily bypassed this small area. Arrows pointed the way to Maine or Georgia. It took some time for me to get the joke.

There were a few more bumps of a few hundred feet each, and then I reached Center Point Knob, at one time the mid-point of the trail. There was a walk through a field, and then into Boiling Springs along the beautiful lake in town. Boiling Springs had a wonderful ice cream shop. This became SOP, Standard Operating Procedure, whenever possible before the drive home.

A week later, I met Bob at Pine Grove Furnace State Park at the small store in the park. Pine Grove Furnace State Park was a hidden gem. It had a nice lake, and nearby cabins seemed interesting. The days that I was there were fun. The small general store is the home of the half-gallon challenge. Since the exact halfway point on the trail is within the state park, they sell half-gallons of ice cream. The idea is to see if a thru-hiker can eat the full half-gallon. It is harder than it sounds. I resisted the temptation, and went for the ice cream sandwich.

Bob took me up to Route 94, and I hiked back to the park. It was easy trail this day. The worst of the rocks were north of the Susquehanna. Much of the trail was on old woods roads, a trail description that usually made for easy hiking. I stopped for lunch at the Tagg Run Shelter. It was a nice spot, and I was starting to enjoy the trail journals. After lunch, there was the easy climb up to Pole Steeple, a beautiful overlook down to Laurel Lake and a YMCA camp. Pole Steeple was .5 miles off the AT, but well worth the time. There were steep trails up from the lake and camp, and many people were up there, even though it was a Tuesday. Some of the rock lookouts seemed dangerous, and young, unsupervised kids were getting too close to the edge for me. I guess I'm a sissy. The side trail on the way to Pole Steeple had orange tape everywhere. I guess there was a lot of damage to the vegetation, and the caretakers were trying to get it to regenerate by shifting the camping areas. On the way down to the park, I passed a wooden sign showing the exact midpoint of the AT. I understand that the sign has since been retired and replaced. It was 1,069 miles to both Katahdin and Springer. There was easy trail and a road walk along a beautiful creek, then through the park itself.

Three days later, on Friday, July 18, I met Bob at the park again, and he took me down to the Shippensburg-Arendtsville Road to start the 8.3 miles. As Bob dropped me off, a thru-hiker came out of the woods. Bob teased him about being behind schedule, since most of the thru-hikers were through Pennsylvania by now. The top of the ridge at the start of the hike was a very pleasant area, with the best-named side trail (snowmobile) that I have ever seen. It was a former roadbed called "Dead Woman's Hollow Road." I wonder what the story was. It was a very easy hike down, partially through a private game preserve. I wondered what the story was for that, too. This was an easy day, all downhill, and back to the park. I understand that since I was there, a new museum for the AT is located at Pine Grove Furnace. I was sad, leaving the park, but have not been back since.

It was a few weeks later, on Thursday July 31, before I got back out. I met Bob at Caledonia State Park. This park is another hidden gem. Off we went up Route 233 for an easy drive to the trailhead at Shippensburg-Arendtsville Road at the top of Big Flat Ridge. It would be 11.4 miles this day, with much of it flat on the top of the ridge, and then a nice, easy, three-mile decline into the park. About a mile in, I arrived at the Birch Run Shelter. There was a large trail crew at the shelter. They were doing extensive maintenance to prevent water runoff from washing out the trail. They were digging trenches on either side of the trail and creating a "roadbed" of small stone that I believe they had crushed themselves from the fragile rock in the area. All of this is done with hand tools. Very few power tools are used on the trail.

I stopped for lunch at the Milesburn Cabin. The cabin was open, which meant someone was using it, but there was no evidence of anyone being around. There was a dirt road that terminated at the cabin, so people could drive to it. This cabin, and several others, were operated by the Potomac Appalachian Trail Conference (PATC), a mega-club out of DC. The cabin could be rented. It was remote and rough, but I thought it could be a great remote spot for a family getting to know the outdoors. It had a wood stove and some pots and pans and some bunks. It was 2 or 3 rooms.

There was a brief, steep climb from the cabin, and I met a lone wolf trail volunteer about my age. He had a pickaxe-type tool, and was cleaning out the water runoff features that you see a lot of. Thank goodness for all the people who volunteer to keep up the trail. Generally, trail maintenance seems better in the south than in the north. To the point that I am writing this, I have not done any trail maintenance or volunteered for anything. I'm starting to feel guilty about this. Except at the power lines, there were not any good views along this section, but it was easy and pretty.

I soon came to the side by side Quarry Gap Shelters. I stopped for a snack, and was getting tired. The hike down to the park seemed long, and the grade more uncomfortable than it looked on the map. On the way down there was a "tunnel" of rhododendron that was fun. There would be a lot of these, some for miles, on the trail in Virginia.

Ben and Michelle got married on August 16, so the activities leading up to the wedding, and helping Ben close out his Brooklyn apartment, took priority. A few days before the wedding, there was a massive power outage in the New York City area that lasted a full day or so. It affected some of the wedding guests who could not get out of the city. Ben and Michelle would live in State College for the next two years while Michelle continued working toward her PhD. Since Ben was on the road doing consulting work in sourcing, mostly in the auto industry, the State College Airport was fine to get him to Detroit every week. He had become an important member of his firm in just three years. His firm really did not care where he lived.

On Wednesday, August 20, I met Bob at Caledonia again. Bob took me 10.7 trail miles south to a little park at Old Forge. From there it was an easy walk to the twin shelters at Tumbling Run. I was starting to read the trail shelter trail journals, although there did not seem to be much activity now. There were not many people on the trail. It was in the middle of the week. There was a strong climb up to Chimney Rocks, where there were great views.

For the rest of the day, the trail seemed easy; but there were many rocky areas, and some unusual rock formations that I got pictures of. Crossing Route 30 at Caledonia seemed like a milestone. Once across the road, there was still a nice easy mile along a creek, passing some pavilions with families out for a picnic. The drives home were getting longer.

The following Friday, I met Bob at Old Forge, and we traveled down to Pen Mar. Pen Mar, as the name implies, is at the border of Pennsylvania and Maryland. It seemed important to me, but I was still not finished with Pennsylvania, since I had a 16-mile gap up north of Boiling Springs. In Pen Mar, the trail went through a little park, although back in the day, there was a large amusement park that people came from miles to see. I understand that Camp David is in this general area, although you will never find it on any map. For fun, you can ask the locals where it is, to see what they say.

In the pavilion at the park there were some large packs and a few long-distance hikers milling around. Bob went over to talk to them for a while, and then he accompanied me a few yards on the trail north and I got a picture of him at the Mason-Dixon Line. He took one of me at the welcome to Pennsylvania sign.

Bob was off, and there was a little down to Falls Creek, and then a climb. It was an uneventful day, with no views. In three hours I was at the Antietam Shelter. Getting over Antietam Creek was not an easy task, but soon I was back at Old Forge.

There was only one section left to complete Pennsylvania.

The following Saturday, September 6, I met Bob at Boiling Springs, and he took me for the approximately one-hour drive to Route 850. There were a lot of back roads, and it was tough to get around the mountain. I told Bob this would be my last day for the year. He indicated that he was more than willing to shuttle me down into Maryland when I got to it. I did not have a plan beyond Pennsylvania. Although it was 16.6 miles on the trail, my longest to date, the last 13 miles was about as flat as it could be, through the farmlands of the Cumberland Valley. I thought even I could do that, although I was still carrying 210 pounds without my pack. A picture someone took of me from a viewpoint this day at the top of Little Mountain was an unkind reminder.

The trail from Route 850 went up through some fields, and then into the woods. For the first time, I was carrying a Sony Walkman because I wanted to listen to the Penn State game during the long day. That did not work that great, and Penn State lost (they went through some bad years and JoePa came close to losing his job.) I somehow lost the trail going up to the Darlington Shelter, but soon found it. After the hike down from Blue

Mountain, as expected there were farm fields, many road walks and crossings, and some of the hikes were along roads just on the other side of a tree line. I rescued a box turtle from a hard-top road. Within a short stretch, I crossed I-81 (for the second time), Harrisburg Pike on a single-lane pedestrian bridge, and the Pennsylvania Turnpike.

The Conodoquinet (obviously an American Indian name) Creek was very high and muddy from a heavy rain that week. It was a pleasant day, and refreshing along the water. The way into Boiling Springs got long, and I was exhausted when I got to the ATC office parking lot. There were some long-distance hikers on the office porch, but I was too timid to talk to them much to see which direction they were going, or what their story was. I would get better at that. I still felt like a novice, though I now had a story to tell. I had hiked the entire AT in Pennsylvania. For 2003, the log said 93 miles in 9 days, not duplicating the Father's Day hike with Bethany to Bake Oven Knob. My cumulative log is all 229 miles of Pennsylvania in 24 days, plus 9 miles in New Jersey in one day.

Total miles are now 238.

The ice cream shop helped to rejuvenate me for the ride home.

It now seems crazy that I was done for the year on September 6, but I had reached my goal, and was not motivated to do any more, despite the coming glorious fall hiking season. I could still not fathom setting a goal of the whole trail. It did not seem within reach. I did believe I would keep going though, to see how far I might get. I figured I might need to relearn how to camp. I stopped at Cabela's on the way home and bought a sleep pad, a mess kit, a stove and some fuel. To date, I have not used the sleep pad, and only used the stove when we had a power outage at home.

Apple opened its iTunes music store. For 99 cents you could download practically any song ever written.

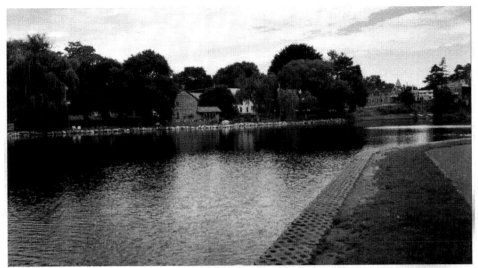

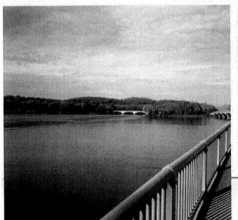
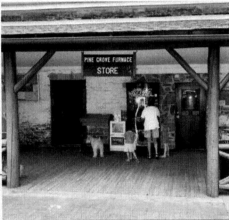

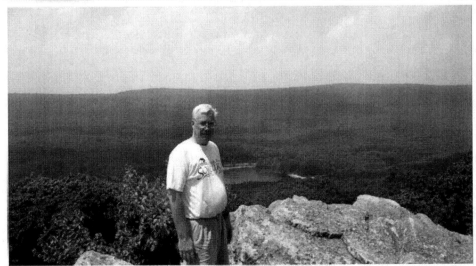

Top: Boiling Springs. Middle: Susquehanna River; Home of the Half Gallon Challenge. Bottom: Pole Steeple.

2004 – South from Pen Mar

Tax season seemed better this winter. The Queen Mary 2 made its maiden voyage, and Janet Jackson had a wardrobe malfunction at the Super Bowl (distracting everyone from the New England Patriots winning over the Carolina Panthers). San Francisco began issuing marriage licenses to same-sex couples. I went on the popular South Beach diet with Virginia's help and lost 32 pounds (2 bowling balls). I felt bad when my local bagel shop closed a few months later. Although I would gain over half of it back over the next few years, at least I would never see 210 again.

I called Bob Freeman, but for some reason he did not explain, he was not taking slack packers below Pen Mar anymore. I wished him the best, and to this day I am grateful to him. I went back to the AT shuttle list. On Saturday, April 24, I met John at Pen Mar Park. He seemed in a hurry, and I was not sure why he had put himself on the shuttle list. We did not connect, and were polar opposites politically; but I appreciated the one ride he gave me for my first hike of the year from Wolfsville Road back up to Pen Mar, 9.6 trail miles.

Starting from Wolfsville Road, in a few hundred yards I arrived at the Ensign Cowall Shelter. Since it was a 3-hour drive from home, I stopped to have a snack and read the trail journal. It was too early for thru-hikers, so there was not much in the journal. This section was partially on private land, and the trail was on a driveway. This was rare, since the ATC has been doing a masterful job of acquiring land in the trail corridor. Perhaps they have acquired this by now. A trail relocation was in the works, according to my guide. There were some steep and rocky, but brief, ups and downs, and some road crossings.

I did not go to the Devils Racecourse Shelter, so did not see the boulder field. Soon I arrived at High Rock. It was a beautiful spring day, but warm, and there were great views to the northwest. High Rock was interesting, and at one point had a pavilion on it. Someone had painted "High Rock" in big red script letters on top of a yellow sun. You can easily drive up there, which might be smart, since the hike up from Pen Mar would be challenging. On my way down, for two miles the trail was steep, and extremely rocky. Since it was a nice Saturday, there were some people out for the day, and some families with young kids, and the dads in tow breathing heavily. Several asked me how far to the top, and they looked crushed when I said I had left High Rock a half an hour before.

There was a short, easy last mile to Pen Mar Park, then off to the ice cream store and the drive home.

I arranged shuttles with Lee, an outfitter from Harpers Ferry, for my next four Maryland hikes. Lee was hard to get hold of, and I'm not sure he owned a watch, but he did always show up, eventually. He met me at Wolfsville Road and took me the 13.4 trail miles to Alternate Route 40 in Turners Gap. Turners Gap was at the top of the hill from Boonsboro. There was a beautiful stone chapel, and the 200-year-old South Mountain Inn, used by several presidents. Food and Drink for all, the sign said. I understand that they have great burgers, but I was not ever there at a good time.

The hike was easy up to the Washington Monument (of Boonsboro), built in 1827. It looked like an old-style milk bottle, about 50 feet tall. A ranger at the park office took my picture. I was looking better with the weight loss. It was Saturday, May 8, so there were people out at the monument. I did not climb to the top of the monument, since I had a long hike ahead. The views were great from the base.

It was an easy trek to the I-70 crossing. A neighbor had a nice welcoming bench and trail journal, just before the wide, fully caged pedestrian bridge over I-70.

A short climb from I-70, and then it was walking along the South Mountain Ridge for the next six miles. There were great views from Annapolis Rocks. It was spring, so there were some wet areas on the trail. It was a long day, but the ice cream stop refreshed for the drive home.

Virginia wanted to go to a weekend conference in Stanford, Connecticut, so I drove up with her and decided to hike up there somewhere on Sunday, May 30. The World War II Memorial had just been dedicated in Washington DC.

It seemed that the nearest AT spot was Bear Mountain in New York. I was able to get a cab at the Bear Mountain Inn, which was still open at the time. The cab took me out to Arden Valley Road to begin my 12.3-mile hike. This whole day would be in Harriman State Park. Near the end of the drive, almost at the trail crossing, I noticed the park at Lake Tiorati, which seemed busy. It was a short, easy walk to the crossing of Seven Lakes Drive. At the crossing I met an older (in their 70s) hiking duo from Philadelphia. I believe they had been out about a week, but did not seem to have gotten very far (about 30 miles). They told me they were out of food, and did not know where they were. They had large packs, and the man in charge of this operation seemed cavalier about their situation. The woman (I don't think they were married, just friends or even acquaintances) seemed a little more concerned. I showed them where they were, and then gave them my map and some excess food. They were headed south, and I was headed north. In the direction they were going, there was not really a resupply point that I could see, but I was not familiar with the area. I told them it was a short road walk to the park (with refreshment stand) at Lake Tiorati, where I had noticed a ranger. They did not want to do the road walk because they had a dog. Off they went on the trail. I was a little concerned for them.

Another two miles and I had lunch at the William Brian Shelter. This shelter was different than most I had seen, since it was made out of stone. It was nice, and well-maintained. This was a popular hiking area, with side trails, and it was a nice Sunday. There were a lot of people out. I actually passed a few hikers, maybe moving more quickly with the weight loss. The area and the trail were rocky. There was a nice view of Silver Mine Lake.

At about the 8-mile mark, I came to the lookout on West Mountain. It was great, since you could see the Hudson River and the summit with the tower on Bear Mountain. I knew I would be crossing over Bear Mountain, but it looked so far away. It was three miles to get there with a big down, and then up. I was discouraged, since I was tired already, and it was getting late. All I could do was suck it up and get going. There was a lot of traffic on the Palisades Parkway, so it took a while to cross. It seemed a while until I was doing a partial road walk up to Bear Mountain, then across some open, flat rock areas to the summit. On the way I met a young man, who asked me how to get back to the Inn. I pulled out a map (one I had picked up at the Inn that morning; I had given my AT map to the older couple) and showed him the shortest route and told him which way to go, and then he argued with me. New Yorkers! I knew I was right, but I wished him well, and headed off. The summit of Bear Mountain was jammed with people and cars. There were great views of the Hudson, and you could just barely make out the New York City skyline in the hazy, late-day sky.

It was still a 2-mile steep and rocky hike down to my car at the Bear Mountain Inn. The beach and lake area were crowded, and there was what seemed to be an important soccer game going on in the lawn between the Inn, and the Pavilion with the merry-go-round. They were out of ice cream. I drove back to Stanford to meet Virginia for dinner.

A few weeks came and went, but on Monday, June 21, I was waiting for Lee next to the Old South Mountain Inn. President Ronald Regan had passed away. A blue jay that had babies in a lamp post did not like the fact that I was hanging around, and was zooming around. Lee drove me down to Weverton Road, about three trail miles north of Harpers Ferry. We got to the parking lot, and there were 20 or so young women milling around the parking lot. They were big girls with big packs, a hiking club from around DC, and they planned to be out most of the week. They were headed north, as I was. Some seemed experienced, and for others it was clearly their first time out. I decided I should get ahead of them for the climb up to Weverton Cliffs. The 500 foot climb was on switchbacks, and not too steep. The climbs were not as tough with my weight loss. The view from Weverton Cliffs is one of the best on the trail that I remember, looking down toward Harpers Ferry along the Potomac and the adjacent railroad tracks, with several trains snaking along. It was a beautiful day, and I lingered a while and took a lot of pictures and did not want to leave. But I was doing 14 miles today, so I had to get going. There was a little more climbing to the top of the South Mountain Ridge, and then I could cruise.

Around lunchtime, at about 3:00 P.M. (I ate several breakfasts on the long drive down), I arrived at Gathland State Park in Crampton Gap. Crampton Gap was the scene of heavy Civil War fighting. This whole area was replete with Civil War references. Right before the park was a private residence, with a beautiful stone arch. Gathland was a beautiful little park with a museum (closed Mondays), several well-maintained barns, and a large pavilion. Jeff was under the pavilion eating lunch, so I joined him. Jeff, from the Midwest, was one of those true slack packers. Jeff, about 60, had recently retired from a large company, and decided to hike the AT. His wife was on the trip with him, and she dropped him off each morning and picked him up at his planned destination each night. They stayed in local B&Bs for 4 or 5 days, and then headed north to a new area. He had started on Springer Mountain the year before, and this was about their fifth trip to the east. His wife would hit the antique stores or outlets while he hiked. The arrangement suited them both well. We talked for quite a while. He was waiting for his wife to arrive.

The Gathland State Park had a memorial to Civil War Newspaper Correspondents. It looked like a rook on the chess board, but one wall, and was a large, imposing structure. I was off, to the north through a nice lawn, past some ruins, and into the woods. I did not stop at the Crampton Gap Shelter, as it was a quarter-mile off the trail.

There were some more nice views down towards Boonsboro, and about a mile from my car, I hit Fox Gap, where there was another Civil War Monument to a battle there and a small, low-walled cemetery.

At a campground near my car, I thought seriously about taking a shower, but opted for the ice cream instead. It was a long ride home, and I was now getting home well after 8:00 P.M. I had hiked for seven hours, and drove about that much.

On Thursday, July 8, I decided to try to meet Lee at his outfitter place. It was zoo, and he was nowhere to be found, even though I had made prior arrangements with him. He seemed to have capable people running it for him. As usual, he showed up without his watch, and I followed him to leave my car at Weverton Road. We drove through Harpers Ferry, and then down to the trailhead at Key's Gap in West Virginia. After today, I would finish my second state, Maryland.

There is some sort of long day hike or race, where hikers and/or runners try to hike in four states along the AT; Virginia, West Virginia, Maryland and Pennsylvania. I think it is about 40 miles, and they try to do it in 24 hours. That would be beyond my comprehension. I will leave that to the younger crowd.

Soon after Lee dropped me at the West Virginia Route 9 trailhead, I heard a noise of a hiker ahead who seemed to be moving strangely. I caught up to him in short order. His trail name was One Legged Wonder. One Leg had lost his leg in a hunting accident about five years earlier. He was hunting alone, fell, and his gun went off. He would have died had his wife not come out to look for him in the Tennessee woods. He had a prosthetic leg on loan from a medical equipment company. One Leg (aka Scott Rogers) had started his hike in Georgia, and was attempting to hike the entire trail this year. If he would make it, he would be the first "above the knee amputee" to do so. This was so interesting. I almost just went around him after a few words, but then decided that I would just fall in behind him, and we talked all the way to Harpers Ferry.

One Leg's wife and family, including all five of their young children, were following along with him. The family was staying in campgrounds in their camper, and they would meet up with him about once a week. Money was very tight for them. He had created a website to garner support for his effort.

Because One Leg could not keep a normal hiker's pace, he was most always alone. Many people knew of him, but none really hiked with him very long. He was not complaining, that was just the fact. The five miles into Harpers Ferry went by quickly, not by the watch, but in interest. He had discarded most of his books and maps. He decided he was better off just to "take the trail as it comes." He had fallen several times, and once rolled down a hill and could not get back up, so he bushwhacked down to a road (luckily) and eventually got a ride back to the trail. He would do a 2-mile road walk for a Mountain Dew. As we approached Harpers Ferry, One Leg's pace quickened, and he practically ran across the US 340 Bridge over the Shenandoah River.

One Leg was headed to the ATC headquarters office in Harpers Ferry.

They were expecting him, having heard about his story. He got a warm reception there, as do all thru-hikers. Their picture is taken on the porch and kept in a book in order of arrival, so that those behind can see the date that each hiker had made it to this "mid-point" of a thru-hike. Of course we know the true mid-point is 100 miles to the north at Pine Grove Furnace. I might have bypassed the office completely had it not been for One Leg. I felt proud to have my picture taken with him on the porch of the ATC Headquarters.

One Leg planned to stay at a hostel in town, and then meet up with his family the next day. He was then going to drive with them up to Maine to do a flip-flop. He would start again at Katahdin, Maine, and then hike back to Harpers Ferry. I followed One Leg on his journey in Maine through his website, but he was having trouble in the difficult Maine terrain, skipped some sections, and then a family emergency terminated his hike for the year. I wonder if he ever tried to finish. His website is down except for a picture of him and his family. A blog indicated he actually was a featured guest (the bionic hiker) at Trail Days in Damascus in 2011.

I left the ATC office before One Leg, and headed toward downtown Harpers Ferry. On the way, I passed Jefferson Rock. Vandalism was an ongoing problem there. Bill Clinton and Al Gore did some "trail maintenance" there a few years later. I had a burger and a beer at a tavern. I was actually decent enough to go into the tavern, since I had not sweated much this day, having hiked slowly. I lingered on the streets, bought some postcards, went to the historic buildings and read history during the Civil War, at John Brown's Fort. It was a great little town, and I pledged to return, but have not. I asked a tourist to take my picture at "The Point" of the Shenandoah flowing into the Potomac. Then I was off across the footbridge to the Chesapeake and Ohio Canal towpath. The trail followed the towpath for an easy and scenic three miles back to my car.

Over a month went by until Tuesday, August 17, when I was out to do the 13.5-mile West Virginia- Virginia Section 2. I met Lee at his store, and we skirted Harpers Ferry on the way to Key's Gap, where I dropped my car. Then we were off to Snickers Gap on Virginia 7. It was almost 11:00 A.M. before I was hiking, even though I had left home at 5:00 A.M. I noted in my trail guide that this was a rugged day hike. Part of this section was nicknamed "the roller coaster." It did not disappoint. With my broken-in, correctly fitting shoes and my weight loss, I could handle it. Not to say I wasn't tired when I was finished, but I did fine. There were steep ups, and uncomfortable grade downs. Most all of this section had a rocky footpath. There were great views west down into the Shenandoah River Valley.

Someone took my picture at The Lookout, and I did not look too much worse for the wear. I passed the junction of the Blackburn Hostel, but did not take the time to stop. It was getting late. I arrived at the David Lesser Shelter after 4:30 P.M. There were a half-dozen long-distance hikers getting ready for dinner at the nice pavilion. The shelter itself had a deck. I chatted a while with Eric from New Jersey. Eric loved camping, but not hiking. I have learned that there are those who "hike to camp" and those who "camp to hike." Outdoor people often like one or the other more. Eric was apparently not shy, as he was very comfortable in his boxers, no shirt and flip flops. I was on my way, and soon encountered a southbound thru-hiker who was on a mission, with his head down and ear pods in. He did stop long enough to tell me he was headed to the Blackburn Hostel and was trying to make it by the time they put on their pasta dinner. Only the first eight to arrive could partake.

I reached my car at about 6:00 P.M., stopped for ice cream right away, and began the long drive home. I was energized by having done this tough section and had no problem driving, even though I rolled in about midnight. I made it to work the next day.

Six days later, on Monday, August 23, I drove all the way down to Front Royal (almost four hours). I had called the local cab company in advance, but because it was my initial contact with them, I did not want them to travel too far to meet me the first time. I was way early and was impatient, but they were right on time for the scheduled meet at Manassas Gap, right on Route 55 near Linden and an I-66 overpass. *Check*, another interstate crossed. The cab drove me up to Ashby Gap. Dirt back roads seemed to be prevalent, though there were some beautiful properties. We saw a large flock of turkeys. The parking lot for the trailhead was on a side road off of US 50.

It was a long, steady climb out of Ashby Gap, but the trail was good.

Since it was a Monday, there were only a few people out on this section. I did a lot of web-walking. In fact, one of the only people I met said he took care of all the spider webs ahead of me. I was not quick enough to say that I did the same for him. After the junction with the trail to Dick's Dome Shelter (which I did not visit), there was some more easy climbing. Generally, this section did not have much to distinguish it. I did stop at the Manassas Gap Shelter for a late-day snack.

On my drive back out to I-81, I stopped in downtown Front Royal for the first of several visits, which I enjoyed. I'm now getting home after midnight, but energized by my progress (another 12.3 miles).

The following week, on Friday September 3, I was down in the area again. I met the cab at Ashby Gap (the cab company seemed adept at finding the trailheads), and the driver took me up to Snickers Gap. There were more remote dirt roads. The driver seemed happy to get out of town for a while, and the fares were actually more reasonable than I would have thought. This would be another long hike, 14.1 miles, and the days were getting shorter, not that I was pushing darkness yet.

I left Virginia Route 7 at about noon and soon arrived at Bears Den Rocks, with great views of the Shenandoah Valley. I walked up to the Bears Den Hostel and came close to going in, but was too shy. There really did not seem to be much activity anyway, although there was a car. This time of year, the northbound thru-hikers are long gone, and the SOBOs (SouthBounds) have not arrived yet, although there are scant few of them.

After Bears Den, the next 13 miles was undoubtedly the section that created the acronym PUDs, short for Pointless Ups and Downs. It was 300 feet up, followed by 400 feet down, followed by 500 feet up, etc., the whole way to Ashby Gap. No ridge hiking here. The trail was not an easy footpath, either. I stopped at the Sam Moore Shelter, which was deserted. It was a very nice shelter area, and had one of those eating pavilions with a picnic table. I read the trail journal. The last entry was from the night before. It was written by a young girl who was alone and lonely in the shelter. She wondered why no one else had come along to stay. It sounded pathetic.

In a few miles, I actually caught up to her, stopped at a junction of a side trail. She was in her mid-20s and in some sort of transition in her life, and wanted to be out for a few months. She had only been out three or four days so far. She had issues with her father. It all came out. She was from New York or New Jersey. Sympathetic, I decided not to rush on, but to hike with her for a while. She seemed to like the company. She had a huge pack, so the weight she carried made up for my age. I just listened for a few miles and tried to give her minor advice without being judgmental or lecturing.

Just before we reached the next shelter junction, a young man caught up to us, and the three of us hiked along. When we reached the junction, the two of them decided to stay there for the night, and I was on my way. I felt better that she had someone to keep her company that night.

By the time I got to my car at almost 7:00 P.M. I was done, and my feet did hurt. I was not in the habit of calling Virginia during the day, so when I did get cell coverage on the drive out, she was relieved to hear from me. Since I hike alone, I do let her know my exact hike and time estimates, and she knows who to call should she not hear from me by dark. I don't know if my being wiped out from this hike was related, but I did not get out for another month.

I'm not sure why I did not get out until Sunday, October 3, but I had developed a goal for this year. I wanted to get to Thornton Gap at US 211, which is one-third of the way down Skyline Drive in Shenandoah National Park. It would take me three more days to do so. I had finished the longer, tougher days of Northern Virginia. I bought the AT book and map set for Shenandoah. Although the AT parallels Skyline Drive for most of the Drive's 100 miles, the northern end is the exception. The drive down I-81 and then I-66 to Front Royal was long. I was on the road by 5:00 A.M. and met a cab at about 10:30 A.M. at Chester Gap, at the trailhead at VA 522. The cab then took me into the park. I had to pay the daily fee, and then down to milepost 17.7 at Gravel Springs.

I was apparently not thinking after the cab pulled away. Since he dropped me in a small parking lot at Gravel Springs where the AT crossed Skyline Drive, I just left the parking lot and headed south. Oops. After about 15 minutes I realized my mistake, turned around, and headed north. Shenandoah National Park is beautiful. Our family had driven the northern section on a college trip to UVA and Duke. Since it was a Sunday, Skyline Drive was busy, and I would cross it three more times after leaving the parking lot at Gravel Springs for the second time. Even when I was not crossing it, I could hear the cars and motorcycles along the drive. There were wonderful views everywhere, the trail was about as easy as I had seen anywhere, and since I was already on the ridge, there was not much climbing. I started at 2,500 feet, had two easy 500 foot ups, and then down to my car at Chester Gap at 1,000 feet. It was still 13.1 miles, though. At Compton Gap, around Skyline Drive Mile Post 10, the trail leaves Skyline Drive and then exits the park altogether.

Soon after I left the park, I arrived at the Floyd Wayside Shelter, had a snack, and then the easy finish down past Lake Front Royal and some marsh areas. After the hike, I visited downtown Front Royal again, and bought a bunch of postcards for my album. I was in love with Shenandoah, and to this day, when people ask me what the nicest part of the trail is, Shenandoah is the answer.

Five days later, on Friday, October 8, I did the long drive again. I drove myself into the park and met the cab at Gravel Springs. He took me all the way down to Thornton Gap at US 211, and then the cab headed down the west side of 211 because it would be much faster than taking the drive back 30 miles to the northern park entrance. The speed limit on Skyline Drive is 45 MPH and it can seem slow after you are on it for a while. The AT would cross Skyline Drive six times this day, and there would be view after view. It was a beautiful fall day. The leaves were starting to turn. At one point, the trail follows a ridge 50 feet above the drive, and you could see the cars and campers down below. At other times the trail would pass just below the pull-off viewpoints on the drive. At about the 8-mile mark on the hike I came to Elkwallow Wayside, a Skyline Drive tourist stop for souvenirs and snacks. I could get a burger and ice cream to nourish for the remaining six miles I had to go.

Out of Elkwallow, a 1,000-foot climb started up to Hogback Mountain. About halfway up, I stopped at Range View Cabin, one of those PATC cabins that you can rent. I was getting tired, and still had four miles to go. Once I got to the top of Hogback, it was an easy three miles down to my car at Gravel Springs. The 18-mile drive out of the park was great, and I stopped a few times at the views. I could not get enough of Shenandoah. I did not realize it at the time, but it would be four years until I would return, or hike south of Pennsylvania at all.

I still had to finish an 8-mile gap in between Chester Gap at US 522 and Manassas Gap at Virginia 50 and I-66. I had let this go for last because it was short (8 miles) and I would not have to worry as much about darkness, since the days were getting shorter. Saturday, October 30 was a beautiful day, and I was still hiking in shorts and a cotton T-shirt. For the last time I would use the Front Royal Cab Co. I decided that cabs were not a bad way to get shuttles. They were not necessarily the cheapest, but they were not horrible either, and they did often have long drives to meet me and get back to their home base. What I was paying seemed fair, and I appreciated that what they were doing for me was out of the box. I was spending a lot on gas with all the driving, but was saving on motels by doing this one long day at a time. I did not know if I had the stamina to hike more than one day anyway, although with the weight loss and my getting started at a gym, I was definitely in better shape than three years earlier.

The hike would be an 800 foot up and down, and then a 400 foot bump to my car at Manassas Gap. About five miles in I arrived at the Denton Shelter, a beautiful one with a separate eating pavilion. The shelter had a deck, and there was a shower of sorts set up a few hundred feet away. It was beautiful. There was a family from the DC area with two teenagers having lunch under the pavilion. They were out just for the weekend, and would stay at the shelter overnight and then head home. We talked quite a while, and they seemed impressed with my "story" of now having hiked from Thornton Gap all the way through Pennsylvania. I was getting impressed myself. They mentioned that they had seen some bear scat (poop) along the trail. Others I had met this nice day seemed to be talking about bears as well. I was on my way, and there was a road crossing in a clearing and then steps (stile) built over a wooden fence.

On the way up the last bump, I passed some bear scat. There was a corral of sorts, with a great view to the west. It was getting late in the day. The corral seemed out of place, but there was an abandoned house nearby. Soon after, I heard a rustling and a thump just to my right. I was eating an apple and almost choked on it. I looked over, and 20 feet to my right, I saw a bear cub that was apparently climbing a sapling to get some berries. I must have startled it, and it fell out of the tree and was wandering away. Then to my left, I heard more rustling. It was Mama Bear. Oops! I was directly in between. All the books said this is not where you want to be. Mama did not threaten, and actually wandered off in the opposite direction from the cub. Since both were slightly ahead of me, and the books say you should not go toward them, I turned around and headed back south. After a minute or two, I decided I was safe enough, and had only a mile to get to my car. I discarded my apple, made a lot of noise and did not see them again.

For the year, I had done 123 contiguous miles south of Pen Mar in 10 days, plus the one day up at Bear Mountain (12 miles), for a total of 135 miles. In the 3 years, I was at 36 days and 372 miles. I must have driven 4,000 miles this year alone. I did not have a plan for the next year, but one would present itself.

The Boston Red Sox came back from a 0-3 game deficit to defeat the Yankees in the American League Championships, and then went on to win the World Series, breaking the curse of trading Babe Ruth.

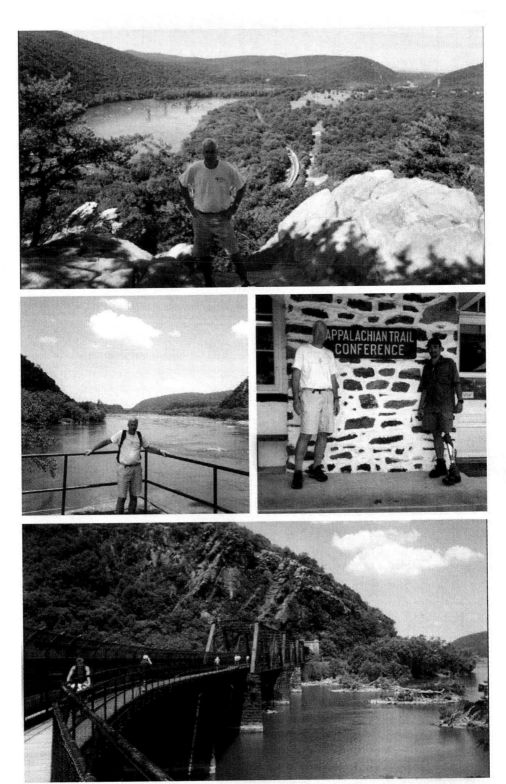

Top: View from Weverton Cliffs. Middle: The Point at Harper's Ferry; Dennis and the One Legged Wonder. Bottom: AT footbridge over the Potomac.

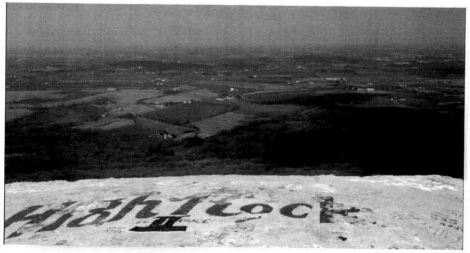

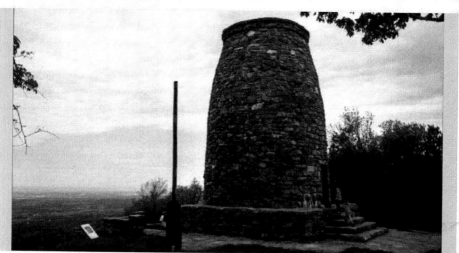

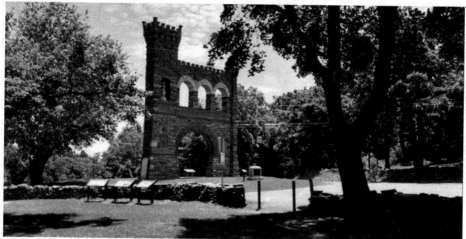

Top: High Rock. Middle: Washington Monument of Boonsboro.
Bottom: Gathland State Park.

2005 – Toward the Hudson

The winter and spring of 2005 were eventful for our family. Our daughter Bethany and her boyfriend Kevin got engaged and were married in June in New York City. Virginia and I decided to downsize from the 5-bedroom, 2-story Colonial in suburbia and found a small house on two wooded acres overlooking the Delaware River just south of Easton, Pennsylvania. The view was as spectacular as any on the trail. It would be a 25-minute commute to work, but we loved the place, which was modeled after a lighthouse in Maryland. Ben's wife Michelle finished her PhD at Penn State, and they were looking to move back to Allentown. Ben and Michelle bought our house. Michelle got a position with a consulting firm in Philadelphia. It would be a 1 ½-hour commute by car and bus. Ben decided to get off the road and got a job with a large local industrial gas company in sourcing.

Condoleezza Rice was sworn in as Secretary of State. New England beat my beloved Eagles in the Super Bowl, YouTube was launched, and the NHL hockey season was cancelled. Michael Jackson was acquitted of molesting a 13-year-old boy at his Neverland Ranch. Lance Armstrong won his seventh consecutive Tour de France.

With the wedding, buying and selling the houses and major outside work to the high-maintenance plant beds, it was Saturday, July 23 when I finally got out to the trail the first time.

Since I could see New Jersey from our new home, it seemed logical to head north on the trail.

I called Ron of the Vernon, New Jersey Taxi. I decided on a section closest to his location, and hiked the 12.5 miles from Quarry Road near Unionville,

New York to New Jersey Route 94 near Vernon. It is maybe the only section of the trail where the southern end of the section is north of the northern end.

After a short climb up from Quarry Road, the trail followed an easy, old road just south of Quarryville, New York, and then came to a paved road and over a bridge. The trail continued in and out of woods and along roads and over streams for the next few miles. I stopped for lunch at the Pochuck Mountain Shelter. A local couple about my age was at the shelter. They were out for a day hike, but soon left so I could read the trail journal.

There was a great view from Pochuck Mountain west to High Point. Although it was raining slightly when I left Quarryville, it had turned into a beautiful day. There was some old puncheon over swampy areas, until I came to County Road 517, where a beautiful, wide boardwalk had been built over the Pochuck Swamp. It went on for almost a mile, and included a suspension bridge. The boardwalk was a popular walking area, and was wheelchair and stroller accessible. Many people were out, and someone took my picture at the bridge. Oops, the weight was starting to come back.

It would be a month on Tuesday, August 23, until I met Ron again at Route 94. Over the next few years, I would spread 200 bags of mulch at our new home, so I did not have a lot of extra time. My drives were not that long this year. I could head up Route 611 and then cross over to New Jersey in Portland, and then up past Blairstown, New Jersey, on Route 94. This year I would be a regular at a sandwich shop in Blairstown to pick up my lunch for the trail. Ron took me up through Warwick, New York, to the trailhead on Route 17A at the top of a ridge just north of Greenwood Lake. I noted the ice cream stand near the trailhead. This would be a day of walking across the top of a ridge, but it would be a long 15 miles. Over the first few miles there were great views down to Greenwood Lake with its island in the middle. Bethany had a customer in Warwick, New York, and actually had an opportunity to get out on the lake with him. I understand it was an exclusive community. Ron of Vernon Taxi had taken Derek Jeter into the city from there. There was a rock climb of sorts, and a wooden ladder up a rock face. Soon I came to the New York/New Jersey border, painted on a rock slab. Sitting at the border was a thru-hiker, maybe in his 70s, with a British accent.

He seemed injured and exhausted, and had a pack that was almost as big as he was. I was not sure if he could make it to the road, let alone to Katahdin. He said he was fine, and headed out. What could I do? I was headed in the opposite direction. It is sometimes a tough call to know what to do when someone seems to be in trouble but insists they are fine.

At the Wawayanda Shelter was one of the first bear boxes that I had seen. The trail journal had various rants from hikers about a guy who had taken peanut butter crackers into his sleeping bag with him at the shelter and was attacked by a bear. He was OK, but the bear had to be put down, and everyone was upset at him about it. The bears are prevalent up in this area, and all precautions are needed.

After going over a dilapidated iron bridge over the Double Kill Stream, there were a series of old woods roads and easy walking until I started the short but steep down to Route 94. Although steep, the difficulty was mitigated by switchbacks and beautiful stone steps. There were a lot of them. *Who does this,* I thought? The construction seemed amazing. After 15 miles I was tired, and taking my time on the steep steps. I soon heard a clatter behind me of hiking poles on the steps. It was Doug from Connecticut. He was in a hurry, but stopped long enough to tell me he was trying to get to the dairy store near the trailhead at Route 94 before closing. Off he went. There was a short, open field walk to my car at the road. I found the dairy store at a farm. Doug was there, and he bought me an ice cream cone. I took him to the hostel at a church in Vernon. He seemed to know exactly where it was, and had been there before.

Doug, it seemed, had been out on the trail for a few years, hiking up and down the AT. He was in his 30s, a big, good-looking guy. He seemed to have some means. He said he liked his life of just being out all the time. I got to thinking that he was hiding from the mob, or maybe his wife's lawyer. Was it my imagination running crazy? Or was I right?

In late August, Hurricane Katrina devastated the Gulf Coast, including New Orleans, when the levy broke.

I had to step it up if I was going to log any miles this year, so I set a tentative goal of trying to finish New Jersey. It was close enough to home, and Ron was working out well for the shuttling. So Friday of Labor Day weekend, on September 2, I met Ron at Culver's Gap trailhead at Route 206, north of Newton and Branchville. The Culver's Lake area seemed nice, and busy with the holiday weekend. Cell coverage was spotty, so we did not connect right away. Eventually we were off to the Highpoint State Park Headquarters north of Sussex to start the 14.3-mile day. Ron took the back roads, which he seemed to know, even though he was a distance from his home base of Vernon. We saw a bear on the way. He dropped me off and I looked around the state park building, but there was not much there. Today's hike was across the flat Kittatinny Ridge. Into the woods behind the HQ building I went.

After about a mile, I snapped a picture of the nice view of Sawmill Lake. Although there were no significant ups or downs, the trail did have some minor rock challenges up and over small humps. New Jersey did have its share of rocky trail. I got a picture of the stone Mashipacong Shelter.

Just before Sunrise Mountain, I encountered a state employee who was recording the trail elevation and mileage on his hand-held GPS. He was taking great care, but did stop to talk. At Sunset Mountain I stopped for lunch near the parking lot, and someone took a picture of me at the benches looking to the east. My cotton shirt was soaked. I did not realize that a few more steps would give me the great 360 degree views at the day shelter.

At the day shelter I met Harvey, from close by the area in New Jersey. He had just started hiking the AT, so it was only his 5th or 6th day out. He seemed impressed with my progress. The day shelter had a roof but no sides, more like a pavilion, with stone columns. It was fairly large, and could have held a dance. You could see the Delaware River to the west. It was a great spot, and anyone could drive up there for the views. This was similar to High Rock down at Pen Mar, where you could drive to a point on the AT with great views. Since I had just taken a break, I did not stay too long.

There was more rocky trail on the way to the Culver Fire Tower. It was built in the 1930s. They permitted climbing on it, but since I'm mostly afraid of heights, I got up no more than one flight of steps to take a few pictures. Soon after, I was doing the 500 foot descent into Culvers Gap and the parking lot.

It would be a few more weeks, on Saturday, September 24, before I could get out again. Mowing my lawn took some work with the banked terraces at our home, and I was still spreading a lot of mulch. I was still doing golf on Sundays, and was still working hard. Ron met me at High Point State Park Headquarters again and took me north to Quarry Road, up near Unionville.

It would be an easy day of only eight miles, and though the elevation gain was 1,000 feet, it was just a gradual up all day. After about a mile in the woods, there was a long, dark section over puncheon through the Vernie Swamp. I stopped and had lunch on the dam of a pond. After lunch, there was an unremarkable, quiet trail through a mixture of woods, farmland and swampy areas. I visited the High Point Shelter, which showed no signs of life, and few recent entries in the log book. It was another stone shelter with a metal roof. Both north and southbound thru-hikers were long gone or had quit because they would not make their goals.

I reached the nice observation platform in High Point State Park. It was about a 2-story deck to get you above the scrub pine tree line so that you could enjoy the views, since by this time you had reached the Kittatinny Ridge. There were people around who had hiked from the nearby monument or park headquarters. Someone took my picture. The weight was coming back more. In another easy one mile up, I was back at my car.

Rather than head home, I drove over to the High Point Monument, which you could see well from the platform. Dumb me, I did not realize what High Point meant; the highest elevation in New Jersey, at 1,803 feet. I came to understand that people have a hobby of getting to the highest point in each state. The beach at the lake of the park was busy for a late September day. The monument parking lot was almost full. The monument very much resembled the Washington Monument in DC. The view from the base of the monument was great, so I did not think it necessary to climb the monument itself. You could see the Delaware River at Port Jervis, New York. Many years before I had started a canoe trip down the Delaware from Port Jervis with the Boy Scouts.

Later that day, Hurricane Rita clobbered the Texas and Louisiana coasts, just a month after Katrina.

I expanded my goals a little, and wanted to fill in all the sections up to the Hudson River. Ron picked me up at the top of the ridge on Route 17A near

Warwick. He took me to a remote trailhead on East Mombasha Road, just off 17A. It was Saturday, October 1. The hike was only nine miles, but there were some challenging ups and downs over small boulders. It was a nice day. I wouldn't be out if it weren't, being the fair-weather hiker that I was. There were good views from the mountain summits.

I hiked down into a ravine next to Fitzgerald Falls. The flow was moderate, as we had not had much rain. The area seemed very remote, and I did not see anyone this day until I got to Cat Rocks, just after the wood-sided Wildcat Shelter. Cat Rocks is a set of boulders that go above tree line, so it afforded 360 degree views. The AT went directly across the top, and I was a little nervous. There were people around, as this was a destination for rock climbers. From there it was an easy hike past the Eastern Pinnacles to my car at 17A. The nearby ice cream store was on my mind all day.

The weather and mulching did not allow me to get out until the end of the month, and I still had three days to fill in all the New York/New Jersey sections to the Hudson. On Saturday, October 29, I met a cab/limo driver out of Greenwood Lake. Ron from Vernon Taxi indicated I was out of his range, but he referred me to this company. I met the driver in town, and he followed me to East Mombasha Road, where I could barely get my car off the road to park. This would be a rewarding day.

On the way to Arden Valley Road at Tiorati Circle, we saw a mother bear followed by five (5) cubs, run across the road right in front of us. What a sight! After being dropped off, I wondered about the older couple that seemed lost, that I had given my map and some food to the previous year on my way to the Bear Mountain Inn. In a short while, I was at the stone Fingerboard Shelter. I got down close enough to it to take a picture. It was in a nice setting, perched on a rock slab. A few snowflakes fell, so I felt I needed to get going. The first part of today would be in Harriman State Park. Harriman is huge, encompassing 100 square miles, 200 miles of hiking trails, and 31 lakes and reservoirs.

The hike was pretty, but the footpath was rocky. There was not much elevation change for the first five miles. There was an extensive signboard at one of the side trail junctions showing 14 short mileages to shelters and roads, and the mileage to Katahdin (793) and Springer (1,365). It must have been old, since it added to only 2158, and the trail is about 2180 or so (my accountants eyes noted). The trail has continual relocations, and today's section had apparently been relocated several times. I went through the "lemon squeezer," where the path goes in between large, high rock formations, and eventually narrows to the point where you must squeeze yourself through.

I met several hiking parties along the way. One was a grandmother with her two teenaged grandsons. They were out for a long weekend. Grandma had a huge pack and was moving very slowly, maybe less than one mile an hour. The two boys seemed very patient. I met another group of four from a hiking club in Maryland. They were motivated AT section-hikers, out for a long weekend, and trying to log about 50 miles or so, with the goal of getting to the Bear Mountain Bridge. At the same time they were disdainful, yet envious of my day-hiking the trail in the manner that I was doing it. Completing the trail is not at all on my radar, or at least I was not admitting it, and said so to them. They were younger and had completed more of the trail, so it was very much their goal.

I had lunch at Island Pond. It was a rain-free day, but cloudy and overcast. There was a chill in the air, and I had to put my golf wind shirt on while I was eating. There was a bridge over the man-made outlet of Island Pond. Soon I was headed down from Green Pond Mountain, and crossed over the New York State Thruway (I-87). *Check.* On I-87, this overpass is marked as Appalachian Trail, so I always looked for it on days that I was headed up to Massachusetts and Vermont in later years.

Once across New York 17 you could see the intimidating cliffs of Arden Mountain. I always looked for those as well, when driving along I-87. Immediately, I began the steep climb called "Agony Grind." It was about 500 feet up in about a third of a mile, and was perhaps my steepest climb to date. The rock steps were big, in some cases 24 inches, making me wonder how shorter people might do it. The view at the top was spectacularly colorful down into the Ramapo River Valley. You could see the ribbons of the Interstate and Route 17 for miles, which made it very interesting. The hardest climbing was over, but still another 200 feet to the Arden Mountain Summit, and then down to Little Dam Lake and over the wood bridge over the lake inlet. My car was right where I left it, and then off to the Greenwood Lake ice cream shop and the 2-hour drive home.

Two weeks later, on Saturday, November 12, Ben offered to come along on my second-to-last hike of the year, from Blue Mountain Lakes Road to Camp Road near Blairstown, New Jersey. Ben was off the road and living at our old house with his wife Michelle. It took only about an hour to get there, so we took two cars. I dropped mine at Camp Road. The trailhead at Camp Road is very near the Mohican Outdoor Center run by the AMC (Appalachian Mountain Club), known mostly for the Highland Center and Huts in the White Mountains of New Hampshire. The AMC's influence runs all through New England, and down into New York and New Jersey. According to the website, the Mohican Outdoor Center offered meals, lodging and outdoor activities during the summer season. It looked nice and at one point, I thought I might stay there on a hike. But it never made sense, since I was only an hour from home. We drove over there, but it was closed for the season.

Ben was driving and I was navigating, and we finally found the trailhead. But we had to leave our car at the bottom of the mountain, in a remote cul-de-sac. The paved road up the mountain was closed off and it was a good thing, because it was not maintained. Once we walked up the steep road, the road on top was fine. The best access would be from the west, but that would have meant a lot more driving.

We found the trail, and this would be a nice, easy day. Ben and I both had jeans and heavy shirts on, which we did not shed at all. It was about as flat a 7-mile day as it could be across the southern part of the Kittatinny Ridge. I have good pictures of Ben and me, each taken toward the views to the east overlooking Fairview Lake and Sand Pond and the Scout camps. On some parts we were walking along a precipitous edge of the side of the mountain.

We arrived at the Catfish Fire Tower. There was a park ranger vehicle parked. I made it up one flight of steps, and decided it was not for me. Luckily, Ben has not inherited my fear of heights, and he climbed to the top of the 80-foot tower and was invited up into the enclosed top by the ranger. I got some good pictures of him at the top of the tower. The views were great from the bottom, and Ben said they were even better from the top. The leaves were all down at the top of the mountain, but there was still a lot of color in the valleys. There was a short but steep descent to Camp Road. A lot of cars jam themselves on the side of the road here, since there is limited parking and it is a popular area for hiking in the state forest. I got a picture of Ben on the same bridge that I had taken one of Bethany and Kevin. It reminded me of a picture we have of Bethany in Yosemite from an overlook down into the valley. In going through some old pictures of my parents, we have one of my sister Melodee, from exactly the same spot taken maybe 40 years earlier on a trip west when we were growing up.

Ben and I retrieved my car, and an hour later we were eating ice cream at the Purple Cow in Easton. Ben headed home after a brief visit with Mom. What a great young man he had become.

There was only one more day to finish everything to the Hudson River. I was out the next Saturday, on November 19. From the AT shuttle list I found George from Newton, who was willing to help me get from the Blue Mountain Lakes Road trailhead up to Culvers Gap at Route 206. George was a teacher, a little younger than I, but talking about retirement. Our politics were not the same. Retiring was not occurring to me.

The hike from Route 206 was an immediate climb of about 400 feet. Once on top, there were many nice views from the ridge looking back to Culvers Lake and then later on, Lake Owassa. All the leaves were down now, and unlike the week before, the color in the valley had vanished. There was no one out in this section today. I did not visit the Brink Road Shelter. The trail was a little rocky. It was not as flat on this part of the Kittatinny Ridge, so I had to work a little. I decided that Pennsylvania had a bum rap for rocks, and that parts of New York and New Jersey were just as much so, but were not as long, only about 70 miles in New Jersey, and 80 miles in New York. This was an 11-mile day. The sky became blue later in the day. I had no concerns about darkness, which would not be until six o'clock or so, and it was still early. All the same, I did not add the extra three miles to see Buttermilk Falls.

After a brief uphill walk on a gravel road, I came to Crater Lake. The AT trail guide said it was a popular cottage community in the early 1900s, but when the government acquired the land, the cottages were razed in the 1970s. I usually wonder about how lakes sustain themselves on the tops of mountains and ridges. It would seem like gravity would drain them, and where does the water come from, with no higher elevation for water to flow from? Could the water table be that high? I'm sure some geologist could explain it. After all, I could see this 16-acre example right in front of me. It was a nice spot, but it was getting late. With about a mile to go, there was a steep rock climb down the face of an escarpment. It seemed safe enough, but I was using all care on the climb down. Once at the bottom, I looked up and took a picture. It was probably about 60 feet straight up, but the trail was well-marked, and there were always good places to put your feet and hold on. Soon I was to the trailhead, and then down the closed road to my car.

Driving home, I felt good about reaching my goal of getting all the sections filled in to the Hudson River; but I had really only hiked 8 days this year, for a total of 86 miles. With buying the new house and Bethany's wedding, we'd had a lot going on. It would have to do.

Total miles are now 458.

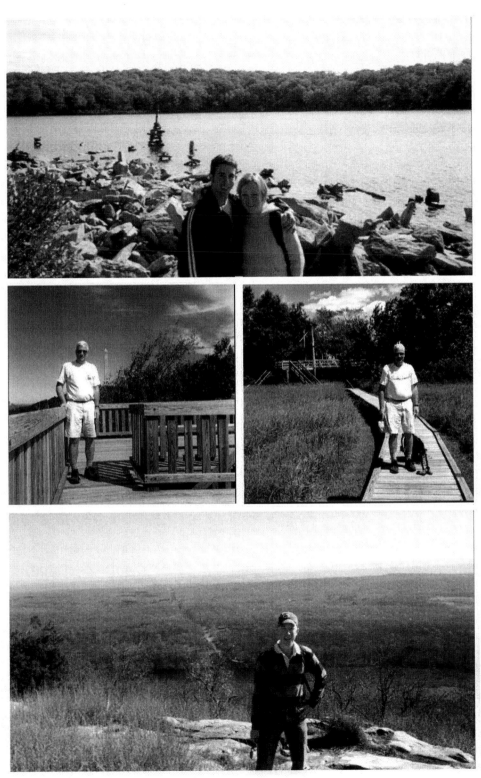

Top: Bethany and Kevin at Sunfish Pond NJ. Middle: Viewing platform near High Point;
Boardwalk of Pochuck Swamp NJ. Bottom: Ben on Kittatinny Ridge NJ.

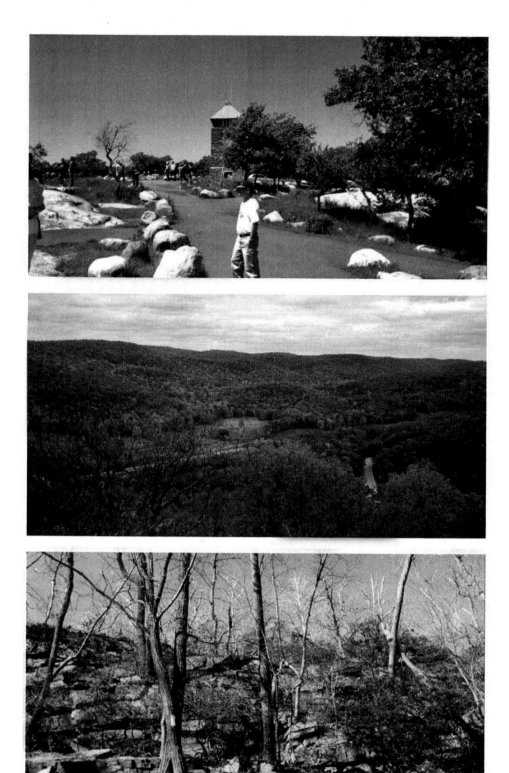

Top: Bear Mountain Summit NY. Middle: Interstate 87 Corridor from top of Agony Grind. Bottom: Escarpment south of Crater Lake NJ.

2006 – Connecticut

I was gaining the weight back. With the move, I got away from going to the gym. I was still playing a lot of golf, and the weeds at the new home were unforgiving. I still had not given up the idea of getting out on the trail, but this year it did not seem to be a priority. It was Monday, June 12, when I got out for the first time.

Western Union was no longer sending telegrams. A winter storm had dropped 27 inches of snow in New York City.

One of my golfing foursome, Al, the father of one of my business partners in the firm, Tom, passed away in February of cancer. He was a wonderful, quiet guy, and we had played many Sundays for the last twenty years. Al had also befriended my father-in-law George, when George moved to town after George's wife Helen passed away. Unfortunately, just as their friendship started to blossom, George passed away suddenly. Tom, Al, George and I and a few others had a great golfing trip to Myrtle Beach one year. George loved it. What happens in Myrtle, stays in Myrtle.

I decided to jump up to Connecticut. I was kind of saving the remaining New York sections for when the kids might want to go with me. The trail in Connecticut is only about 50 miles and carves a tiny slice out of the far northwest corner of the state.

I found Greg Peters on the AT shuttle list, and since he lived in Torrington, I thought I would try to accommodate him for my first day and pick a section close to him. Greg was a retired Army NCO and also a retired prison guard, and to keep busy, was driving a school bus. Greg had a passion for the trail, and he loved being a part of it so much, he would never take any money for his time or gas. I'm glad that I was able to reciprocate for him when he came down to Pennsylvania. He is still shuttling as of this writing, and I contacted him recently. He is still working on the trail down in Tennessee and Virginia.

Greg's trail name was Ridgerunner. Soon after starting my hiking, I had adopted a trail name as well. Some people make up a trail name on their own. I find the best ones are often assigned by others due to an event or something in their makeup or personality.

I chose my name based on a family vacation event years earlier when we visited Colonial Williamsburg. Ben and Bethany were about twelve and ten. One of the activities was "joining the Continental Army." Trying to embarrass my children, I was cracking jokes in the ranks and the drill instructor yelled at me, "Shape up, Snowhead!" I never forgot that, and since my hair had been turning (and still is) grayish-white, it seemed to fit. I don't use it often, but I do sign trail journals "Snowhead from PA."

To get up into Connecticut, I was driving up through the Delaware Water Gap, and then up along the Delaware on Route 209, which is a long, slow, but pleasant drive to Milford. Then across I-84 to the Taconic State Parkway, and then cross-country on US 44 through Millbrook, New York and on to northwest Connecticut.

I met Greg at the Route 4 trailhead near Cornwall Bridge. Greg was very knowledgeable about the trail in all of New England, and would talk of "The Whites" and "Mahoosucs" and the Green Mountains, none of which were on my radar. Greg took me up to the trailhead at Route 112. It would be an 11.5-mile day.

From the road, I was into the woods and climbing from the get-go. It was not particularly steep, but I was out of shape, and the 800 foot up in 2 ½ miles was a struggle. Over the first two miles I kept hearing the roar of car engines racing around. When I got to the Hang Glider View I saw the reason. The Lime Rock Park, a resort of sorts for auto racing enthusiasts, was only a mile away down in the valley to the west. I thought it was interesting, and it did not and still does not particularly bother me. I think it horrifies the purists that the serene and quiet nature of the trail is disturbed. They are the same ones who think you should never go beyond the 18-inch footpath.

That is hard to do.

For years I was reading the Allentown, Pennsylvania newspaper and the *AT Journeys* magazine that a similar auto racing resort was being planned up in the Blue Mountains north of Wind Gap, Pennsylvania. The ATC and local township officials have been fighting it for years, but the last I saw, it is not dead. To be continued.

On the way up to Hang Glider View there were nice views both east and west, including a spectacular large, white house that was new, but almost looked like a castle. The Connecticut hills were pretty in the early summer. The spring and early summer vegetation always looks so much greener and nicer than in the later summer. The streams in the mountains in Connecticut seemed to be running full, much better than the dry hiking in Pennsylvania a few years before. The trail was nice, but no ridge walking here. There were many PUDs (pointless ups and downs).

I got a picture of Roger's Ramp, which squeezed you in between two large boulders.

I was very tired when I got to Old Sharon Road, so skipped the last two-tenths of a mile to get to Route 4, the technical end of the section. I would make it up when I did the next section to the south, I thought. There were some nice homes along Old Sharon Road, which seemed to be a summer community out in this remote part of Connecticut. It was a half-mile from the trail crossing to my car at US 7 and Connecticut 4. Cornwall Bridge did not have an ice cream store, but there was a convenience store which would do. It was three hours home.

Two months would go by until I found the time to go out again. Was I losing interest? It was just hard to find the time. Virginia and I had power of attorney for an aunt of mine, so we would share the weekly one-hour trek to visit her in the nursing home. Feeling responsible for our old house that Ben and Michelle had purchased from us, I helped Ben with some lawn and mulching projects. Stuff just got in the way.

Wednesday, August 23, would be my first of four days over the next three weeks. Greg had been away hiking, but now he was back, and willing and able to help me, after his bus driving duties in the morning. He was early, as usual, when I met him at the Route 112 trailhead. I got in the habit of stopping ten minutes before our meeting place, just so that I could go over my checklist and have my pack and poles set to go. Greg drove me over to Salisbury, Connecticut, at the Connecticut 41 trailhead. The trail does not go directly into Salisbury, but kind of skirts around it. I think the townspeople like it that way. I don't think they like the hikers coming into town that much, being so dirty and smelly, but many do anyway. A sign at the grocery says to keep the packs outside the store.

The first half-mile of the section was on streets on the outskirts of town, and then a nice little climb, including a ladder or two, up to Barrack Mantif. Then a gradual uphill to Billy's View. Just before Billy's View there was a coed group of incoming college freshmen, doing a pre-orientation thing before the actual orientation. There were about 15 or so, and they were doing 20 miles on the trail over 3 days. They had just started, and were getting to know each other. They seemed very disorganized and leaderless. I think they were just dropped off and were going to be picked up at the end. They all had huge packs with equipment supplied by the college. I don't think many had done something like this before. I took a group photo of them with about 10 cameras, and I was off.

I arrived at Giant's Thumb, which looked exactly like that, and about 10 feet high. The footpath was easy, and I had done all the climbing for the day. Someone took my picture at Rand's View. Then I started the long down to the Housatonic River. At the river there was a dam, and then came the Great Falls. I might have walked out on the rocks at the falls but there was a young couple there, who I thought I should not disturb. The Falls were really quite nice, and I got some good pictures. The trail then followed along or near the river, and was very pleasant in the shade.

The last mile and a half was a road walk to my car. It was a hot day, so I was glad for the air conditioning in the car when I got there, drenched in sweat.

Exactly one week later I met Greg near Cornwall Bridge again, and he took me south this time to the trailhead near Kent, Connecticut, at Route 341. I would hike the 11 miles back to Cornwall Bridge.

From the road, I walked through a cow pasture, where I had to watch my step; but the cows had seen hikers before, so they were not bothered.

A significant climb up from the pasture got me to Fuller Mountain. Along the ridge there were many views down into Kent, and the Housatonic River Valley to the east. It was clear, but another hot day. I was still wearing cotton shirts and only had one pair of cotton hiking shorts that I had worn virtually every day out since I had started this venture. It was a tough 400-foot climb up to Caleb's Peak, with more wonderful views to the east. Then there was a little down to St John's Ledges. Someone had defaced the sign, to make it Uncle John's. I was not sure why. The tough down was mitigated by 90 rock steps built by AMC from the White Mountains. These trail builders amaze me.

Once at the bottom, there was a five-mile dirt road walk next to the river. It was serene and picturesque. Even though I knew I was next to the river, the thick vegetation did not offer many views of it. At the end of the road walk I only had a mile and a half to go. It was up 500 feet in the first mile. It seemed endless, and the trail was very rocky. I started to get cranky and annoyed. Once at the top of Silver Hill, there was a tough 400-foot, half-mile descent down to Route 4. I was more annoyed. I wanted no part of making up that two-tenths of a mile up to Sharon Road. I kind of forgot about it until I am writing this, so now I feel obligated to fill it in sometime.

Bethany and Kevin asked about getting out for another hike with me this year, so on the Sunday after Labor Day, we met at the Bear Mountain Inn, which was now closed for renovation. We wanted to hike the section east of the Hudson, which was less than seven miles back to the inn. We left their car at the inn and drove over to Route 9 and parked at the old, closed gas station on the corner.

Bethany led off, and a half-mile in, we missed a left turn and continued on the Carriage Connector Trail. It was about a mile until we realized it, but Kevin figured we should just continue on to the Osborn Loop Trail, which would take us back to the AT. Usually, you are better off retracing your steps if you lose the white blazes, but in this case, we knew where we were. This is a reason to always have a map, trail book and compass, which I always carry. We had gone about two miles out of our way, but it did not matter, since it was a short day.

We stopped along Manitou Road to eat the sandwiches we had purchased in Fort Montgomery just north of the Bear Mountain Bridge. A little farther north is West Point. West Point became a piano customer of Bethany's a few years later, so she has gotten back to the area.

A short but steep climb down took us to the road and the impressive Bear Mountain Bridge. The hike over the bridge was spectacular, but a little nerve-racking for Bethany and me, who have the fear of heights. They led off with Kevin on the outside of Bethany. I followed them fifty feet behind, and just looked straight ahead while hiking, pausing every now and then to enjoy the view. There were many boats out on this weekend day and it was a beautiful sight, looking down to the Hudson. It was a half-mile across the bridge. Once over the bridge, the AT turns into the Bear Mountain State Park, and runs directly through a zoo, which was neat. It then tunnels under Route 9W and heads up into the park and past Hessian Lake. It was a busy day at the lake.

After retrieving my car, we drove up to the summit of Bear Mountain, which was mobbed. Of course I had hiked over the summit two years earlier, but Bethany and Kevin enjoyed seeing the New York City skyline from there. We all headed home.

Three days later, I headed back to Connecticut to hike Section 1 from the Massachusetts/Connecticut border back to Salisbury. I met Greg at the Route 41 trailhead near Salisbury, and he shuttled me up the trailhead of the Undermountain Trail, which is one of the most popular in the state. It was only a five-mile drive and very bikeable (if I owned a bike). Since there is no road or trailhead at the Massachusetts/Connecticut border, my plan was to hike up the Undermountain Trail, pick up the Paradise Lane Trail, and head over to Sages Ravine, pick up the AT there, and then head south on the AT to Salisbury. That was the plan.

The trail was easy, with a few hundred feet of climbing. On my left I heard a noise, and spotted a large bear running. I panicked and started to run too, and soon realized that he was running parallel to me, and soon disappeared. I continued on, yelling, "Bear!" every minute or so, to keep him away. Soon I arrived at Riga Junction, the intersection of the Undermountain Trail and the AT. Oops. In my panic, I somehow had missed Paradise Lane Trail junction.

No problem, I would just head north on the AT to Sages Ravine, complete the section, and then turn around and head back south. I climbed up to the summit of Bear Mountain (the Connecticut Bear Mountain) and started to eat lunch. It was a little bit cold, and out of the cloudy sky there came a little snow squall. It was September 13, for goodness sake! I looked at my map and elevation profile and realized it was 800 feet down in a mile to Sages Ravine. Then I would have to turn around and climb back up. I was discouraged, turned around, and headed south. I promised myself I would make up the seven-tenths of a mile when I did the Massachusetts section to the north, which would be easy.

I passed Riga Junction and headed along the ridge past a few campsites, and encountered a group of about a dozen young people ages 10-15. It was a Wednesday, so I thought it strange. They were from a close-by private day school, out for an overnight camp-out as part of their curriculum. There was only one teacher among them, and he seemed to be about 25. The student-teacher ratio seemed odd by today's standards. I thought I would mention the bear, but did not want to panic the group. Surely the leader knew the area?

There was a steep, 150-foot bump up to Lions Head. I have some pictures of the rich farm valley below, and the Wononskopomuc and Wononpakook Lakes (what names!) in the distance, just past the town of Lakeville. There was still a chill in the air, clear, but with a solid cloud cover.

It was steep at first, climbing down from Lions Head; but then an easy down to my car. It seemed warmer. I had hiked over 10 miles I figured, but was done ahead of schedule, and was mad at myself for not going down into Sages Ravine.

I stopped at the ice cream shop in Salisbury and took some pictures around this quaint little town. It seemed like it came straight out of a romance novel (not that I've ever read one).

I did not plan to quit this early in the year, but somehow I never made it out again. I ended up doing only 47 AT miles this year in 5 days. I was now up to 505 AT miles in 49 hiking days. It would be a fantasy to complete the trail. At this rate, it would be 22 total years, and I would be 76 when I finished. I had never hiked more than one day at a time. I had never stayed away from home, since I had always driven to and from the trail on the days that I hiked. The days were getting longer as both north and south, I was hundreds of miles from home. I figured I would have to learn to camp out. I had purchased a sleeping pad and a stove and some fuel, but never used them. I told people I would have to "step it up" if I would have a chance to hike the whole thing. It did not seem possible. I would just keep going. It was a part of what I did now.

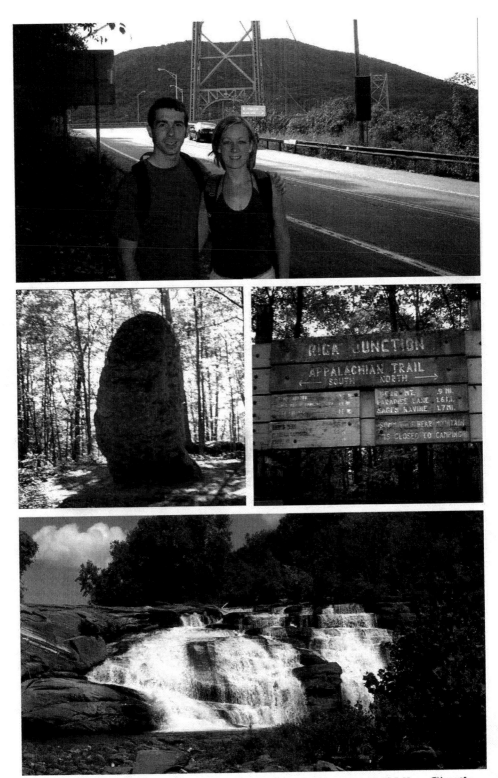

Top: Bethany and Kevin at Bear Mountain Bridge NY. **Middle:** Giant's Thumb; Riga Junction. **Bottom:** Great Falls on the Housatonic River.

2007 – Massachusetts

I got back to the gym over the winter, but it was not helping the weight situation. Even though I ate healthily at home (Virginia is a vegetarian), my big lunch "specials" with my partner Tom, and snacking, were not doing me any favors. I was in better shape, though.

Apple CEO Steve Jobs announced the iPhone. A Virginia Tech student murdered 32 people and injured 23 others before committing suicide.

I did not have any plans for Memorial Day weekend, and Virginia did not mind, so I decided, for the first time, to hike more than one day at a time. Greg was out hiking and not available for shuttles, so I decided to jump up to northern Massachusetts, and wait for him to return to finish Connecticut. Greg had offered to help me with southern Massachusetts, and even down into New York. I decided to use North Adams, Massachusetts as home base. The AT runs right through the town. I did learn that nearby Mount Greylock was closed for the next two years due to road construction. The AT goes directly over Mount Greylock, the highest point in Massachusetts. The AT was open, but I decided to defer those sections. I would go up anyway and hike the section north of North Adams, and then hike down through Cheshire and Dalton.

I got up early on Saturday, May 26, and drove up to North Adams. Around noon, I got a cab from town to take me up to the County Road trailhead in Southern Vermont. I was getting a late start, but it was only seven miles on the AT back to town. The cab driver was a young kid who hiked a lot up in the area and knew the trailhead, even though he did bushwhack hikes (not on any trail). I generally think I have a good sense of direction, but I could not imagine going out into woods, especially ones I did not know, and just climb a mountain. County Road turned into a dirt road, and was remote.

The hike was level and easy, on a nice footpath. At one point the trail passed a boulder the size of a pickup truck that was balanced on another rock. Curious that it was not mentioned in the guide. I reached the Massachusetts/Vermont border. The southbound side sign said welcome to Massachusetts. The northbound sign said welcome to the Green Mountain National Forest. It also described how the AT and Vermont's Long Trail coincide for the next 75 miles. At that point, near Killington, the Long Trail heads north and the AT heads east toward New Hampshire. In Vermont, it is all about the Long Trail, which runs the length of the state, north to south.

Past Eph's Lookout there was a rocky knoll at the junction of the Pine Cobble Trail which heads a few miles to Williamstown, home of Williams College. The knoll had a large cairn. I would get used to those in the New England states. The cairns are a clear marker for the trail, when snow might cover up the blazes.

It was a nice downhill past Sherman's Brook, and then the footbridge over the slowly flowing Hoosic River. A few blocks on Massachusetts Route 2 and I was back at my car at the Greylock Community Club, and then off to the Holiday Inn.

I was up early the next day. I had made some pre-arrangements with a cab company near Dalton, but they just seemed to want me to call when I got to the trailhead there at the intersection of Routes 8 and 9. I parked at a church on the corner. The cab driver made fun of my pronunciation of Cheshire. It was easy to find the trailhead there. It would be nine miles on the AT back to Dalton.

The first mile was through a field, and then on some quiet streets in town. Then I headed up about 800 feet in a mile to the Cobbles. I had to retrace my steps several times at the top until I found the trail. That would be most of the climbing for the day. From the Cobbles there was a nice view down into the quiet town and its large reservoir. Mount Greylock was impressive on the other side of the Cheshire Valley.

It was a level walk across North Mountain, and then a gradual down to

Dalton. A mile of street walking got me to my car. What an easy day. I was done by 1:30 P.M., a first for me, since all my previous hikes involved driving distances of up to hundreds of miles before and after my hike.

I drove back to the Holiday Inn in North Adams, cleaned up and then explored the area. I drove over to Williamstown and visited the MASS MoCA, a contemporary art museum in North Adams. I dined at the Italian restaurant in town. It was nice to get to know the area, although briefly.

When I got back to the room, I checked the weather, and it looked horrible for the next day. I cancelled the cab and my hike, and got up early on Memorial Day and drove home.

Greg was still not available, but I wanted to finish Connecticut, so I got a cab out of Kent on Wednesday, June 6. The older, pleasant gentleman picked me up at the Kent trailhead on Route 341. We were headed down to Hoyt Road at the Connecticut/New York border, where the trail crosses (by design) Hoyt Road (in the middle of nowhere). Rather than crossing the Housatonic River over to Kent and then down US 7, the gentleman chose the long dirt Schaghticoke Road on the western side of the river, so that we could pass through and he could tell me about the local Schaghticoke Indian Reservation. This was all unsolicited.

The Schaghticoke Tribe was a small, aging tribe, living in not the greatest circumstances. They had not enjoyed any benefits that other larger tribes in Connecticut (think Foxwoods) had come to know. I'm not sure why, but looking at their website, in a rambling manner, they seem to blame each other and the state and federal governments. It was interesting. We drove past the chief's house along the dirt road. The rest of the drive was pleasant enough, past covered bridges on winding roads.

From Hoyt Road, it was a pleasant walk through a semi-forest and field, across Route 55 and then 500 steep feet up to Ten Mile Hill. Then it was 700 gradual feet down from Ten Mile Hill. Once down, there was a short walk along Ten Mile River. I stopped long enough to get a picture of Ten Mile Shelter.

I was in the digital age of the 90s now that Ben and Michelle had given us a new camera for Christmas of 2005. I was not that adept at using it, and somehow failed to get a picture of the steel Anderson Bridge, which crossed the Ten Mile River right at the point it flowed into the Housatonic. The Housatonic and US 7 parallels most of the AT in Connecticut. A short one mile along the river and then near Bulls Bridge. I got briefly lost, walking along the edge of a field. I retraced my steps and found my way.

I started a gradual 900-foot climb up Schaghticoke Mountain. The trail veers back into, and then out of New York, either to get near the summit of Schaghticoke, or to stay out of the reservation. I'm not sure which. On the far side of Schaghticoke Mountain there were nice views west, and then once I reached Indian Rocks, the views were back east, looking down at the Housatonic. It was a steep climb down from Mount Algonquin to my car at Route 341.

This 11-mile day finished Connecticut. I drove into Kent for the ice cream. It was not quite the quintessential town of New England like Salisbury to the north, but nice. Hiking the AT in Connecticut and Massachusetts could be done almost bed and breakfast-style, with plenty of nice, picturesque towns along the trail to stay over, I thought.

My kids and I were looking for an outing. We had done some whitewater rafting on the Lehigh River in the Jim Thorpe area. It was mostly Class I and II. Most of us were looking to step up for some more excitement. Some friends of mine in the firm had gone down to West Virginia on the New River and the Gauley River. They almost lost their dad in the Class IV rapids. Maybe that was a little too much excitement. A smaller step up would be some Class II and Class III rapids on the headwaters of the Hudson up in the New York Adirondacks. It would be 10 in a raft, with a guide and helmets. We rented a house for a long weekend. Bethany, Kevin, Ben, Michelle and I, and two of Bethany and Kevin's friends, took a long weekend and rafted on a Sunday in early June. I don't know if we ever got to Class III, but it was a blast.

Greg was back and willing to help me again. Exactly two weeks later, on June 20, Greg drove all the way down to the New York trailhead at Route 55. I planned the 14.5 miles of New York Sections 2 and 3. It was to be a long day, but the elevation did not look difficult. Greg took me to Hoyt Road.

About 100 feet from Hoyt Road, I was soaking wet, walking through the tall grass that had grown up along the narrow trail. I was still in the only hiking shorts I owned, and still in a cotton T-shirt. In a mile I was at the Wiley Shelter, but there was no way to get dry. A few more miles and I reached the undeveloped Pawling Nature Reserve, which I knew only because of the sign, with a trail journal in a box. The reserve had open fields, and the footpath was often on puncheon over swampy areas. I left the reserve and hiked down through some fields, picturesque with grazing cows. A feed silo looked like a rocket ship ready to take off. I arrived at Route 22, the end of the section, but I was only halfway through the day.

Just across Route 22 was the often-photographed platform of the Appalachian Trail rail station. It is a small, blue deck, with a bench and yellow railings. A train to New York stops there on weekends and holidays. I ate my lunch on the platform, and a train went whizzing by. A couple came out of the swampy area where I was headed, and took my picture on the platform.

I entered the high grass area on wooden puncheon and crossed the Swamp River. The last mile to County Road 20 was down through an open field. Coming down through the field, the imposing West Mountain was staring me in the face. I had now hiked about nine miles, and was getting tired. It did not seem like it had been that difficult a day, but I had left home about 6:00 A.M., driven 200 miles, and hiked since 11:00 A.M. It was now about 3:30 P.M. I got down to the road and took a picture of Dover Oak. It must have been eight feet in diameter. I sat down and seriously thought about calling Greg to pick me up, but there was no cell service. I figured I could make it to my car.

I crossed the road and took a picture of a little orange reptile in the middle of the trail, and started the 700-foot climb up West Mountain. I got about 50 yards and started to get lightheaded, and could not catch my breath. I stopped to rest. I walked a few more steps, and began to think I was in trouble. I'm not sure why, but I had just run out of gas. I sat down and ate what food I had left, and drank a lot of water. In about 20 minutes, I started to move again, but was making slow progress. Should I go back to the road and try to get a ride? I decided to go forward. This is what hikers do, but it's not always the best decision. It took me well over an hour to nurse myself up the hill. I was recovering a little more, and actually took a picture at the view back down into the valley.

Fortunately, the remaining four miles along Nuclear Lake and out to my car were very flat, with easy trail. I was lucky. I stopped at a convenience store and bought two sports drinks, and I'm not sure how, but I was able to drive home.

In July there were worldwide musical performances by charity event Live Earth. On August 7, Barry Bonds hit his 756th home run, breaking Hank Aaron's record.

It would not be until August 16 that I got back to the trail. I planned two days on the trail on the southernmost sections of Massachusetts. I would stay overnight in Salisbury, Connecticut.

Greg met me about noon at unpaved Jug End Road, which was easy to find just off Route 41. I was only doing 5.5 easy miles today after the drive. My car was equipped with a well-stocked cooler for when I would arrive after the hike. Greg dropped me at Kellogg Road. I got a picture of Greg, not being sure if I might see him again (I have), and he took one of me.

It was an easy one mile along the west side of the Housatonic out to Route 7. The trailhead there was only two miles from Great Barrington. It was easy walking through the valley on some bog bridges, crossing roads, through corn fields. The imposing Jug End could be seen in the distance. There was a 3-foot stone monument showing the site of the last battle of Shay's Rebellion in 1787 at the South Egremont Road crossing.

There were more bog bridges over some low areas, and then a clean footpath through the woods to my car. I enjoyed the contents of the cooler, and stayed at the trailhead a while. I had done 5.5 miles in a little over two hours.

I had a reservation at an inn right on the green in Salisbury. It was a Thursday, so the price was not too bad. It seemed a little snooty. The rooms each had their own names, and were too frilly for my taste. I felt silly walking into the lobby in my smelly hiking clothes. The place was almost always booked on weekends in the summer, and especially the fall foliage season, by seniors who came back year after year. I showered up and looked around town for a dinner spot, but settled for a seat at the bar at the inn, where I could watch a game on TV.

The next morning, it was a short drive up to the Undermountain Trailhead. Greg was early as usual, and it did not take long to get up to Jug End

Road. It would be easy for one to use a bicycle to shuttle this section.

Unlike the day before, I knew this would be a tough day, and from the beginning, and it did not disappoint. The climb up Jug End was almost 1,000 feet in a little over a mile. Steep. On the way up and at the summit, there were great views north to the Berkshires. There were some PUDs across the rocky, open ridge crest. The sun was bright, and it was tough going.

I passed the Guilder Pond Trail, but did not walk over to the pond. The hike continued, with more open rocky ridges. Low scrub pines, bushes and grassy knolls and rock faces dominated the ridge. There was no protection from the sun, so I stopped to eat my lunch where some thru-hikers had stopped for a break. We were at the summit of Mount Everett. They were two men and a woman in their 30s. That is a little unusual, since thru-hikers tended to be in their early 20s, or just beginning retirement. People who thru-hike are often in a transition stage of their life. Their main topic of conversation was would they be able to make it to Katahdin before winter set in up there. They planned a zero day in Great Barrington. I didn't think they would make it, since it was getting too late in the season.

The sun was draining, and I realized I was not making very good time. There was one more climb up to Race Mountain, and then I could escape the sun back in the woods on the hike down to Sages Ravine. I sat in the coolness of Sages Ravine, tormented by my next decision about whether to hike up to Bear Mountain to pick up that seven-tenths of a mile that I had missed the year before. It would be an 800-foot climb up, and then the steep down to Riga Junction. The mileage was not that different, adding only a few tenths.

I was just too tired, and took the Paradise Lane Trail cutoff to the Undermountain Trail and down to my car. I decided not to drive home, and was lucky to get a room on a Friday night at the inn in Salisbury. Once I had my shower and a cold beer, I had rallied and was mad at myself for being a wimp. I got up early the next morning, and was home by ten o'clock.

A few weeks later, on Sunday of Labor Day weekend, I drove up to New York and met a woman cab driver at the Route 52 trailhead near where the Taconic Parkway intersects with I-84. She was a flower child from the '60s (maybe I was too). She may have smoked a little too much pot. I had to help her find the way down to Fahnestock State Park at the Route 301 trailhead. I wonder if she ever found her way home.

The park was busy on the holiday weekend. The parking lots were full, but it was after eleven o'clock. From the road, I did not have to climb much, but was soon overlooking Canopus Lake and its full beach. There were a lot of families out on the trails in the park this nice day. The trail was rocky, but the ups and downs were gradual and before I knew it, I was at the summit of Shenandoah Mountain (in New York, no less). The summit was open, and someone had painted an American flag on the rock face as a memorial to 9/11.

It was a gradual down to the RHP Shelter. This shelter was different from most. It was actually a house at some point (although a small one). It had windows and a covered patio off the open front. It looked like a doll house. It was unusual that it was so close to a few different roads. I would think vandalism would be a problem, but I saw no evidence of any. A sign with mileages to Springer and Katahdin totaled 2,173. The trail is living and breathing all the time, with relocations. A little climb, up a steep bank, and I would be crossing under the Taconic Parkway.

After a short, hot road walk, I was back in the woods on a gradual climb up to Hosner Mountain. The trail became rocky, but there were nice views of farms down in the valleys. There were switchbacks down Stormville Mountain to my car.

A few days later, Virginia agreed to go along with me up into the Berkshires in Massachusetts. I would hike three days, and she had an interest in the Shaker Village near Pittsfield, Massachusetts.

We got up early on September 6 and drove up to the area. We explored around a little, and then we stopped off at the Dalton trailhead, so that Virginia would know where to pick me up. We drove south down Pittsfield Road, and easily found the trailhead. Off she went to check in to our Pittsfield Motel. It was about noon.

The hike back north to Dalton was initially very flat, with easy trail along the Berkshire Plateau. I met a brother and sister who were southbound thru-hikers. Since each of the sections I was doing this time I was hiking north, I would see them each of the next two days. We laughed when we saw each other on the third day.

At the end of the day there was a steep climb down Day Mountain on steps. I met a northbound thru-hiker with a big pack who was struggling to come up. I was struggling on the down. My knees felt the pounding. At one of the road crossings, I talked to a New York City-area couple who had a rustic vacation home nearby. As I neared the outskirts of Dalton, a man had a grill set up and was feeding thru-hikers hot dogs and hamburgers, and had coolers with cold drinks. He offered me some, but I would be meeting Virginia shortly.

I reached the quiet Depot Street in Dalton. There were nice homes, and I wondered what it would be like to live on the AT like that. I crossed the Housatonic River, and Virginia was waiting. She had been out to the Shaker Village west of Pittsfield, and enjoyed her day. I got cleaned up, and we had a late dinner at a nice place on Route 7 south of Pittsfield. When we got back to the motel, I tripped and fell in the parking lot, ripped my pants, and banged up my knee. We laughed that I could hike for three days and not get hurt, but fall in a motel parking lot.

The next morning we found a quiet breakfast joint, and then headed south on Route 7 through Lee, Massachusetts, and then across to the Route 20 trailhead. I would hike the nine miles north to Pittsfield Road.

From the highway, I was climbing immediately into the October Mountain State Forest. The trail was good, and it was not too steep. Greenwater Pond, which ran next to Route 20, was visible on the way up. There were houses along the pond, and it looked nice for recreation. The climbing went on to the summit of Becker Mountain. Everything was green, and the forest was lush.

Across the ridge to the summit of Walling Mountain, staying above 2,000 feet, I went. Then it was a slight down to Finerty Pond. The trail followed the shore for a few hundred yards before heading away. There was no activity in the area. I was booking it, with easy trail on top of the ridge. There were some swampy areas over puncheon. Puncheon are usually two wooden planks nailed onto support logs or lumber. Puncheon can go on for long sections to protect fragile areas, and to make the trail hikeable.

After County Road, here came the brother, and then 10 minutes later the sister, whom I stopped to speak to. They were going to get a ride into Lee to resupply once they got down to Route 20. They would have to hitchhike, as it would be a long road walk to town.

After County Road it was level, quiet and easy to the October Mountain Shelter. I stopped there for lunch. No one was around. There might have been some late northbound thru-hikers, but since I was also hiking northbound, I was less likely to see them.

From the shelter, it was another easy two miles to the road. Virginia was there waiting. She found the trailhead, but was very nervous about it. Driving out into these remote places was just not her thing.

Virginia has always had an interest in natural foods and alternative health modalities. She had been reading about the Kripalu Yoga Center for years, so wanted to drive down there to visit the place. It was only about 10 miles from Pittsfield, where we were staying. We decided to have dinner there in the cafeteria. It was a great place to explore and get to know what they offered. The food was served buffet-style, and was excellent. There were many healthy choices.

On the way out to Kripalu from Lenox we passed Tanglewood, the summer home of the Boston Symphony Orchestra, the Boston Pops. Their season had just ended. The Berkshires have a lot to offer, with a lot of nice resorts and places to visit. Their leaf-peeping season would begin in about a month.

The next day we were up early, and headed down to Lee. We drove around the outlet mall there, which Virginia might visit while I was hiking, and then we did the short drive down to Tyringham. Tyringham had a post office, but no other services for hikers. It was a quiet Saturday morning.

Virginia drove off back to Pittsfield to spend a quiet morning reading in the motel room before she had to check out.

It would be an easy nine miles back up to Route 20, AFTER the sometimes-steep, 800-foot climb up from Tyringham to Baldy Mountain. Once on top, the trail was easy all the way to Upper Goose Pond. Along came brother, followed by sister. We laughed. I got a picture of an old chimney, which was all that remained of a fishing and hunting club. Since it was a Saturday, there was activity in the area. There were kayakers out on the water, and young families roaming around. I did not walk over to the cabin that is run by AMC. I knew Virginia would be waiting.

I took a lot of pictures when I crossed Interstate 90. *Check*. It was scenic in all directions. A beautiful sign simply said, "The Berkshires." The trail seemed to wind around to get to Route 20. Virginia was there in the big parking lot, which seemed to be a jumping-off point for a few other trails in the area. I changed my clothes, and we headed home.

A week or so later, I drove up to New York to hike a few sections north of the Hudson. It was September 19, a Wednesday. I parked my car on a dirt road between Route 9 and Route 403 near the Route 9 trailhead, and walked back to the closed gas station, which seemed to be under some sort of renovation now, and I did not think I should park there. I called an area cab company, and called again, and finally one showed up. I'm not sure if cab companies take hikers very seriously. I guess they figure we will wait.

It was a long drive out to Fahnestock Park at Canopus Lake. The cab driver got mad at me when I misunderstood him mumbling about the fare. I fixed it and I thought I was generous, but he drove off in a huff. I had trouble extending my hiking poles. One did not seem to want to tighten.

As I entered the woods from the road, I met a local couple who were headed my way, so we hiked together and talked along a mine railway bed. The bed was interesting, narrow and elevated through the woods. The AT left the railway bed, which continued on to Dennytown, NY. I was still in Fahnestock Park, and there were a lot of hiking trails in the area.

The couple told me about the area, and the history of the iron foundry that made the large chain that was strung across the Hudson during the Revolutionary War to stop British ships.

After leaving the railway bed the trail became rocky, and throughout the rest of the day, there were PUDs. The AT would intersect with other trails in the park and cross roads.

I got some pictures of the boulder fields at the southern end of the park. It was a gradual down to Canopus Hill Road. I still had five miles to go, and was weary and a little lightheaded. I ate lunch along the road.

I started to recover a little, but the trail was not easy here in New York. There were some short but steep climbs up and down, and very rocky. Finally

I got to the top of Denning Hill, and could start going down. It was still not easy going. I was really tired, and there was one last little up over a hill before the Graymoor Friary. I was glad to reach the trailhead, but I still had a little road walk to get to my car. I had hiked 12.4 miles, but it seemed longer.

My last day for the year would be a month later, on October 22, a Monday. The Dow Jones Industrial Average closed at an all-time high a week before. I was feeling good about the old 401k. Oops...

I had the short 7.2-mile New York Section 4 between Route 52 and Route 55 to fill in. It was my last New York section. I had called a cab company out of East Fishkill, and they said it would be no problem to come out to get me that day. They were right, and a cool young woman driver picked me up at Route 52 and drove me up through Stormville to the Route 55 trailhead. The last time I was there was the day I'd had some physical difficulties coming up West Mountain.

As at many trailheads, boulders block the trailhead entrance to prevent ATVs from using the trail. There was always room to get by. It was an easy first three-tenths of a mile until crossing old Route 55. After that, it was a gradual climb up Depot Hill. The trail was rocky, with brief scrambles up and down. On the top of Depot Hill there were nice views to the north. The leaves were turning bright colors down in the valleys. On the top of the hill, many leaves were down, so while hiking there was the constant *whish* of walking through the ankle-deep leaves.

I arrived at the Morgan Stewart Shelter and ate my lunch. I would usually pick up a sandwich on the road, and Virginia had packed my snacks, including a trail mix that she always made. Whole wheat peanut butter crackers had become a staple. The shelter was quiet, with few recent entries in the trail journal. A sign on the side of the shelter indicated 734 miles to Katahdin, and 1,376 to Springer. Wow, that must have been really old, since it only totaled 2,110. The trail, as I am working on it, is 2,181. Ever-changing.

From the shelter, it was a gradual downhill, but still a rocky path. I soon arrived at I-84. There were steep rock steps to climb to get up to the road overpass. Two women on bikes had paused there, and they took my picture with I-84 in the background. *Check.* On the other side of I-84, there was a road walk on a dead-end road. When I got to the dead end, I just could not find the trail, and floundered in the woods a while. I turned around and walked down towards I-84 until I found a blaze and tried again. I still had no luck, and got to the dead-end, and the blazes had disappeared. I turned around again, and finally found the spot where the trail climbed up a little bank. All the leaves had hidden the path. It was an easy last mile to my car.

Having finished New York, it seemed like a good stopping point. For the year I had done 117 miles in 12 hiking days, and was now up to 622 total miles. I had finished Pennsylvania, New Jersey, New York, Connecticut, Maryland and West Virginia. I was well into Massachusetts, and had just started Virginia. I was still under thirty percent of the trail completed, and at the rate I was going, I still was not admitting that I was trying to accomplish the whole trail. *Just keep going.*

I was getting too far from home now to do this one day at a time thing. My new strategy would be to hike three days at a time, and stay over two nights. I could drive to the area, hike a short section on day one, pick a longer or tougher section on day two, and then hike a shorter section on day three, and drive home. That would work for a while. I still would not camp. I also decided that I would head south next year, in addition to going north. I would do the south in the spring and fall, and the north in the summer. It would not work out exactly that way, but that was the plan. How would it work?

The Mitchell report released the names of 89 major league baseball players who had used performance-enhancing drugs, and Boston finally finished the "Big Dig."

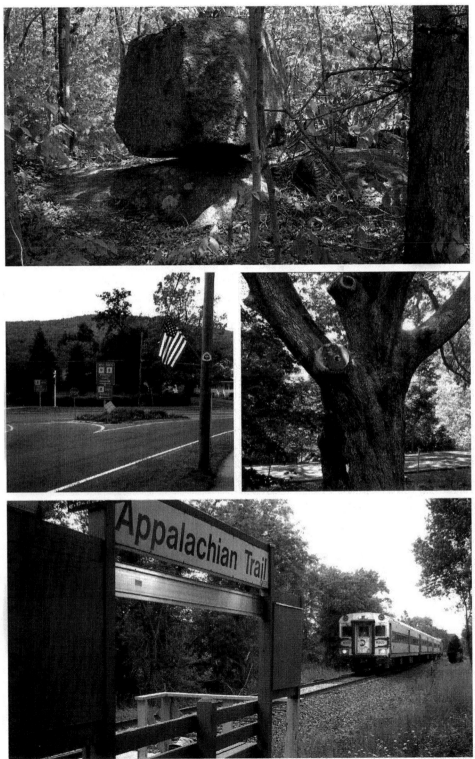

Top: Balanced boulder near VT/MA border. Middle: Dalton MA AT crossing; Dover Oak NY. Bottom: AT RR Station NY.

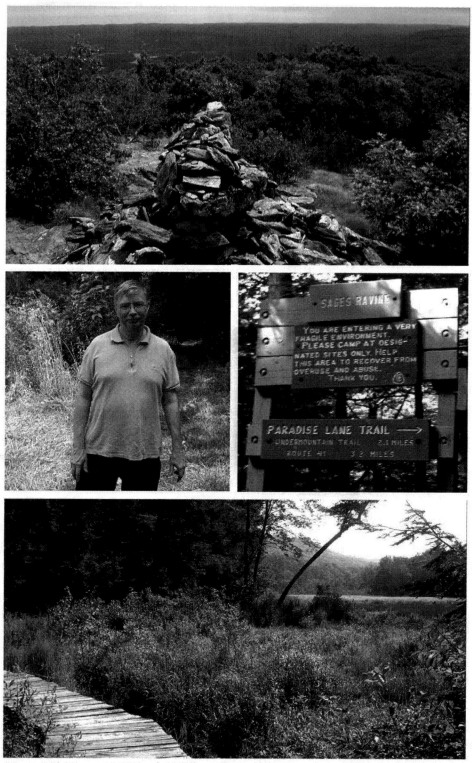

Top: Mt Everett MA. Middle: Greg "Ridgerunner" from CT; Sages Ravine. Bottom: Massachusettes wetlands.

2008 - North - Into Vermont

Although I loved going down to Shenandoah, I wanted to work north on the AT as well. I had a little bit to finish in Massachusetts, even though I couldn't because of Mount Greylock being closed, and then I thought I would work into Vermont.

On Saturday, August 17, I drove up to Great Barrington in southern Massachusetts. I had arranged for a cab to pick me up at the Route 23 trailhead, about four miles east of town. There was a large swinging wooden sign at the trailhead which was good, since the parking lot was hidden. I waited at the road. When the cab arrived at mid-day, the driver took me up to Tyringham.

From Tyringham, the trail ran through a low, wet area before an easy 200-foot climb up to Cobble Hill. From Cobble Hill you could see across to the next set of mountains, but the trees blocked the view down into the valley. It was a clear day, with a gray sky. Down from Cobble Hill, I crossed over a low, barbed-wire fence which was on top of a stone wall, and then through a series of fields.

At about the 3-mile mark, I would climb up 1,000 feet over the next 1 ½ miles. I was definitely out of shape. Once on top, there were great views down into the Tyringham Valley. There were people around some of the viewpoints in an open area, and a group of women asked me to take their picture, and then they used my camera to take one of me. I had actually bought a synthetic shirt. It was soaked from the climb, and my weight was at its worst.

After two miles of walking along the ridge on easy trail, I skirted a pond created by a long beaver dam. The dam looked to have been 100 feet across, and the trail crossed below the level of the pond. This was interesting, and a little unnerving. Water was leaking from the dam the whole way, so the trail was wet. Around the far side of the dam I could see a beaver lodge in the pond, but no actual beaver were visible. I don't know about their habits. Around the far side of the pond, I stopped to take some pictures. The pond had a glassy surface, and the reflections of the sky and tree line in the water were amazing.

I was only halfway through my 12-mile day, and was tired already. I had been up early and driven over 200 miles to get up there, and it was around 3:00 P.M. now. I ate a snack in a hemlock grove. I was still walking across the ridge. I passed the side trails to the two shelters. I was not interested in adding any more miles. There were some easy, but hard on me, climbs up and down from the ledges where I stopped to rest.

The last 2 ½ miles down to my car seemed endless. A lot of the hike was easy trail, but dark in the hemlock forest. I arrived after 6:30 P.M., but had the cooler well stocked. I was beginning to like arriving at the car and enjoying the adult beverage and lingering for a while. I put on some fresh clothes. Changing here was not a problem, since the parking lot was hidden from the road. I was off to the motel for a shower and dinner.

The next morning, it took a while to find a breakfast spot that opened early. I started to ask cab drivers for the best early breakfast in town. I met the cab at the same remote Route 23 trailhead. I would hike from south to north today, from Kellogg Road, where Greg had dropped me off the year before on my way to Jug End. It would only be 7 ½ miles today, and I was getting an early start.

I had about a half a mile of road walk to get to the woods at Boardman Road. Then I started a 500-foot climb up to June Mountain. It was a level mile to Homes Road where I stopped for a snack, and realized I'd forgotten my watch somehow. It did not matter, since I had my phone. I had plenty of time. It was a big, 700-foot up to the summit of East Mountain. From the top there were nice views down into the Housatonic Valley. Across the top of East Mountain, there were flat rock ledges to walk across.

Somewhere around the Tom Leonard Shelter, I lost my SPOT GPS locator that I had just purchased this year. Since there is not always cell service, it would be another way to let Virginia know that I was OK from time to time. It had a 9-1-1 button on it, but I just used the "I'm OK" button, which would send Virginia an email or text with my GPS coordinates. It did not seem like they always went through due to tree cover, and other unexplained reasons. I felt like I was becoming a slave to it. I was glad it was gone. When I got home, I cancelled my subscription, so that if someone found it, they would not be playing a joke on emergency people.

The Tom Leonard Shelter was quiet. As I passed above it, I notice the roof had a big white square painted on it, I guess to locate it from the air. From the shelter, it was an easy downhill to Lake Buel and across the short, broken, cement dam, and past a marshy area with tall reeds, to get to my car. I got cleaned up and changed for the ride home, and even had a beer. That was a mistake, since I would normally stay and relax for an hour if I did that, and I never did that again before driving home. I was now done with Massachusetts, except for hiking up and over Mount Greylock.

I still wanted to head north this year, but did not get up again until October. For whatever reason, I did not go north or south in September. I had bought the books and maps for Vermont/New Hampshire, and studied them endlessly. Vermont looked remote, with some long sections with no road crossings in the southern end. Trailheads were out of the way, and there were slim pickings on the AT shuttle list. The towns that were close by did not seem to have cab companies.

I decided I would jump up to the middle of the state and do the hikes around Killington, and planned three days beginning October 3. The trailheads near Killington seemed accessible, and there were a few cab companies around. I was up early, and drove the 300 miles to the trailhead on River Road, past the charming little town of Killington. The town is removed from the busy road to the main resort ski area, which has many shops and restaurants.

I had made arrangements for the three days with a one-woman cab company out of Rutland. Once she answered the phone, she proved to be dependable. She met me at the River Road trailhead, and took me back to my Route 4 starting point. It was already past 1:00 P.M., but the hike was only six miles.

From the US 4 highway, I was climbing in rough terrain. I had become spoiled, with the mostly easy footpath in Virginia and Massachusetts. After about a mile and 500 up, I came to Maine Junction, which seemed like a big deal, since this is where the AT leaves the Long Trail. The Long Trail heads north to Canada, and the AT runs east to Hanover, New Hampshire. I lingered a while and took pictures of the various signs. After passing several side trails, there were great views back towards Sherburne Pass and the ski slopes on the other side of US 4. The hills were in full color. A lot of leaves were down at elevation. From this point, the trail continued to be rugged, although there was not much climbing. But the trail was not flat either, just little ups and downs.

At Gifford Woods State Park, after another rugged mile, I passed through an area of campsites, cabins and shelters. It was a small area, but people were arriving for a weekend of camping and enjoying the color and the fall season. The trail became easier, and I soon crossed Route 100. After having a little difficulty finding the trail on the other side, I was at Kent Pond. Someone took my picture with Kent Pond in the background. On the far shore was a little hill with beautiful fall colors. I was in jeans and a sweatshirt. I was still not wearing sophisticated hiking clothes.

The trail became much easier, along dirt roads, and I passed Mountain Meadows Lodge. I had considered staying there on subsequent trips, but never did. From the lodge it was a very easy walk on well-maintained trail to Thundering Falls. A boardwalk took you to a decked viewpoint of the falls, which were wonderful. There were a few houses and other buildings close by, and I got lots of pictures. From the falls, the AT is on a three-tenths of a mile boardwalk over the Ottauquechee Flood Plain, all the way to River Road. None of this was in my old book and map, since the boardwalk had just recently been completed in 2007. I would get the new books for New Hampshire/Vermont later. It was nice that visitors to the area could take advantage of the boardwalk to get up to see the falls. It would be a nice outing for families or anyone. I lingered at my car before driving back to a motel in Rutland about 10 miles away.

The next morning, I would meet my driver at the large parking area at

US 4, and she would drive me around the mountain. I would be hiking the 12 miles over Killington. She would drop me at the Upper Cold River Road trailhead on the south side of Killington. The elevation profile on the map looked intimidating. It would be a five-mile and 2,500-foot climb to the summit of Killington. I was getting in better shape from the hiking that I had done so far this year, but this would be my toughest climb since I had started hiking.

It started off easily enough, along a dirt road and over a bridge with a full flowing stream, and past the stone Governor Clement Shelter. Heavy, colorful, undisturbed leaves surrounded the shelter area. Then it got serious. There was nothing to see or do but climb the mountain. The trail was rugged. There were no easy footpaths or stone steps built by those wonderful trail builders. Just a tough climb that was endless and unforgiving. I was breathing heavily and had to stop now and again, but pressed on. Except for taking a drink every half an hour or so, I did not stop. I'd had a big breakfast, so had plenty of fuel. Several times, I thought I must be at the top, only to see more ups around the next corner. Three hours after I was dropped at the road, I was at the high point of Little Killington Ridge. I lingered a while but it was cold, and I was wet with perspiration. I headed down to Cooper Lodge, an enclosed shelter with big swinging wooden windows that were open, but could be closed in bad weather.

I went inside. My jeans and sweatshirt were drenched with sweat. I don't know why, but I had packed extra clothes, so I stripped down and put on another pair of jeans and a heavy windshirt. It felt great, because just then it started to snow a little. It was a Saturday, and there were a few people around. Many had hiked up, but none had come up the south side. I wanted no part of taking the side trail up to the summit of Mount Killington, since it would be another 300 tough feet up.

I ate my lunch at the shelter, and then started down the AT on the north side of the mountain. The little snow squall had ended, and it was turning into a nice day. The sun peeked through the socked-in clouds, and there were great views from open areas when crossing over or along the actual ski slopes of Killington. After a little while, the trail entered the woods. The trail was somewhat easier, and not as steep going down, and there were switchbacks to take away the grade.

On the way down, I met a couple who I caught up to. They were doing a loop hike from their condo that they had in the area. They were actually from the Lehighton area, which was near me in Pennsylvania. They were big skiers, and came up to the area a lot. Almost as an afterthought, they said that they had learned of an event at Killington the next day, Sunday morning. They had gotten an email from their condo association. ABC's *Good Morning America* program was doing a "Fifty States in Fifty Days" thing, in connection with the upcoming election. The next morning, *GMA* would be at the lodge at the top of Killington. They were offering a free ski lift ride and free breakfast to get a lot of people up there early in the morning. It sounded interesting. Later that month, *GMA* would be in Lee, Massachusetts, where Virginia and I had been the year before.

I finished my hike down. The trail continued to be easy, but I was spent from the 12-mile day, and especially the tough climb up. I got back to my car and took a lot of pictures around the trailhead at US 4. It was warmer now that I was off the mountain, and a bright day now. I headed back to Rutland for a warming shower.

I started to think about the next day, and figured the next hike would always be there; but it might be fun to go up to the summit the next morning to see the goings-on before driving home. Virginia thought so, too. I called the cab to cancel my Sunday hike.

I was up and out at 5:00 A.M. and started to drive out US 4. I thought I knew where ski lift was, since I'd passed something on the highway called Skyship. Oops, that wasn't it. I circled back to the actual ski area thanks to the navigation system in my new SUV, and found the lift. A lot of people were there on this early Sunday morning. It was foggy. I took the enclosed lift up, and walked over to the lodge. Many people were up there. The TV trucks and vans with the satellite antennae were all over. Obama signs outnumbered McCain signs. Every half-hour or so, Marysol Castro would do a live report, and the people would cheer. Marysol had a bright-green coat on, and you couldn't miss her. I went into the lodge to get some breakfast, but only got some slim pickings, as the locusts had been through.

As people started to thin out, I decided to hike up to the Killington

Summit. It was on wooden steps for a while, and then a short but tough climb up some rock steps. Then there was a little more climbing through some scrub pines to the open, rocky summit. In all it was less than half a mile. I was glad I had not hiked to the summit the day before. It had turned into a beautiful morning, and I stayed at the top a while. There was still fog in the valleys, but the mountains stuck out above, making the valleys look like lakes. The sun had just risen, but you could not see it with the cloud cover. There were layers of dark and light clouds, with some brighter sky mixed in. It was wonderful, and even an inferior photographer like me could not mess this up.

I headed down from the summit and took the lift down, and drove back to the motel in Rutland. I showered, packed up and headed home. On the drive I was listening to the World Series game on the radio. My beloved Phillies kicked butt that day, and went on to win the World Championship of Baseball.

That would be it for the north this year. I really did not know how I could do Vermont. In the south there was a 23-mile section, and a 17-mile section that seemed beyond my limits. Other sections in the north did, too. I guess I would have to break down and buy a sleeping bag. Oh well, that was a next-year problem. Solutions would begin to present themselves.

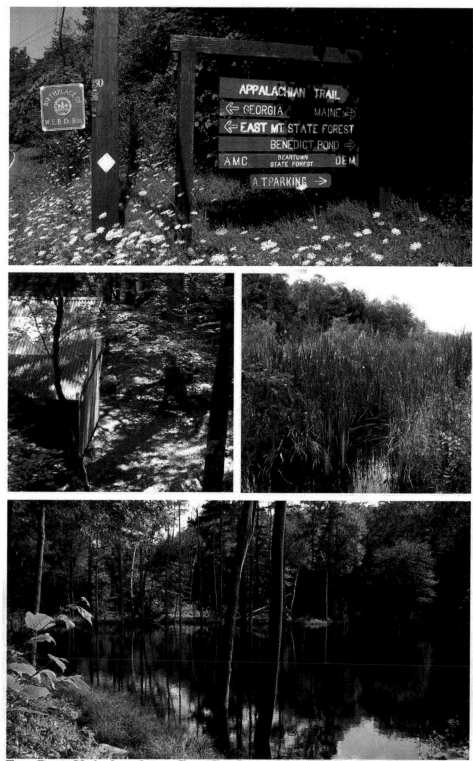

Top: Route 23 signboard near Great Barrington MA. Middle: Tom Leonard Shelter; Marsh near Lake Buel MA. Bottom: Beaver Pond near Great Barrington MA.

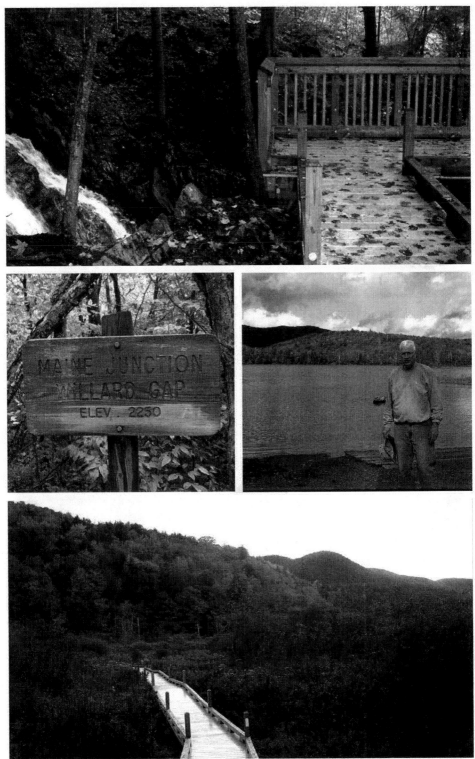

Top: Platform at Thundering Falls near Town of Killington. Middle: Maine Junction-AT & Long Trail in VT; Dennis at Kent Pond VT. Bottom: Boardwalk over Ottauquechee Flood Plain.

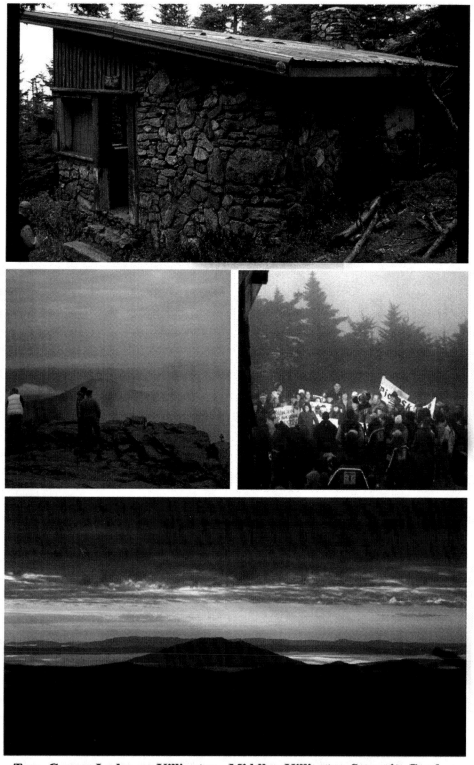

Top: Cooper Lodge on Killington. Middle: Killington Summit; Good Morning America on Killington. Bottom: Sunrise from Killington.

2008 – South - Shenandoah

The first part of 2008 was not great. In fact, it sucked.

Tom, my partner, my best friend in the firm, and part of my Sunday golf foursome, died of cancer. The first two weeks in January, he thought he had the flu. The doctors eventually figured out what was going on, and two years to the day of his father's passing, on February 23, he was gone. Tom was nine years younger than I, but was a smoker until he gave it up cold turkey when he lost his dad to cancer. Sadly, it was too late.

We were in the middle of tax season, and it was tough. Heroically, Tom tried to work, but he couldn't. Now, not only did we all have our own busy schedules, we had to figure out his work and assign it to others in the firm. He had the largest client list, and was a key partner in the firm. Fortunately, with six other partners and a professional staff totaling twenty-two, it could be done. Everyone had to step up, which they did. We tried our best to support his wife of almost thirty years. They did not have any children. In the middle of all this, my mother ended up in the hospital for five days, but she recovered nicely. The stock market was crashing, and our financial system seemed to be falling apart. It all sucked.

There was just a lot to do, but by July, I could think about hiking. I was ready for a break, and was looking forward to getting back down to Shenandoah National Park, which I had not been to since 2004. I had already finished the northern third of the park. Shenandoah can be divided into three sections by road crossings over the mountains, east to west. I had accessed the northern part via a cab out of Front Royal. The AT paralleled Skyline Drive through almost all the rest of the park, and there were multiple crossings all the way to Waynesboro at I-64 at Rockfish Gap. There was a shuttle service out of Luray, but it would be expensive, fairly so because it was a long way for them to go. They were actually the only ones authorized and licensed to provide this type of service in the park. The license cost them something. With hindsight, had I owned a bike, it would have been easy to shuttle myself in Shenandoah. I called Jim from Mountain and Valley Shuttle, and he would help me four or five times.

I decided to stay at Skyland, one of the two lodges in the park, and planned to hike three days. I got up early and drove down to Skyland and met Jim at about 11:00 A.M. on July 17, a Thursday. He took me down to US 211 at Thornton Gap. It would be 9.5 miles south back to Skyland. The Panorama Restaurant was closed, with fencing all around. I doubt it has reopened. As much as I like Shenandoah, I don't think the park got much use. I'm not sure why, because it is beautiful.

With the difficult winter, I was not getting to the gym much, and the weight was as bad as it had been since I lost the two bowling balls on the South Beach diet. I could figure this out immediately on the 1,200-foot climb out of Thornton Gap. By the time I got to Mary's Rock two miles later, I was spent. The views in Shenandoah, however, are unsurpassed everywhere, and soon perked me up. It was very hot and humid, and the sky was hazy. I continued on another mile, and stopped for lunch at the Byrd's Nest #3 day shelter. It was a beautiful stone structure. I still had six miles to go.

The footpath was easy for most of the day, but now I had another 600-foot climb up to the Pinnacle. After a gradual down, I entered the Pinnacles Picnic Area. I had stopped there in the morning to use the restroom facility. There were several campers parked there and the grills were fired up, and it smelled good. One family offered me a burger, but I declined. In this area, the trail runs very close to, but never crosses, Skyline Drive. At one point you were up high looking down at the ribbon of the drive, and also US 211 running down into the valley toward Luray. At other times, the trail ran directly below the Skyline Drive viewpoints with their three-foot rock walls.

Deer are plentiful in Shenandoah, and unlike everywhere else, they are not shy or threatened. You could get close to them and take pictures easily. As you passed the numerous viewpoints, the valleys were spectacular, and the distant mountains seemed to go on and on. It was very green everywhere.

The last two miles and 800 feet up were a real chore. I was really out of shape. My feet were getting blisters, too. I was really soft from the winter. I finally reached the paved entrance road to Skyland, and to my car in the parking lot. It was nice to check in and get a shower, and a beer and dinner at the lodge.

The next morning, after a big, early breakfast (I opened the place), I met Jim at the US 33 trailhead in Swift Run Gap. There is an entrance station to Shenandoah there, but the rangers did not seem to mind me leaving my car there along the road. Jim drove me north on Skyline Drive to the Bearfence Mountain parking area.

From the parking area it was a downhill to the hut side trail, which I did not take. Shortly past the hut, I spotted a bear. It startled me at first. It was standing on a fallen tree, which was hung up and a few feet off the ground, but level. I was only 25 feet away, but it was not concerned. I was not threatened now. It took me a minute, but I pulled out the camera and took half a dozen pictures. I swear the little guy was posing for me. The deer and bear in Shenandoah could not be more tame.

There were few views on the way to Swift Run Gap. The trail was not difficult, and once I hiked the 500 feet up to Bald Face Mountain over two miles, it was downhill to Fishers Gap. Despite my being out of shape, I made great time on the easy path and reached my car in four hours. It was ten miles, so it was well ahead of my two mile an hour normal pace. I had not even stopped to eat lunch. I ate it in my car on the way back to Skyland. My feet were killing me. The blisters were all opened now, and after my shower, I decided to cancel the next day, got up early and drove home.

The following weekend, my sister and I and some of our old friends from high school hiked the New Jersey side of the Delaware Water Gap up to Sunfish Pond. We looked like drowned rats in the few pictures that I took. We got caught in a severe thunderstorm at the pond. It was frightening.

I decided to take a few days off from work, which to that point had been few and far between. I tried to get a reservation at Big Meadows, but it was full, so I was back at Skyland. I planned another three days, which I would complete this time. It would mean more driving along Skyline Drive, but I did not mind. Around every turn in the road was another magnificent viewpoint. It was hard not to stop at all of them.

On Monday, August 4, I met Jim at Skyland again, and he took me south on Skyline Drive, the few miles to Fishers Gap. I really should have bought a bike. I really could have walked the drive or hitchhiked, which would be easy to get to Fishers Gap. The hike would only be 6.5 miles back to Skyland.

From the Fishers Gap parking area, there were great views west, down into the populated valley. It was hazy, but you could still see the mountain range on the other side. It was a 500-foot climb over two miles to Hawksbill Mountain. On the way up the trail, though not steep, was rugged, and at times you came out to viewpoints with steep drop-offs. The tops of the trees were below the viewpoint. On the way to Rock Spring Hut, the trail became much easier. I'm sure the thru-hikers in Pennsylvania, New Jersey, and New York think fondly of the easy trail here. The trail crossed over an old lava field, acres of white-ish rocks that you could spot every now and then on the far mountains. At one point, you could look back east and see the drive about a half a mile away.

At Hawksbill Gap, the AT was back in touch with the drive. At Timber Hollow, the trail ran directly below the drive's overlook, and you could see the cars and the people out with their cameras. Just before Skyland, the trail ran along another steep ridge, with big drop-offs. I hugged the inside path. I passed the Skyland stables. There were about 20 horses eating from a big pile of hay.

That night in the lodge, a group of women from Luray put on a clogging show. They were all shapes, ages and sizes, but they loved it. They practiced all winter and performed once a week at the lodge during the season. Shenandoah closes in the winter.

The next morning, I made the 20-mile drive down to Swift Run Gap again to meet Jim. The rangers seemed indifferent about where I parked. Jim would take me south this time, to Simmons Gap. It would be a 9.5-mile hike back to my car. It was a gray day, and a few sprinkles were on my windshield. In this section, the AT would cross the drive three times between Simmons Gap and Swift Run Gap, but it did not run too close to it for much of the hike. It felt a little more isolated.

From Simmons Gap, it was a gradual 600-foot climb after passing the ranger station. It started to drizzle. The fair-weather hiker that I was, hiking in rain was new to me. I left my camera in the pack once I reached the top. I could barely see the summit of Flattop Mountain to the east. It was now an easy 600 feet down to Powell Gap. Wow, the trail in Virginia is nice. There are rocks in spots, but generally easy. By the time I reached Powell Gap, it was a full-fledged rain. I sent a signal with my new spot GPS locator at the open drive crossing, but it did not go through, Virginia would tell me later. Maybe I did not wait long enough. I broke out my golf rain jacket and my Tilley hat. I usually did not wear hats while hiking, since I sweated too much.

At Smith Roach Gap, the rain started to let up, and it got a little brighter. The AT crossed the drive again, and we were back on the eastern side, climbing 900 feet up to Hightop Mountain. As the sun came out, it was very humid from the moisture in the woods. I was drenched and breathing heavily on the climb. Just past the tree-covered summit of Hightop, there were views south where you could see Skyline Drive snaking around a mountain. US 33 was visible through the hazy sky. The trail switchbacked west and crossed the drive yet again. In the last mile of easy trail, I swear I spotted a bear peeking at me over some scrub bushes. Brazenly, I went toward it with my camera, but it must have been my imagination.

When I reached my car, I headed north toward Skyland, but pulled over at a more private lookout area to change. It was only early afternoon.

I ate my lunch, and then stopped at the South River Falls parking area. I decided since it was early, I'd hike down to the base of the falls. It was a steep hike down. On the way, I spotted several deer along the trail. They showed no concern. I got to the base of the falls and there were a dozen or so people down there, including a family that included a teenage girl with her boyfriend tagging along. There was a lot of angst between the young couple and the parents. Young kids were actually hiking up the waterfall. Several adults were wading in the pool below the falls. Someone took my picture in my clean, dry shirt. The hike back up to the car was strenuous. I'm still not in very good shape, but getting better.

On the drive to Skyland, there was a young bear posing for pictures along the road for a half a dozen cars that had stopped. After dinner that evening, I drove over to Big Meadows Lodge. It was similar to Skyland. People were out on the back porch to watch the sunset.

The next morning I packed up, had an early breakfast at Skyland for the last time, and headed south to meet Jim at Fishers Gap. He would take me down to Bearfence Parking Area. It would be an easy 8-mile hike back to Fishers Gap. The shuttles were getting expensive, but Jim was on the road from Luray for 2 or more hours to shuttle me for 15 minutes. There had to be a better way. If you pulled up to one of the trailhead overlooks, many cars would stop, and it would be an easy conversation to get a ride 10 miles north or south. After today, I would finish the central section of Shenandoah.

From the Bearfence Parking Area, it was an easy downhill to Bootens Gap, and then a climb up to Hazletop. I'm dense, but I have begun to notice that summits of mountains on the trail often seem to be marked by a large tree across the trail, with a section cut out to allow you to get by. Was this intentional, or just because trees on the summits are felled by lightning? I have never seen any reference to it in any book. The downed tree often provides a seat to rest after climbing the mountain.

It was a very easy downhill to Milan Gap. The sun was getting stronger. Milan Gap is the only actual AT crossing of Skyline Drive in the central section of Shenandoah, but there are many other access places.

Past Milan Gap, there was an open area with a small cemetery. In another mile, with the trail becoming more rocky with easy climbing, I was in the Big Meadows area. The trail circled around the western side of the lodge. There was a great spot under the Blackrock Viewpoint along the steep ledges above the trees looking west, but with a long perpendicular mountain ridge to the immediate south. There were additional rocky ledge viewpoints. I hugged the inside with my sweaty palms.

I never saw the lodge on the hike, but the trail passed directly through the Big Meadows campground. Families were out for their summer vacations. It was nice for them, I thought, but it would not have been my family's style. To us, roughing it was staying in a hotel rated less than three stars. We were spoiled.

I reached Fishers Gap and drove back to the Big Meadows campground, where I had learned that anyone could stop and use the public showers for a small fee. It was great. I ate at the Big Meadows Wayside, got gasoline, and drove home.

After a two-day trip up to Massachusetts, I was waiting for a cab at Rockfish Gap on Sunday, August 24. I would hike 8 days in August. I had jumped down to the southern end of Shenandoah. Rockfish Gap is where the AT crosses Interstate 64, and is the southern terminus of Skyline Drive and the northern terminus of the Blue Ridge Parkway. Shenandoah is a closed park with gated admissions, but the Blue Ridge Parkway is open, and more easily accessible. I would hike three days and almost finish Shenandoah. I stayed at a motel in Waynesboro because of the proximity to the south district of the park. On this first day, I would leave my car at an old, closed, orange-roofed Howard Johnson, and the cab took me up into the park to Sawmill Run. It was about noon. I was up really early, and had driven 300 miles to get down there. I-81 was becoming very familiar. The same pleasant but overweight cab driver would help me over the next few days. He loved driving up into Shenandoah, since it was a real diversion to him. He lived in Waynesboro, but had never been in the park. We spotted turkeys and other wildlife along the way.

At the park entrance, there seemed to be no problem with the cab going onto the drive, as long as I paid the fee at the gate. Jim would be horrified, since I think he was actually the only one licensed to go in there. It worked out for me each of the next three days, and the fares were not as high as I had been paying. The driver dropped me off at Sawmill Run. It would be 10 miles back to my car in Rockfish Gap, and it was almost 1:00 P.M.

After the driver dropped me at the Overlook, I took some pictures of the view across the mountains. Beyond the next mountain was Waynesboro. I actually had a little trouble finding where the trail crossed at the viewpoint, and then had to think about which way to go. Once settled, I started a little climb on easy trail, and then headed down into Jarman Gap. The end of the down was through an open field, and you could see across the gap where it crossed the drive. There, on the far hill, you could see where the trail went up through a meadow on the other side. Much of the trail south of Jarman

Gap was open area, including the summit of Calf Mountain. From Jarman Gap it was two miles and 1,000 feet up, but easy trail. Then I headed down to Beagle Gap, crossing the drive again.

From Beagle Gap it was another 700-foot climb to the police radio towers on the summit of Bears Den Mountain. At the summit, there was a group of incoming college freshmen doing their pre-orientation thing. Oh, it was that "back to college" time of year. I hiked down to McCormick Gap, crossing the drive again. After a short, steep climb, I cruised downhill for four gradual miles to Rockfish Gap. There were several gates and old roads to cross, and then a side trail to the entrance station. Thru-hikers were encouraged to walk over there to pay the entrance fee to the park. I had already done that. In a few minutes, I was crossing Interstate 64. *Check.*

Waynesboro was a trail town that hikers looked forward too. I think it was because there really had not been any significant town since Daleville, 135 miles to the south. It seemed pretty dead to me. The dinner place was an okay buffet of sorts. I did find a good greasy spoon breakfast spot the next morning. I met the cab at Rockfish Gap again, and he followed me up into the park. The ranger station was not even open yet, which seemed strange, since it was after 8:00 A.M.

I dropped my car at Sawmill Run, and then the driver took me north to Jones Run. It would be 12 miles south to my car. Although a more remote area of Shenandoah, the trail still never was far from Skyline Drive, and crossed it four times in between Sawmill Run and Jones Run.

After about a mile in through the woods, I was at Blackrock, "a tumbled mass of large lichen-covered blocks of stone" according to the guide. Even the trail across the rock field was not bad. It was very open, but the views were nice across the ridge and down toward Waynesboro Valley. Coming down from Blackrock, I bypassed the hut. I really did not see many of the huts in Shenandoah, since most all were a little off the trail.

I cruised through the day, crossing the drive multiple times. The park was quiet on this Monday. I felt like I had the place to myself. The southern end of Shenandoah is the least-used part. It was all easy trail, with little climbing, and the last five miles were very flat at first, and then a gradual downhill to my car at Sawmill Run. I was at my car in less than 5 hours, and it was not yet 2:00 P.M. I was often hitting the dinner hour when finishing my hikes. The only solution would be a beer and a nap before dinner.

I had made arrangements for the cab driver to meet me early the next morning at Jones Run. He took me up to the Loft Mountain Camp Store. There was still no indication that he'd had any trouble getting into the park. The entrance station was closed when I went through.

I went in the quiet store and bought a few snacks, just to justify my being there. It was early, and I had plenty of time. I was only hiking 6 miles today, but I still had a 300-mile drive home. I picked up the AT just east of the store, and followed it as it circled around the Loft Mountain Camp Ground. There were only a few campers and tents around. There was a side trail to a nice amphitheater for summer shows.

It was a gradual but rocky down from Loft Mountain. I crossed the drive at Doyles River Overlook, which was empty of cars. In another easy mile I was at Brown Gap, crossing the drive again. Between Brown Gap and Jones Run it was an easy climb on nice trail. At one point there was a ravine of sorts, looking across to a cliff wall of stone.

I drove back to the Loft Mountain Camp Store, where they had showers. Then I went back out to the drive and had a burger at the Loft Mountain Wayside, and headed north to Swift Run Gap. From there I exited the park and drove down US 33 to Harrisonburg and I-81. Harrisonburg is the home of James Madison University. Bethany was heavily recruited by JMU to go to college there after her piano audition, but she chose Indiana University at Bloomington.

I did not hike in September at all. Ben scored great tickets to see a game at the old Yankee Stadium in its final season. The following year, he took me to see the Phillies play at the new Yankee Stadium. We entered the park just as Jimmy Rollins hit a leadoff home run. The Phillies won. Phillies fans in the center field bleachers annoyed the Yankees fans no end.

Bethany, Kevin, Ben and I rented canoes and paddled downstream on the Delaware from Easton to Riegelsville, past our house. Virginia and Michelle (who had to work on a project for her company) could spot us using our telescope, lunching on an island, 400 feet down and a half-mile away.

I did a weekend in early October up in Vermont and could have stopped there, but I had one small section to finish Shenandoah. I could not let it go. So on Friday, October 17, I was sitting at Rockfish Gap again. I planned to hike two sections south of there, and then on my last day I would go back up into the park, hike the remaining eight miles in Shenandoah, and drive home.

I called the cab company I had used back in August, and was horrified when the dispatcher told me they were not allowed to go up onto the Blue Ridge Parkway. I asked for the driver I had used the month before, but he was in the hospital. It did not make sense that they would go into the closed park of Shenandoah, but would not go up on the open Blue Ridge Parkway. It was noon. How would I get a shuttle in time to allow me to hike today? There was a visitor's center in Rockfish Gap. My guidebook indicated they would even make shuttle arrangements. There were a few volunteers in there, and I described my plight. None got the message that I needed a ride up to the Humpback Rocks parking area, only a crummy six miles south on the Blue Ridge Parkway. I thought about road walking up there, and then back down the trail. I thought about hitch hiking, but it was too risky.

I was desperate, and pulled out my AT shuttle list that I only had for the cab company's phone number. There was a person listed, but they were near Charlottesville, 40 miles away. I called anyway, and a nice gentleman answered and said I was lucky, and they were just leaving to come to Waynesboro, and they would be happy to help me, and they would be there in half an hour. Wow, trail magic!

Bill and Charlotte were a delightful couple in their early 70s. Charlotte had section-hiked almost all of the AT in the summers with a group of other women. They would go for a month or so each year. Her advice to me was to do New Hampshire and Maine before I got too old and my knees could not take it. I already knew what she meant. They did not even want to take any money, but I insisted that I give them a nice contribution to their local hiking club, and that seemed to make it all right. I was forward and asked if they would help me the next morning too, and they would. Boy was I lucky.

Charlotte shuttled quite a bit in the area, and was even known to the Shenandoah Park rangers. She told me of driving up a side road to rescue some hikers who had gotten caught in a freak winter storm. A year or so later, I saw a story on the history channel about a father and grown son who started a hike over Christmas break from Waynesboro, hiking up into Shenandoah. It snowed over 30 inches in a day, and they got caught in it. They made their way to the Loft Mountain Camp Store, where they broke in to use the phone and hunker down with candy bars until they could be rescued. The Park Rangers could get them to the point where someone (maybe Charlotte) could pick them up at a side road. It all fit.

Bill and Charlotte shuttled me up to the Humpback Parking Area on the Blue Ridge Parkway. It would be 7.4 miles back to Rockfish Gap on the AT. It was 1:30 P.M., but I had plenty of time, even though the days were getting shorter.

It was a two-tenths-of-a-mile access trail to get to the AT from the parking area. I found the maps and trails here confusing. It did not help that there was a Humpback Parking Area and a Humpback *Rocks* Parking area. It would ultimately lead me to missing a section, which of course I feel compelled to make up. At the Glass Hollow Overlook, the leaves at elevation were starting to turn, but the valley was still green. At Cross Mill Creek I met a young man and we swapped cameras for a photo op. I was in those same shorts and a sweatshirt.

We hiked to the shelter together, only a tenth of a mile away. At the shelter was a bench with a memorial plaque to John Donovan, a local adventurer who had died while hiking the Pacific Crest Trail in 2005. Cross Mill Creek ran right in front of the shelter. It seemed unusual that the shelter would be placed so near the creek. Planners are often worried about water contamination.

From the shelter it was easy "old woods road" for a few miles. I was going up a slight rise, and a deer was coming down toward me. I stopped and took some pictures, but tried not to move. It did not spot me right away and kept coming. At the last minute, he spooked and ran.

The trail had wandered quite a distance from the parkway, but was now approaching it again, and I could hear the cars above. The trail continued to be easy, but the last two miles of each day always seem long. I hiked up a little rise to get to the parkway, crossed over, and was at my car at the closed HoJo. I was off to my Waynesboro motel.

I was to meet Bill and Charlotte at Reeds Gap, where Virginia 664 crosses the Blue Ridge Parkway, at nine the next morning. They could not have been more helpful. Although the AT crosses the Blue Ridge Parkway north of the James River and even a little bit south of there, it is nothing like the AT and Skyline Drive, which run right next to each other for 90 miles. I was early, so on my way down the parkway to Reeds Gap, I stopped at Humpback Rocks Visitors Center. It was a tiny building, with only a few exhibits and limited books and candy bars for sale. The surrounding area was beautiful. There were many split-rail fences and rock walls along the drive, with nice lawns.

Reeds Gap was busy when I arrived. There was a Boy Scout troop ready to head out for an overnight. All the parents were dropping them off. The parking lot could handle all the cars. Bill and Charlotte were right on time, and took me back up to the Humpback Parking Area so I could hike the 12 miles back to my car.

I'm not sure what I was thinking, but instead of taking the access trail that I had taken the day before, I took the direct route up to Humpback Rocks. That meant I would bypass several miles of the AT. I had forgotten about that, and now think I will have to make it up. There is that pledge, "that I will pass every white blaze." My pledge does not include road walks, but everything else. It was a beautiful Saturday. The one-mile hike up to Humpback Rocks was not easy. On the way I passed a dad with his little daughter. She was a gamer, but I was a little concerned that she might fall and get hurt. Was I becoming a sissy?

Humpback Rocks was a treacherous place. It was early, but there were people all over. I talked to a few students from UVA in Charlottesville, and we swapped cameras. Our family had visited UVA on the college visit trips, and Ben was accepted to the honors program there, but chose Penn State. The views west were great. It was peak color here in Virginia. When the little girl and her dad arrived, I had to leave as she started to scramble on the rock ledges, because her dad was not paying close enough attention. I continued the climb of over 1,000 feet up Humpback Mountain after I reached the AT. I was done climbing for the day, so I thought I had it made.

I passed through a picnic area which was vacant. Leaves covered the grounds, and the restrooms were locked up tight. Before crossing the parkway at Dripping Rocks, the AT hugged ledges with steep drop-offs and a great view across the valley to the next ridge. Across the way were the towering (they were only 4-5 floors) condos of the Wintergreen Ski Resort. I would learn about it later. The buildings were lined up near the top of the ridge. It seemed dramatic. The resort was at the top of the mountain, and the ski slopes could easily be seen. It was about four miles away.

The next four miles paralleled the parkway, but below it. There were nice views into the Sherando Valley below, along Virginia 664. The trail became difficult in this section. There were minor ups and downs, but it was mostly unrelenting rocks on the trail. I had become spoiled with the nice footpaths in Virginia. I passed two large men carrying a huge chainsaw. They had cleared a large blowdown on the trail. I would see their handiwork a mile later. I was constantly hearing the cars on the parkway above, and kept anticipating arriving at the crossing at Three Ridges, but it just was not coming. The trail was tough.

When I got to the crossing, I wimped out. Rather than crossing the road to continue on the AT, I walked down the parkway to my car. That is another half-mile I will need to make up. It is too bad, because I believe there were nice views at Three Ledges, possibly including the Wintergreen Ski Resort, which was just below. I will catch it sometime.

Rather than drive the parkway again, I headed out Route 664 through Sherando to Waynesboro.

For my third day, I had arranged with Jim of Mountain and Valley Shuttle to meet me at Simmons Gap. He was there waiting when I arrived a half an hour before our scheduled meet. It would be the most I ever paid for a shuttle. Jim would have three hours of driving today. I thanked him for his help. Jim drove me south to the Loft Mountain Camp store lot, so I could start my 8-mile hike. The store was abandoned for the winter. After this day, I had completed Shenandoah.

From the store, I headed north toward Loft Mountain. It was another beautiful fall day. The colors were not peak yet. From Loft Mountain you could see the drive on an adjacent ridge about a mile away. The next few miles were an easy downhill to Ivy Creek. Hiking down and then up from Ivy Creek was beautiful and peaceful. I did not see a soul. From the Trayfoot

Mountain, I could look directly down at Skyline Drive, 100 feet below. The trail walked across the Ivy Creek Overlook, but did not cross the drive at this point. The trail headed down toward Pinefield Gap through a thick forest of young scrub trees that formed a solid low canopy, so it was like walking through a tunnel in spots.

At Pinefield Gap, the trail crossed the drive for what would be my last time. On the way up from the gap, I encountered an antlered deer on the trail that showed no interest in giving way. I took some pictures and moved forward, and he grudgingly meandered into the woods. The last mile was an easy 500-foot descent to my car at Simmons Gap. There was actually another vehicle there, but I did not see a sign of anyone.

I lingered for a while, changing clothes for the drive home. I had some melancholy about leaving Shenandoah, but have not been back since.

My Phillies won the World Series on a cold night in Philadelphia. Ben would go down to the victory parade.

By any measure I had put in a good year on the trail, and I was at a good stopping point. I'm not sure why, but I was compelled to get out one more time, and two weeks later, on Friday, October 31, I was waiting for Bill and Charlotte at the Tye River trailhead on Virginia 56. It was in the middle of nowhere. I had left at 4:00 A.M. and driven over 350 miles to get there. It was about noon. Bill and Charlotte were right on time. It was a long drive around the east side of the mountain to Reeds Gap. A couple from DC were there getting ready for an overnight loop hike.

The hike started out easily enough, up through a clearing, and even the climb up Meadow Mountain was not difficult. I lost a baseball cap that a client had given me. I got to the junction of the Mau-Har Trail. It was tempting to take Mau-Har which would be much easier (I think) along Campbells Creek. It would rejoin the AT in three miles, rather than the 4.6 over Three Ridges. That would be cheating, not that I hadn't done that before, but I will clean up my mistakes.

The climb up started easily enough, but soon became steep and tough. It was rock scrambling. There were views, some through the trees, and some on open viewpoints on ledges. It was way past peak leaf season on the mountain tops, but there was a little color left in the valleys. One view to the south was across to the Priest, with the Ty River Valley below. I would later hear a story of the Ty River Valley. The steepest part of the climb was 500 feet in half a mile.

I made it to the top of the north ridge of Three Ridges, but with all the leaves down, I lost the trail. I retraced my steps several times. The white blazes just seemed to stop once I hit the top of the ridge. I decided to stop to eat, and then just took my best guess and started down from the ridge, and luckily hit the trail. There were just too many leaves on top, and the AT was not well marked.

The hike down was also steep and rocky. It was becoming a tough day. I was doing this section the easiest way, from north to south, and was actually losing 2,000 feet of elevation, but it sure did not seem like it. I usually did not choose my direction based on elevation, but I had today, and was glad. I finally got to the Mau-Har Trail junction. I was tired, but glad I did not take the easy way out. I still had two miles to go, but the trail became easier on nice switchbacks down to the Tye River. The river crossing was on a narrow wooden engineered suspension bridge that must have cost a fortune to build. I think it was necessary, since the Tye River could really run high.

I had made a reservation at the Wintergreen Ski Resort. I knew nothing of it, but in this remote area of Virginia, there were no nearby towns, and the Wintergreen entrance was two miles from Reeds Gap. Since it was not summer or winter, the rates were reasonable. I felt silly in a 2-story loft condo with two bathrooms and a kitchen, but it was the smallest they had. All the units were owned, but it was operated like a hotel. It was a big, nice place. I took the same long drive around the mountain that we had done that morning, and drove up the long entrance road. It was dark when I was checking in. I had dinner at the sports bar.

Bill and Charlotte could not help me on Saturday morning. I jumped south a few sections to get close to a town with a cab company. I drove down the parkway to US 60, and then east to the Long Mountain Wayside trailhead. The wayside was about three acres, with parking and picnic tables. It was jammed with school buses, cars and people. There was some sort of a running race in progress, and this was the finish line. I crammed my car in a spot and went down to the road to wait for the cab. The cab took me on some back roads, and eventually on the parkway again to the Punchbowl trailhead.

At road crossings during the morning, there were people posted as part of the race, so the race route on roads must have more or less paralleled the AT. The hike up and down several peaks of Rice Mountain was on easy footpath. It was a pretty area. Leaving Rice Mountain, there was a two-mile, 1,200-foot descent down to Pedlar River Dam. The descent used switchbacks and rock steps, and was not difficult.

The crossing of the Pedlar River was on a narrow wooden suspension bridge, just like the one over the Ty River. There were a lot of people around on this beautiful 1st of November Saturday. A family took my picture at the bridge. On the other side of the bridge there was a little climb up to get on the hill overlooking Pedlar Lake. There were views through the trees down to some houses and the road along the lake. The lake is the Lynchburg Reservoir. Lynchburg was a distance east. Lynchburg, apparently, is the largest city in the country without an interstate highway. The trail followed the ridge overlooking the lake for a time, but eventually moved away.

After Swapping Camp Creek, the trail climbed some rock steps, and the gradual climb of 1,000 feet over the next four miles. There was a pleasant walk along Brown Mountain Creek. At both ends of the creek walk was a sign describing the area as the former site of a freed slave community that existed in the early 1900s. A former member of the community described life as he remembered it.

I stopped at the Brown Mountain Creek Shelter. There were two men my age from Virginia who were section-hiking the AT. They were staying there for the night. It seemed early in the day to be stopping, I thought, but it was their hike. I never had to worry about the next shelter. As I approached US 60, the trail got steeper, but still on an easy path. The wayside was abandoned when I arrived. All the runners had made it.

I enjoyed the drive back up the parkway to Reeds Gap and stopped several times, including the viewpoint of the Irish Creek Valley and 20-Minute Cliff. Twenty minutes after the sunlight struck the rock face, the residents below knew dusk would fall on the valley floor. It was still bright, and even though it was past peak color, the mountains and valleys were still beautiful.

After showering in my condo, I drove around Wintergreen. It was new, and seemed to have a lot to offer. There were ski slopes, golf courses, indoor and outdoor pools in several areas of condos and home sites. A sign overlooking the hotel was posted at Founders Vision Overlook. When I googled Wintergreen when I got home, I was disappointed to see that the developer, which was some sort of Nature Foundation, was in financial difficulty, and they may need to sell some of their undeveloped land.

The next morning, I would meet Bill and Charlotte for the last time. They picked me up at the Tye River Trailhead at the foot of the Priest on Virginia 56. A tragic event took place in this area in August of 1969. The remnants of Hurricane Camille, which devastated the Gulf Coast, stalled directly over the Tye River Valley one night. Without any warning, while the residents were sleeping, heavy rains caused mudslides and flooding. Hundreds of residents lost their lives, and entire communities were lost. In the dramatic drive down Virginia 56, one could see how steep it was, both down into the valley from the west, and on either side of the valley with Three Ridges to the North and the Priest to the south.

Bill and Charlotte drove me down to the Fish Hatchery and dropped me there. It would be a tough, steep walk up Fish Hatchery Road to get to the AT. Although it could be driven, there was a locked gate that residents along the road opened and closed when they entered and exited. The road was just too rough for the public. The trailhead was one long mile up. On the way up, four local guys who I had seen getting organized in the parking lot below passed me like I was standing still. They were early twenty-somethings and were out for a few days of camping.

I finally reached the trailhead, and it was a short walk to a gate and then steep climbing to Spy Rock. Spy Rock was supposedly used as a lookout by the confederates during the Civil War. Spy Rock was a massive dome, about 40 feet tall, and an acre on top. The four packs were set in a clearing, and I could hear the voices of the four young guys. I put my pack down and started to walk around the rock, but I had a long day ahead and a long drive. I continued on to Main Top Mountain. I had climbed 600 feet in the mile since I'd left the road. There were limited views through the trees on Main Top.

I started to descend down toward Cash Hollow and Crabtree Farm. At Crabtree Farm Road there were some old campers and old cars in the area. The campers appeared occupied, but I did not see any activity. The road could be taken to the Crabtree Campground. The area gave me the creeps, so I just moved ahead and came to a sign for the Priest Wilderness. The trail up the Priest was a wide old woods road, and easy. I was climbing again now, and would go up 700 feet in a mile and a half, but it did not seem hard. The trail circled around and up Cone Mountain. You could see the ledges of the Priest summit from the road.

On this beautiful fall Sunday, there were quite a few people milling around at the top of the Priest. There were some side trails to make the Priest more accessible than the massive climb coming up from the Tye River. I bypassed the Priest Shelter and headed toward the summit. The trail did not actually get to the rocky open viewpoints, but stayed in the woods. The leaves were thick on the trail, and there was the *whoosh* as you moved them out of the way. I went over to the view where the most people seemed to be. I did the usual camera swap. I was in shorts and a cotton T-shirt, sitting on rock with my back to the view of brown mountains that went on forever to the west.

There was a little chill in the air, so I put on my sweatshirt for the long 3,100-foot descent over 4.5 miles using 37 switchbacks. I kept thinking that I was glad not to have had to climb this thing. After a mile, there were great views east down into the Tye River Valley. It was 2,000 feet down, so everything looked tiny. I passed a trail volunteer coming up carrying a hedge trimmer of sorts. He was keeping the vegetation back on this well-maintained section of the trail. *Wow*, I thought, *four miles of uphill hedge trimming.*

There was a beautiful log bridge over Cripple Creek, and in another mile, I was at the parking lot. It was a long drive out to Interstate 81, and another 300-plus miles home.

2008 started out terribly for the firm, but both the firm and I recovered, and life goes on. Amazingly, 2008 was my biggest year of hiking to that point; 166 miles in 18 days. The trips were getting longer, and I was now in a remote area of Virginia. Vermont looked problematic for the day-hiker that I was. It was not going to be easy from this point on.

To that date, I had completed 788 miles in 79 days in 7 years. I was over a third completed. It was still not a pace to get me to any goal line. I had to remember it was the journey, not the goal.

Barack Obama was elected president. The stock market would continue to hit lows. Bernard Madoff was charged with a $50 billion (with a B) Ponzi scheme. The Detroit Lions went 0-16.

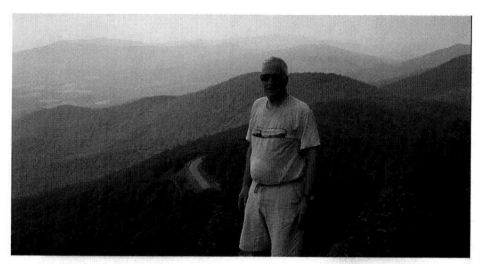

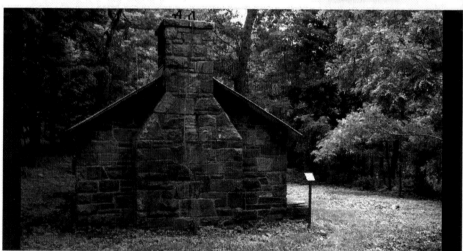

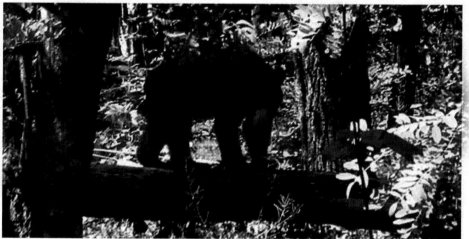

Top: Dennis above Skyline Drive. Middle: Bird's Nest # 3 in Shenandoah. Bottom: Posing Bear in Shenandoah.

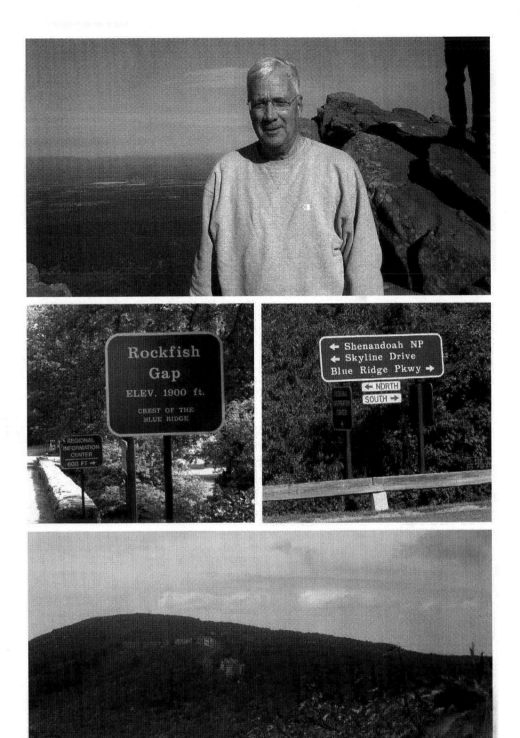

Top: Dennis at Humpback Rocks. Middle: Rockfish Gap at Interstate 64. Bottom: Wintergreen Ski Resort from Dripping Rocks.

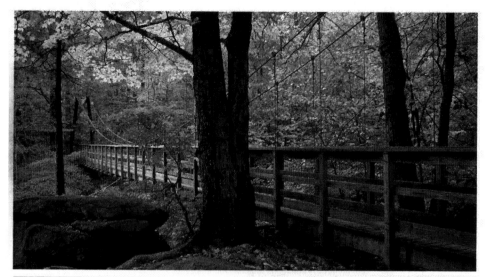

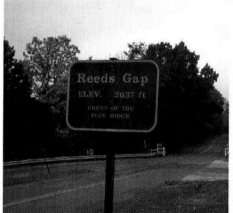
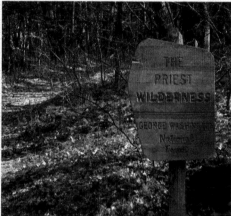

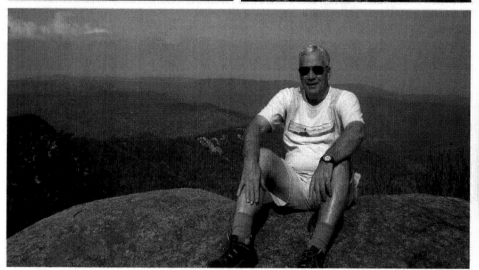

Top: Suspension bridge over Tye River. Middle: Reeds Gap VA; Priest Wilderness. Bottom: Dennis from the Priest.

2009 – North - Vermont Conference

I had been a member of the Appalachian Trail Conference, which had changed its name to the Appalachian Trail Conservancy at some point, since I had started hiking back in 2002. I had gotten the magazine *Journeys,* and enjoyed reading the articles about the trail towns, etc. I was getting familiar first-hand with more of the trail towns. I knew there was a biannual meeting, but had not paid much attention.

Over the winter of 2009 an issue showed up, and to my luck, the 2009 meeting would be held in Vermont. Further, there were hikes scheduled for most of the days, and many of them were on the AT. These would be group hikes, with six to twenty people, and driver-hikers would shuttle between trailheads. Most all of Vermont would be covered. This was a major break for me, since I was getting discouraged about the logistics of day-hiking Vermont.

After tax season was over, I wasted no time in registering for the conference. To my dismay, all the AT section hikes were "full," but the hike registrar said not to worry. I could get on them when I got there, since many people changed their minds, and I would have no problem, he said. That turned out to be true.

Chrysler and then GM filed for bankruptcy, reflecting the still-poor state of the economy after the stock market would reach its lows in March. My 401k had become a 201k.

The conference was held at a small college in Castleton, Vermont, near Rutland. Many of the attendees were about my age, and attended year after year. Many were section-hiking the trail, just like me. Who knew? Breakfast and dinner were served in the campus dining halls, trail lunches could be purchased, and I stayed in the dorm; but many tented on the campus green. It was great to meet all the people and hear their stories about hiking. About 300 people attended at least part of the conference. Since I was trying it out, I decided on four of the conference's seven days.

I drove up on Friday, July 17, registered, and was able to get on a hike for the next day.

The hike was only seven miles, but we had to drive across Vermont to get there. I drove and took Julian, who would become a friend, and Wanda and Carolyn, part of a group from Williamsport, Pennsylvania. Wanda was an organic farmer and lab technician at Bucknell University. Carolyn was a courageous young woman who was a transplant recipient. Julian was a teacher from Maryland. There was another car of women, and we met our hike leader, Dave, in West Hartford. West Hartford was a tiny little burg with a one-room library and a general store. Hanover, New Hampshire was only ten trail miles to the east, but nonetheless, West Hartford would be a nice little respite for the thru-hiker. Dave left his car in West Hartford for the afternoon shuttle, and we drove out to the Cloudland Road trailhead. It took us a good half-hour and twenty miles to drive around.

The hiking was easy, but slow because of the group. I did not mind. It was nice to hike at a leisurely pace and get to know the others one at a time. There was Ellen from Boston, Cheryl from Tennessee, and Maggie from Virginia. All of their stories were interesting. All were members of their local hiking clubs and hiked all year long, much of it not on the AT. The only place I did hike was on the AT.

There was an easy climb up to Thistle Hill, then across to Arms Hill for lunch, in an open, grassy area with a nice view south to another ridge. After lunch it was across to Bunker Hill, and then downhill all the way, steep at the end, crossing the White River to West Hartford. On the way down we passed through Red Pine Plantation, an area of very tall Norway spruce. Dave took the drivers (me and Ellen) back to Cloudland Road to get our cars, while the others chilled at the West Hartford general store.

Cloudland Road was a gravel road with sharp stones and my new SUV picked up one of them, which gave me a slow leak. I got air and was fine to get back to the campus, but did not want to take my car the next day until I got it fixed. The drive back was fun. Julian and Wanda were a riot in the back seat. We easily arrived in time to shower for dinner.

I was able to get a hike for the next day due to cancellations. It would be eight miles, and we would hike from Stony Brook Road to Lookout Farm Road. Both trailheads were very remote, and were accessed from the north. I did not see these roads in my old book and map set, but new maps had been published, which I bought at the conference.

There were seven of us in three cars. I drove with Janie, our hike leader, from Altoona, Pennsylvania. Janie was not a strong leader, and talked about issues she had with her group the day before going over Killington. I saw her a day later, and she said she was going home early because things were not working out. She had been scheduled to be a leader on an overnight backpacking hike.

It was a good group, and everyone helped Janie be the leader. The group included Dan, an attorney from New Jersey, who was with his daughter, Andrea. It was their third or fourth AT conference together. Andrea was in her twenties, and worked as a medical researcher in New York City and was married to a doctor who was doing his residency. Dan and Andrea were both experienced hikers, and the previous year had hiked in the White Mountains in New Hampshire using the hut system, which they described to me. This was not on my radar yet, but I found it interesting and useful. Dan had apparently fallen, hit his head on a rock, and they had to cut the "hut" hike short. Dan and Andrea were very nice, and we often had meals together. John, Wendy and Alice were also part of the group. Wendy was a gamer, and was trying to log as many AT miles as possible this week, and was doing one of the overnight hikes that were too long for a day hike down in the southern part of Vermont.

We started out from Stony Brook Road at Notown Clearing, just behind another group from the conference who was doing a 12-mile section. We caught them at the first viewpoint, which was jammed due to limited space, so they moved on quickly. We were climbing about 1,000 feet over the first two miles. I felt like I was constantly on someone's heels, so I had to learn to stop and wait for the person in front of me to get ahead before climbing at my pace. I was learning this group-hike thing.

The area we hiked was part of the Les Newell Wildlife Management Area, which was 50,000 undeveloped acres, 8,000 of which were owned by the state. There were two 500-foot bumps. In between we crossed Chateauguay Road. When I was up in the area the year before on the weekend I hiked Killington, I had tried to get to the road from the south. After driving endlessly, I gave up. The road at that time was too washed out.

We reached Lakota Lake Lookout, and you could still see the White Mountains in the distance, even though it was a slightly hazy day. In another mile and a half we reached The Lookout, a private cabin, used by the hikers with permission. The cabin was a one-room empty thing, looking like it would fall down any minute. It did have a viewing platform built on top of it, with a side ladder to climb up there. Most did, but I did not, due to my fear of heights. I could see just fine from the porch, thank you very much.

In another mile we were at our side trail at Lookout Farm Road, which wasn't a road at all, but a steep, rocky third-of-a-mile trail down to our cars at Green Gate Road. We still had to shuttle ourselves around and up the long, remote Stony Brook Road. Janie talked the whole way home.

That night, the entertainment was a slide show of a family from Hawk Mountain, Pennsylvania, who went on a hiking adventure every summer. The mom was a writer, and this was her research. Years before, she and her husband had hiked the Pacific Crest Trail with their one-year-old daughter, four-year-old son, and six llamas to carry their gear, food and water. Wow.

There were no scheduled hikes on Monday so that people would attend the afternoon annual meeting of the ATC. I had decided to try to hike a short section that I had cancelled the year before when I went up to the summit of Killington for the *Good Morning America* program. I recruited Julian to go along, since he had an interest. Virginia called around for me, and she found a garage to get my flat tire fixed. It had picked up a sharp stone on Cloudland Road two days before.

Julian and I drove to the Vermont 103 trailhead just south of Rutland, which was not far from campus. I had made arrangements with Killington Cab Co. for a shuttle. At the trailhead, we met Steve, another conference attendee who planned to hike the same section by doing it in and out. He would hike to Upper Cold River Road and then back to his car, retracing his steps. He decided to join us. We waited for the cab that was long overdue and did not answer his cell. We did not need the cab at this point since we had two cars now. We started out and after the first turn, the cab called to say he would be there in five minutes, so we went back to meet him. It was frustrating, and was getting late.

Finally, we were hiking south from Cold River Road. We had only hiked about half a mile and Julian decided he was hungry. I was too, but thought we should have gotten a little further. We did find a nice spot along Gould Brook. Julian was a talker, which made it fun. He would stop hiking to tell a story which could go on.

The first three miles were flat and easy, and then a little rise to Beacon Hill. The pace was slow and I started to move ahead and then wait. Steve stayed back with Julian. Steve was from Michigan, and a retired Ford engineer. He was a great guy, a good hiker and in good shape. He clearly had a lot more patience than I did. We got to Beacon Hill and met four older (late sixties early seventies) women (including the Trekking Twins). They were from the conference, and were doing the same section that we were.

The Trekking Twins were fabulous, and actual twins. They had been section-hiking the AT ever since they each lost their husbands within a year of each other. They had hiked a lot of the AT, and were expecting to complete it. They had not done much of Pennsylvania, but most of the north, including Maine, and a lot of the south, too. They were working on Vermont before, during and after the conference. They were from Virginia, and had gone to the University of Virginia, where one met and married a doctor, and the other a lawyer. They lived separate lives in separate cities, but reunited when they both were widowed. They bought hiking poles and shoes, and never looked back. They were slight, but powerful hikers. They lived in Florida in the winter and Virginia in the summer. They complained that it was difficult to stay in shape in Florida over the winter since there were no hills, but they just walked fast every day.

Like me, they only day-hiked, did not camp, and arranged for shuttles. They said they even hired a guide in Maine's 100-mile wilderness to take them in and out of logging roads to access the trail. I asked them about the

23-mile section in southern Vermont, and one said it was their token back-pack, the only time they had slept on the ground.

The women took a picture of Julian, Steve and me from the summit of Beacon Hill. There were great views down to Vermont 103 and the Rutland Airport. We headed down. The 600-foot descent was steep and challenging. I led the way down. The four women blew by us on the descent, which was a little embarrassing, I thought. The women were having a ball on the tough descent, and were really hiking with joy and purpose.

I did wait several times for Julian and Steve, but then quickly got ahead, and finally just continued on to the cars. They showed up about 20 minutes later. There was really a lesson for me in all this. We were hiking as a group. There was no time limit or deadline. We could easily make dinner. When you are hiking in a group or even one other person, the slow one should be in front, and just go at that pace.

It is very different for thru-hikers, who, even though they might be hiking together, they are never actually together, sometimes a mile or more apart. Since they are going for miles, they all need to hike at their own pace, and they do.

I have since felt bad about my lack of patience, and vowed to do better. Julian continued to be a friend, and I would see him two years later at the Virginia conference, where we often ate together.

The next day would be my last at the conference, and I was able to get on a 12-mile hike further to the south in Vermont. There were 10 of us in four cars. Karen from Harrisburg, Pennsylvania was the hike leader. Rob from the same hiking club was the co-leader. The Trekking Twins and Dan and Andrea were also on the hike. Pete from California drove out to the trailhead with me. He was originally from York, Pennsylvania, and he came back to all the AT conferences as a reunion of sorts with his parents and family. He had thru-hiked the AT some 15 years earlier, and hiked a lot in California.

Karen was a strong leader, and actually told an older woman that she could not go on today's hike. The woman had an apparent reputation among the hike leaders as being very slow, which would not be good on a 12-mile day, since it was already drizzling, and rain was in the forecast. Karen said she would set a good 2.25-mile an hour pace, which was slow for Karen. Karen was very experienced, and had actually hiked to Everest base camp. When she was not hiking, she was an attorney in the Harrisburg area. By chance, I would run into her a few years later.

We dropped two cars at the USFS 10 (United States Forest Service) Road trailhead, and the 10 of us piled into 2 cars (including mine), and we wound our way to Mad Tom Notch. Mad Tom Notch Road was remote and very poorly maintained, but we made it to the large trailhead parking lot.

Karen set out at the strong pace she promised, but the group was up to it. I fell in near the end and Rob, the co-leader and I talked a lot of the day. Throughout the day there was a chance to talk to almost everyone, including the Twins, to hear their story. I did not get a chance to talk to Dave from Ohio, since he always wanted to be right on Karen's ass. Rob acted as sweep, with the idea that all in the group had to remain between Karen in front and Rob in the back. The group did spread out some, especially on the immediate climb from Mad Tom Notch to Styles Peak. Rob was from Harrisburg, and was involved in a family plumbing supply business. He and I decided we might be the only Rs at the conference. I usually did not talk politics with hikers, so as not too start any arguments. It was never worth it to me.

The trail ran across the ridge to Peru Peak, and then down to the Peru Peak Shelter, where we had a break. I was able to break out my camera for the first time, to get pictures of everyone. Karen kept us moving, which was a good thing. After the break, we ran into another hiker group from the conference who were hiking around Griffith Lake. There was a level two miles, and then a one-mile climb up 400 feet to Baker Peak. It was not difficult until right at the top, where there was a pretty technical climb up a 100-yard rock face. I was impressed with how the Trekking Twins and Nan attacked it, especially since it had started to rain heavily just before we started up. I would have taken some pictures on the climb up, but I would have fallen behind.

We stopped for a brief lunch, but with the rain, it was not that pleasant. Nan refused to sit on the downed tree log, having had a bad experience with ants at some time in her life. We then cruised downhill to Big Branch and its wooden suspension bridge. A sign said only one person on the bridge at a time. It seemed secure enough. We made another stop at the Big Branch

Shelter, but it was brief, since a handwritten sign indicated it was infested with mice. Many shelters have mice issues. It was an easy mile out to the cars.

Karen, always thinking and taking advantage of her experience as a hike leader, sent Rob back to campus with four hikers, and the other five of us piled in Dan's car to retrieve the two cars at Mad Tom Notch. I drove back to campus alone, which made it a good time to call Virginia.

The conference was a great time. I got to meet a lot of people with common interests, found other section hikers just like me, and also found seven new trailheads in Vermont, which would help me this summer. I also learned that the biannual conference in two years would be in southwest Virginia, right at the point I might be then. Had I known what it would be like, I would have stayed the full seven days; but on Wednesday morning, I drove home.

That Saturday I was in my first triathlon, and came in 890th out of 1,119 finishers, and solid middle of the pack in my age group (6th out of 11). I was strong in the swim (500 meters) and the bike (11.1 miles) but I mostly walked the 5K, and my transition times were terrible.

Virginia wanted to attend a conference at the Kripalu Yoga Center in southwestern Massachusetts, so I dropped her there on August 7 and headed up to Mount Greylock. The roads to the summit were now open after a two-year construction project. The lodge at the summit had just re-opened. I arrived at the summit around lunchtime, and did not have a plan for a shuttle that day. I just sat with my pack near the path where people were heading back to their cars after climbing the summit tower. I asked each group in turn if they could give me a ride down to North Adams if they were going that way. It only took about ten minutes for a father/son tandem to say they would.

They dropped me at Massachusetts 2 but were headed east, so I had a two-mile road walk to get the trailhead at the Greylock Community Center. Once there, it would only be a six-mile hike, but 3,000 feet uphill to the summit. Mount Greylock is the highest point in Massachusetts. From the Community Center, I walked along some streets until entering the woods off Pattison Road. Then it was 1,500 feet straight up in a mile and a half. I was weary, since we had gotten up early to drive up here that morning. I got a little lightheaded on the climb, but persevered. I finally made it to the junction with the Mount Prospect Trail, where you could see down into Williamstown's Green River Valley and west to New York. It was a clear but hot day. Toward the north, the Green Mountains were in view.

Then there was another steep 700-foot climb to the summit of Mount Williams. It was rocky, and the trail was filled with roots. No easy Massachusetts hiking here. In the saddle between Mount Williams and Mount Fitch, I passed a group of thru-hikers, including three very pretty young girls who smiled, but kept on moving.

There was actually a flat trail for over a mile around the side of the mountain before the last steep 500 feet to the summit of Greylock. The steepness at the top was mitigated by some boulder rock steps that were quite an engineering feat. Some new concrete steps were in place as you approached the new, beautiful road. I was exhausted from the long day of driving and hiking.

I had a reservation at Bascom Lodge at the summit. The lodge had gone through some renovation, and had just opened. The first-floor living area had a polished floor, but no furniture yet. I checked in to the second-floor Spartan bedroom. It had showers and bathrooms down the hall. The lodge also had a bunkroom where I met a section-hiker. Josh was a teacher in his 40s, and was from Connecticut. His section-hike had been all of Massachusetts this year. He had done Connecticut the year before. We ended up having dinner together at the lodge.

Dinner was about 15 people, and the lodge operator (a white guy with dreadlocks extending below his rump), doubled as the chef. He did have some inexperienced help, including his wife. Dinner was served family-style. We ate with a couple from New York City who had driven up on a motorcycle for the day. It got too late for them to ride home, so they got a room at the lodge. The wife was a singer/songwriter who had a website and played in some small coffeehouses, etc.

After dinner, I walked over to the tower and around the summit. The nighttime views were great looking down to the south toward Cheshire. There were fireworks that evening, and it was strange to be looking down at them.

The next morning I was up early, and headed down to North Adams for a breakfast at a restaurant I had been to several years before. I had made a shuttle arrangement with Dot McDonald. Dot lived in Brattleboro, about 45 minutes away. She said that she kept her name on the AT shuttle list because the ATC needed her, since there was a dearth of others in the area willing to do it. I was grateful to her.

Dot is an amazing woman. She grew up in New York City and as a child, she and her family vacationed in the Vermont/New Hampshire mountains. She was bitten by the outdoor bug, and always knew she would move up there. When she finished college, she got in her car and started driving, stopped in Brattleboro, and never left there. She had been at the ATC conference the month before, and was actually one of the main organizers, although I did not meet her there. She had offered a free shuttle as part of a silent auction fundraiser, which I bid on, but did not win. Dot would not only help me today, but also two years later, so we spent time in her car together. I enjoyed getting to know her and hear some of her experiences.

Dot is a single mother of an adopted special needs son, Michael, who was now in his 30s. Dot was a teacher, which allowed her to spend summers enjoying her outdoor passions. She had section-hiked the AT, finishing years earlier. She had done the Long Trail several times. She section-"bicycled" across the US over several summers, doing the Rocky Mountains twice since she liked it so much. She was a significant contributor in trail maintenance, and years earlier, was a leader in relocating sections of the AT in southern Vermont. She had been a long-time board member and leader of the Green Mountain Club.

She had taken a youth group on a backpacking trip and a close friend's son was stricken with a health issue (not related to the hike) that ultimately caused his death. She saw a friend get killed by an 18-wheeler on a bike ride. She had stories of assisting more inexperienced hikers that would be very interesting. What a gal.

I met Dot at the remote County Road trailhead in southern Vermont, about 25 minutes from North Adams. Since County Road did not go through to the west (at least not passable enough), Dot knew to drive back around through North Adams, Williamstown and up to Bennington to get to the Vermont 9 trailhead. It took a good hour. Dot would spend 2 ½ hours on the road for me, so I tried to be generous. When she objected, I asked her to just make a contribution to her hiking club, which she liked.

The deep gap where Vermont 9 ran in between the mountains created a VERY steep climb heading south. It was 700 feet in about half a mile, which might have been one of the steepest sections that I had hiked to that point. It was rocky and full of roots, but there were some rock steps which helped. I was sweating when the grade leveled off. That climb from Vermont 9 would be the hardest part of the day.

On top of Harmon Hill, I rousted a local tent camper who did not expect to see anyone this early. He did take my picture with Bennington and its tower in the background. The trail got much easier and level. I met three section-hikers from New Jersey. They were in their 50s and were backpacking for five days. Dot had shuttled them a few days earlier. We all talked about our respect for Dot. I stopped for a snack at the dirt Old Bennington-Heartwellville Road. Just as I was getting ready to depart, those three pretty girls I had seen the day before on the way up Greylock, and a guy with them, came out of the woods. We laughed at seeing each other two days in a row.

The girls were from Connecticut and were thru-hiking together. They were two sisters in their 20s and their 30-something married cousin. They were the bird girls they said, with trail names of Hummingbird, Mockingbird, and the cousin was Lady Bird. They were fun to talk to, especially the cousin, who was a blast. It would be tough for them to make it to Katahdin this year by October 15. The guy had met them a few weeks before and was pink-blazing. Pink-blazing is conducted by male hikers who seem to have more of an interest in the female hikers than the hike itself. I could not blame him.

Shortly, I came to the Congdon Shelter, where I took a few minutes to read the trail journal. It was active with the tail end of the thru-hikers. I had to rock hop across the full-flowing Stamford Stream. An immense beaver dam ran next to the trail. The trail was on puncheon, and the area was very wet with the leaking-but-secure (I hope) dam. The water level was about four feet above the trail, which could be unnerving. A long-bearded thru-hiker came along and he asked about the bird girls. He was another pink-blazer. The trail skirted Sucker Pond.

With about a mile to go, there was a great viewpoint to the south toward Greylock, but I could not pick out the tower. I was at my car at County Road at about 3:30 P.M., about six hours after leaving Vermont 9. I drove back to the Greylock Lodge for a shower, and got ready for dinner. Greylock was busy on this summer Saturday, and at dinner there were about 30 people, including families and senior couples. There were no thru-hikers staying that I was aware of. Many of the dinner guests were not staying at the lodge.

I spent the evening talking to people, trying to figure out how to do the next day's hike down (or up) Greylock, to or from Cheshire. I had no luck.

I did not sleep much and at first light, I just decided to go on faith, and headed down the AT toward Route 8. I did not even pack up, and left my car at the lodge. I would figure something out when I got down to Cheshire.

I had plenty of snacks. I ate some for breakfast. It was very steep and rocky at first, and trail crossed Rockwell Road several times. After the first mile, the trail became a gradual down, and almost level in spots the rest of the day. The grade was easy, but it was rocky on the descent. Closer to the bottom, the trail became easier. An owl buzzed me and landed in a close-by tree. I could get a picture of her, but she was not happy about my presence. A southbound thru-hiker caught up to me near Route 8 in an open field. We chatted and came to Route 8. It seemed confusing about where to pick up the trail. I thought I knew, since I had been there two years earlier, but I confused him more than helped. It was only about 9:30 A.M. I had hiked down in 3 ½ hours.

I had now completed Massachusetts.

The southbounder headed up to the Cobbles, not needing to stop in town, and I started my road walk into Cheshire. I picked up Lanesborough Mountain Road, but it would be six miles to the Greylock Visitors Center at the bottom of the mountain. I had no luck with my thumb out, and the street became a dirt road. After walking at least halfway, or about three miles, the last car that I would have seen stopped to pick me up. The local man drove me to the visitor's center on the dirt road, which became very badly maintained. That was a break. I went into the visitor's center to inquire of the few patrons about a ride, but no one responded, either because they had full cars, or were not going to the summit. It had become foggy, and there would be nothing to see. It was about 11:00 A.M., and I was getting concerned about the noon checkout. I walked out to the road and there were only a few cars headed up this early on a Sunday. After about 30 minutes, a yuppie couple (about my age) in a BMW picked me up and took me to the top. It was great for me, but not so good for them, since the summit was totally socked in with fog.

I took a quick shower, packed the car, settled my bill (which I had to tell them about since they did not seem to know I had even been there or ate dinner twice), called Virginia and headed down to pick her up at Kripalu. We drove home that afternoon.

On Labor Day, September 7, I drove up to the Vermont 103 trailhead. I had made arrangements with the Killington Cab Co. that was late a few months earlier. The owner sent one of his part-time drivers, who was on time. It was about 1:00 P.M. I was up early to get up there by then. He drove around the mountain to Vermont 140. It would only be a six-mile hike. After he dropped me at the large parking lot, I immediately met two women section-hikers who were just finishing the section I would be doing back up to Vermont 103. They had done it north to south, and I would be doing south to north. They had two cars. We talked about possibly trying to help each other with shuttles, but this was their last day.

The climb up to Bear Mountain (yes, another one) was 1,200 feet, but over two miles, so was not steep. The trail was not difficult. There were no views at the summit, and I started down the 700 feet over a mile and a half to Minerva Hinchey Shelter. Minerva was a long-time Green Mountain Club volunteer. It was an easy two miles to Airport Lookout, and then a fairly steep down to Clarendon Gorge. The area before the suspension bridge at the Clarendon Gorge was used for camping, but seemed strange because it was bare dirt underneath a pine forest canopy. There was no one around. *Who had cleaned up the pine needles?*

The suspension bridge was a one lane thing. If someone came the other way, one would have to back up. It had a wood floor and high green fence sides. There were large green steel towers on either bank supported by cables. The bridge itself was about 60 feet long and about 30 feet above the water in the gorge. Julian and I had actually walked down to the bridge back in July while we were waiting for that cab. It was only one-tenth of a mile from the Vermont 103 trailhead. The water in the gorge was flowing strongly, despite the recent dry spell. Vermont was still in good shape with water, as it had been a very wet spring. In fact, at the ATC conference, many of the trails were still muddy. It was really that way most of this year. The books about Vermont hiking indicate that you should not even get out on the trails until after Memorial Day. Hikers often refer to Vermont as *Vermudd*.

I drove down to my motel in Manchester. Manchester was a very nice, high-end town. It had beautiful shops and restaurants. I would not have the sense that it was that friendly. Some towns just do not like dirty, smelly hikers.

The next morning I met Dick Andrews at the USFS 10 trailhead that I had been to back in July with Karen's hike. At the conference, Dick had also offered a shuttle as part of a silent auction fund raiser. I did not win, but a month or so later, I got a call that if I would pay my last bid, Dick would be willing to offer the same deal to me that he had given the winner. I jumped at it, and sent a check off. I had called him and made arrangements with him for today and tomorrow. Dick was a great guy, a retired newspaper man. He was an officer and board member of the Green Mountain Club. It was a great contact. Dick drove me over to the same Vermont 140 trailhead that I had started from the day before. I would head south this time, and hike the eight miles to my car.

Right at the road I crossed Roaring Brook, which had a pretty waterfall coming from the west. It would be a 1,500-foot climb up to White Rocks Mountain. Some was a little steep, but most of it was a comfortable grade, since it was a total of three miles to get up there. The trail had some rocky sections, but most was easy. At the junction with the White Rocks Cliff Trail there were thousands of "white rocks" that had been made into hundreds of cairns over an area of about half an acre. It was spectacular.

It was an easy rest of the day down to USFS 10. The shelters and camping area around Little Rock Pond were empty. At the pond there were some benches to sit and enjoy the peace of the overcast but nice day. I did not see a soul this day.

The next day, I met Dick at the trailhead nearest Manchester. We did not meet until 10:00 A.M., since that suited Dick better, and I did not mind, since I had to check out of my room and then could get a good breakfast at the "Upstairs" breakfast spot. Dick never said where he lived in Vermont, but he did say this Vermont 11/30 trailhead was the closest to his home. He drove me up to Mad Tom Notch. He did not want to go all the way to the trailhead, since the road was so bad. I could not blame him, and did not mind, since I was only hiking 5.5 miles. I did end up with about a mile and a half road walk. In lieu of my paying him for this second day's shuttle, Dick asked me to join the Green Mountain Club, which I was glad to do. I filled out the application on the spot and gave him a check.

After the road walk, there was a 700-foot climb up Bromley Mountain. It was spread over two and a half-miles, so it was not steep. The summit of Bromley Mountain was the top of one of the ski lifts for Bromley Mountain Ski Area. It was kind of neat. There was a ski patrol hut and a large observation deck that was about 40 feet high. I went up about 20 feet, but that was it for me. There were great views south toward Stratton Mountain.

The hike down started right down the middle of one of the wide ski slopes, but soon entered the woods to the west of the ski area. It would be 1,500 feet down to the road, steep at first, but then very gradual and easy. I stopped at the beautiful Bromley Shelter.

The shelter had a handicapped accessible composting privy. I was not sure why it would need to be handicapped accessible. I understand that many new facilities, even in remote areas, are built with this in mind. I understand a crew of people carried a wheelchair bound "hiker" up a tough 4-mile trail in New Hampshire so that he could use a ramp at a rebuilt accessible hut.

When I was about a mile from the road, I met a young girl who was a Green Mountain Club intern volunteer. She had a huge pack, including some type of mulch of sorts that she was going to use in some sort of maintenance at the shelter. She must have been carrying 60 pounds. There was a beautiful new bridge over Bromley Brook with gorgeous rock steps built on the bank of both sides of the stream.

I was back at my car in a total of about three hours, including the road walk. My being in better shape was paying off. I ate my lunch as I started the drive home.

I was motivated to "finish" Vermont. My interpretation was conveniently ignoring 40 miles north of Bennington, which included a 23-mile and a 17-mile section in the Green Mountains. I had no idea how I would do those sections without camping.

About two weeks later, on September 19, Bethany was in an Olympic Distance Triathlon at Lake George, New York. I got up early and drove up there in time for the 8:00 A.M. start. She had her wet suit on and was getting ready for the one-mile swim in Lake George. It was a clear but blustery day. The buoys marking the swim course were blowing all over. Undaunted, Bethany dove in when her wave was called. Kevin and I looked at each other, as neither of us would have chosen to do this. Many swimmers were blown off course. We were both relieved when she came out of the water 45 minutes later. She headed out on the 25-mile bike in the New York mountains. On the 10K run, she passed many of those who may have passed her on the swim or bike. She did great, and placed well in the race.

After she got cleaned up at their room in town, we went to lunch at a place overlooking the lake. They were staying in town and had plans for dinner that night. I headed out to a White River Junction motel in Vermont to hike the next three days.

On Sunday, I was up in Hanover, New Hampshire, waiting at the Ben & Jerry's (which is no longer a Ben & Jerry's ice cream store, but an independent one) for a cab out of White River Junction. There were no cab companies in Hanover. The motel in White River Junction was all I could get because of a parents' weekend at Dartmouth College in Hanover, so the town was busy. I had a ten-mile hike this day, but the elevation and trail descriptions did not seem tough. The cab took me back into Vermont to that cute little burg of West Hartford.

I'd already had my breakfast, but stopped in the West Hartford General Store anyway. I bought a few snacks that I really did not need. From town it was a road walk up Tigertown Road, under Interstate 89, *check*, and on to

Podunk (another Indian name) Road, and into the woods. After I entered the woods, I startled (or he startled me) a thru-hiker who had tented right next to the trail the night before. He was south-bounding and asked if the store in Hartford was open. I assured him they had breakfast waiting. He said a moose had aroused him that morning, snorting.

I would climb 1,000 feet, to Griggs Mountain, but it was very gradual, over four miles. At the Happy Hill Shelter, I met a few day-hikers who took my picture there. I was in my same shorts and sweatshirt, but had not broken a sweat this day, with the easy trail. It was now downhill all the way to Hanover.

About halfway to Hanover I overtook Michigan. Michigan was section-hiking the trail, and he had started near Woodstock, Vermont this time, so it was only his second day out. Michigan was north-bounding the AT and had started at Springer about 4 years earlier, and would do 3-4 weeks at a time, a couple of times a year. There is no one way to hike the trail. He was about my age, and had retired early. He had gone to Michigan University and was from Michigan, so his trail name fit. His kids were out of the house. For some personal reasons, it worked out well for him to get away from time to time. He had a big pack, and even though he was in good shape, he did not have his trail legs yet, and was moving slowly.

I just fell in behind him and we talked all the way to town. I was not in a hurry, and was trying to learn patience. He was very interesting, and had a good career in corporate finance. We got to Norwich, and wound our way through the streets. We crossed under Interstate 91, *check*, and started across the bridge over the Connecticut River. We stopped in the middle of the bridge and took some pictures. It seemed like a milestone crossing into New Hampshire. It was a sunny and pleasant day. We walked through the town, and I took his picture for him at the lawn of Dartmouth College.

Our family had visited Dartmouth on the college trips. Ben did not like it that much, and never applied. Bethany did like it, but she did not apply, either.

Michigan had a beer with me at my car, but headed out. He wanted to get to the next shelter. I was surprised he did not stay in town to get supplies, but I guess he had what he needed.

The next morning would be logistically tough, with two remote trailheads. I was a little surprised that the White River Junction Cab Company would meet me out in the middle of nowhere. I did not even ask them to meet me at the trailhead, but told them to meet me on Vermont 12 at a crossroad where I knew there was cell phone reception. I was actually surprised when the driver showed up. I told him to follow me and he hung tough, heading up Green Gate Road. It really helped that I was familiar with these trailheads from the conference.

I dropped my car, and he drove me around to the Cloudland Road (a gravel road where I had gotten the flat) trailhead. It would be an 11-mile hike. The cab cost a fortune, but I understood, and was thankful to have gotten anyone at all.

From the road, it was an easy hike up through a wooded meadow to Dupris Hill. There were a few leaves down, but the colors had not really started to change yet on this nice, late-September day. Dupris Hill was a bald summit in a meadow. You could see the Suicide Six Ski Area down toward Woodstock. On the way down there were several road crossings. All the roads lead to Woodstock.

At the four-mile mark there was a steep, 600-foot climb on easy trail up Dana Hill, and then 600 feet down to Vermont 12. Some of the hike was in the woods, but there were open fields and pastures, though I did not see any farm animals.

After crossing Vermont 12, I headed up toward Don's Rock. Except for the last half-mile, it was a gradual climb, although very muddy. At several points, I was in over my hiking shoes. At Don's Rock you could see Killington and Pico Peaks. From there I only had a mile to go. I was very careful from here on, as I passed each landmark in the book. By time, I measured each tenth of a mile at six minutes, and kept an eye on my watch. I did not want to miss the junction with Lookout Farm Road. I found it with no problem. It was three-tenths of a mile down to my car.

On the way back to White River Junction, I stopped in Woodstock, Vermont. Woodstock is one of those picture-perfect New England towns. I took some pictures on the town green, and at the beautiful Woodstock Inn and Resort. I did not stay long, as I felt too dirty and smelly.

I also stopped at Quechee Gorge. You can see the gorge well right from the bridge on Route 4, but I hiked down both sides of the gorge from the road. It is a spectacular, deep gorge, and was interesting and great to see.

I got up early the next morning, checked out of my motel and drove to Killington, about forty miles away. I had one section to "fill in" Vermont, and it was only five miles. I found a restaurant for breakfast that was barely open on the way to the ski resort. After breakfast, I headed out to the trailhead at River Road, at the Thundering Falls boardwalk that I had hiked the year before. I had made arrangements with the Killington Cab Co. The owner came late and apologized, but I knew that was how he operated. Even though I was only hiking 5 miles, it would be a 20-mile drive to get to the Stony Brook Road trailhead, which was very remote.

The cab company owner had never been to the trailhead before, and seemed to be getting more and more antsy the longer it was taking and the more remote it got. He kept asking me if I was sure I knew where I was going. Cell coverage was long gone, which made him more nervous. Finally he said he had to get back for another pickup, for which he was already late. I knew we were close to the trailhead, so we stopped, and he headed out after I paid him. A minute or so later, I heard a backfire from his van. I always wondered what happened.

It was less than a mile up the road to the trailhead. From Notown Clearing, it was a good climb up to Quimby Mountain. It was over 1,000 feet, with some very steep sections. There was a rock face with a 20-foot aluminum ladder that had to be negotiated. I was shaky on it, but had no choice. I was getting some experience on ladders at home cleaning my gutters. The ladder was secured and protected from theft. I stopped at the Stony Brook Shelter.

Once on top of Quimby Mountain, it was a flat 2.5 miles across the summit. At a power line clearing you could see across to the Killington or Pico ski area. The last mile and a half was a steep 1,200 feet down to River Road. There were a few switchbacks, but it was tough on the knees. I drove home that day.

For the north this year, the scorecard said 104 miles in 13 days and 4 trips. There were short days, either because of driving and hiking on the same day, or the easier hikes at the conference. Eighty-nine of the miles were in Vermont, 14 in Massachusetts and less than a mile in New Hampshire.

For now, and even next year, I was done with Vermont. I would always think about the 40 miles in the south, but did not address it. At the conference, Dan and Andrea had piqued my interest about the hut-to-hut hiking in New Hampshire, so I was moving on to that. I made myself an aggressive New Hampshire plan that I would do next year, I thought. Oops.

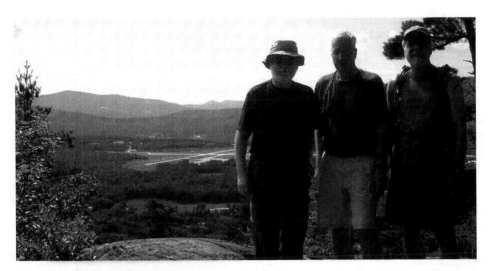

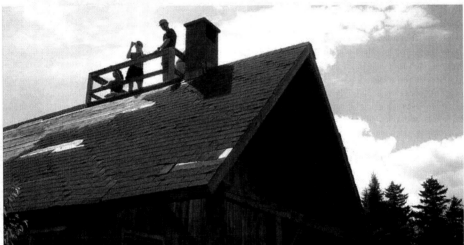

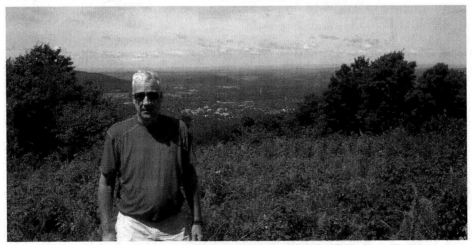

Top: Julian, Dennis, and Steve on Beacon Hill. Middle: Lakota Lake Lookout. Bottom: Dennis from Harmon Hill over Bennington.

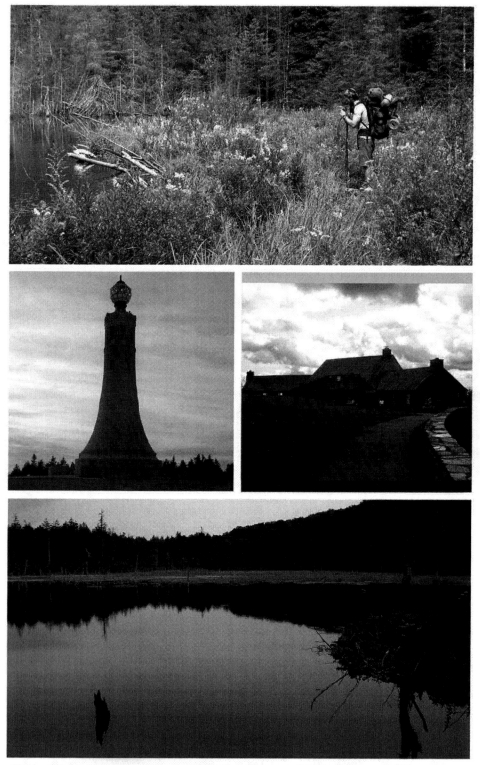

Top: "Secure" Beaver Dam. Middle: Veteran's War Memorial Tower on Mt Greylock; Bascom Lodge on Mt Greylock. Bottom: Beaver Pond.

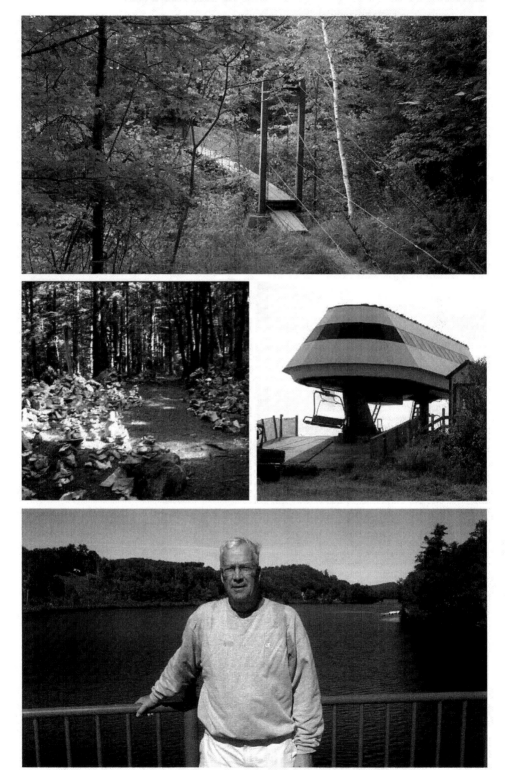

Top: Bridge over Clarendon Gorge. Middle: White Rocks; Bromley Mountain Ski Area. Bottom: Connecticut River at Hanover.

2009 – South - Along the Blue Ridge

US Airways pilot hero "Sullie" Sullivan made an emergency landing into the Hudson River shortly after taking off from LaGuardia. All survived.

It was still another rough tax season without Tom, but it was clear we would make it. I learned that no one is indispensable, and in crisis, some people step up.

Bethany decided she was interested in doing some triathlons, and started to train. She asked me if I wanted to do them with her. This really made no sense. I hadn't owned a bike since the kids were little. I had not run for twenty years. I had not done a lap in a pool for thirty years. Nonetheless, I started to train, and it gave me a reason (other than hiking) to go to the gym. My gym had a pool and a track. After tax season, I bought a bike. Over the winter, I dropped most of the weight I had gained back since the South Beach diet. I went to watch Bethany's first event at the end of April, and got hooked. I registered for the New Jersey State event in July. The New Jersey State is a large, beginner-friendly event on a flat course. It would be a 500-meter swim in a lake, an 11.5-mile bike and a 5K run. My goal was to not finish last.

The muscle soreness in my hamstrings and glutes from the training (mostly the running) made driving the next year or so an issue. I was in a lot of pain, and had to stop often to stretch those muscles that I had not used in a long time.

I was getting down into a very remote area of Virginia. The trail was still a reasonable distance from I-81. It was still running near the Blue Ridge

Parkway. On Friday, May 29, I drove down to Montebello Virginia, and met Earl Arnold at Fish Hatchery Road.

Earl and Lois Arnold operated The Dutch House, a bed and breakfast in town. They were originally from the Philadelphia area, but had moved to Texas and, as they approached retirement, they decided to head back east. They had purchased the Dutch House about five years before. In addition to regular guests, Earl and Lois catered to hikers, provided shuttles and slack packs, and were a big help to the hiking community in this out of the way place. I had decided to stay with them for the two nights I would be there. I left my car at the parking lot at the bottom of Fish Hatchery Road, and Earl shuttled me south to Salt Log Gap.

Although it was only 8 miles on the trail, it was 20 miles and 40 minutes navigating the washed-out dirt roads to get to Salt Log Gap. We were high in the mountains of the Mount Pleasant National Scenic Area, and on the hike I was never below 3,200' or above 3,900'.

It would be a very easy hiking day. Even though it was high elevation, the trail was nice, and the grades up and down were very gradual. Cell phone service did not exist, and I had not called Virginia since I left the interstate. I ended up carrying my phone in my hand the whole hike, just checking for coverage. It was annoying. There were no views this day, and I took no pictures, a first and last.

About halfway through the hike, there was a group of six hikers who had stopped for a break. There was a group of 3, with 2 dogs. They were from the DC area. John was thru-hiking, and his girlfriend Kate had joined him for a few weeks, along with John's friend Mike. They did not seem that friendly. There were two youngish grandmothers, Graham Cracker from Florida, and Grammemie from Tennessee. They had met through an outfitter, and were distance-hiking the AT together. Grammemie had started out the year before, and had skipped a lot of the middle of the trail and was finishing her hike. Once she got to Bear Mountain Bridge in New York, she would be completed. Graham Cracker was attempting a full northbound thru-hike.

The group also included Sundance, a recently retired federal government worker who was doing a thru-hike, raising money in honor of his dad who had recently passed away from diabetes. Sundance was planning to stay at the Dutch House that night, so we ended up hiking the rest of the way together. The grandmothers were going to stay at the Dutch House also, but not until the next night. They would be stopping at the next shelter for this evening, and then hiking over The Priest to the Tye River, and had made arrangements with Earl to pick them up there.

Sundance and I made our way to Fish Hatchery Road, and started down its steep descent. I was just glad I was not climbing up like the year before, on my way to Spy Rock. On the way down, we met two slow-moving (by their own admission) women in their 40s. One was Panama Slow, a thru-hiker, and the other was Jersey Girl. Jersey Girl was a teacher, who worked on the trail a little bit every summer, doing a few hundred miles. She talked a great hike.

Earl was waiting for Sundance and the girls, since they had reservations at the Dutch House, too. I took Sundance in my car. The girls had gotten a ride down the road on the back of a pickup by one of the neighbors up the hill. It was a short two miles to the Dutch House.

Thru-hiker season was a busy time for the Dutch House. In addition to 5 typical B&B rooms, where I was staying, there was a bunk house that could accommodate about 12 hikers. I stayed in one of the rooms on the first floor. I actually had never stayed in a B&B before, so I asked Lois to tell me if I did something stupid. I got showered up for dinner. Lois did laundry for the hikers (I did not need her to do mine), so everyone sat around in fluffy bathrobes until they got their clothes back. Thru-hikers often only have one set of clothes, and when they do their laundry, they put on their rain gear in the laundromat. There was no cell service at the Dutch House, so all had to use the house phone to call home. They had internet, which was phone line and slow. No high-speed lines here.

There were about eight guests for dinner. One was Mother Earth from Indiana, another grandmother who was thru-hiking. She asked me what I liked most about hiking. Was it the flora, or fauna, she asked? I really did not know how to answer, but I just said, "I like getting from point A to point B." The views, and flora and fauna are all great, but I think it comes down to that for me.

Another guest was Citation, a twenty-something thru-hiker, who was clearly on a budget. The young hikers always are on a budget, and the older ones mostly have some money saved up. I heard later in the summer (from the Bird Girls) that Citation could not finish his hike when he contracted a water-borne illness.

Lois prepared a wonderful dinner served on individual plates, with some leftovers family-style.

In the middle of the night, the local emergency alarm went off. Lois, who was part of the squad, was out for part of the night. There was a car crash down along the Tye River near Crabtree Falls.

The next morning, the guests all sat for an early breakfast, and then all were off to the trail. Earl had subcontracted out my shuttle for the day to someone down at the James River. I was to drive down to my starting point at the Punchbowl crossing of the Blue Ridge Parkway, and Ken Wallace would met me at my expected finish time. I was mildly uncomfortable, not wanting someone to wait for me if I was running behind schedule, but Earl assured me it was not an issue.

I parked my car in a little cutout right on the parkway and headed out. Lois had packed a lunch for me. I had to climb from the start, past the Punchbowl Shelter, and a total of two miles and 1,000 feet up to the summit of Bluff Mountain. At the clear summit there were the concrete footer remains of a long-ago taken-down fire tower. It was at about 3,300 feet, and many of the surrounding mountains were not that tall, so the views for miles were terrific. I was looking down at everything, it seemed. There was blue sky, but it was a little hazy.

From Bluff Mountain it was mostly down for the rest of the day on easy, graded trail. In another two miles I was at Saltlog (one word) Gap, and making good time. It was confusing, but I had been at Salt Log (two words) Gap on my hike the day before. It was an easy grade up to Big Rocky Row, with views down into Glasgow, Virginia. It was a brief, steep, rocky down to Little Rocky Row, where I could catch my first glimpses of the James River. A young male thru-hiker took my picture. In a few minutes, his mother came out of the woods. They were thru-hiking together. I had seen a lot of thru-hikers this day, and I asked them all if they had planned to stay at the

Dutch House. Most did, especially the older ones.

From Little Rocky Row it was all downhill, with beautifully designed switchbacks, and an easy, graded trail. I passed Johns Hollow Shelter, which was in a pretty setting. One of the local hikers I met tried to tell me a story about a blind hiker and fire in the area, but it did not really make much sense. The last level mile of the trail before the road was next to Rocky Row Run, a pretty little stream in a nice setting.

I walked along the road and found Ken Wallace waiting for me. Ken lived at a campground in Big Island, a town about six miles east. That was in the summer. Ken headed for Florida in the winter. He was a very pleasant retired gentleman, and put himself on some shuttle lists to supplement his income, and because he loved it. He had a cold soda in his hand for me. He took my picture on the James River AT footbridge. We drove west on Virginia 130 to pick up the Blue Ridge Parkway, and were soon back at my car. I got Ken's business card, and he would help me on my next two trips.

I drove back to the Dutch House and when I got there, Earl seemed flustered, because he had several shuttles to do, and two hikers needed a ride out to the interstate. I volunteered to take them. It turned out to be Kate and Mike, whom I had met the day before with their two dogs. Kate was injured, and decided to abandon her hike with John. Mike accompanied her, but would join John further up the trail. It was a long and winding road down off the mountain back to the interstate, and took 35 minutes. They each held their dog in their lap, which was considerate. I left them at the Burger King at the I-81 exit near Raphine. They were trying to reach friends in Roanoke to come up to get them. I liked the idea of helping the hikers, and do it every chance I get.

Back at the Dutch House, things were getting busy. Graham Cracker and Grammemie were there. I met Circuit Rider. He was a minister from the Midwest who was doing his tenth thru-hike in a row. It was part of his ministry. He had an associate, Carlos. Circuit Rider planned every day's hike before he left home, and stuck to his schedule. He never hiked on Sundays, and was always on the computer taking care of some business back home. Since the next day was a Sunday, he and Carlos would stay two nights at the Dutch House. They were all sitting around in bathrobes. A retired couple came in on a motorcycle. There were half a dozen thru-hikers, mostly young, in the bunkhouse. Some had dinner with us on the porch, and some ate out of their packs to save money.

Getting to actually talk to thru-hikers for an extended period of time, when they were not focused on mileage, was fun. Staying at the Dutch House and going to the AT conference later in July opened my eyes to the community of people that was the AT. I'm not sure I realized it until this year. It was a minor revelation that it was not just about the hiking and the trail, but about the people who enjoyed it.

It was a busy morning again, with Lois settling up everyone's bills, and Earl arranging for transportation. He had some local retired guys to help. Ken and Lois liked to arrange for hikers to "slack pack," and they would end up staying at the B&B an extra day or more. The grandmothers were doing this, as was Melvin, who Earl shuttled along with me to the south. I was leaving my car at the Long Mountain Wayside at Route 60. Melvin was starting his hike from there, and headed north all the way to Fish Hatchery Road. He was doing my hike of today, plus my hike of Friday, or a total of 16 miles. Ken took me to Salt Log Gap to head south. I would pass Melvin today, but we just laughed, and he did not even take his iPod earbuds out to talk. He just kept his head down and went on.

It was a great and interesting section, with easy, 500-foot bumps up to Tar Jacket Ridge, then Cold Mountain, followed by Bald Knob. The switchbacks were generous, and made the grades easy. In between the mountains were Hog Camp Gap and Cow Camp Gap. From Bald Knob it was a 2,000-foot descent over three miles to Route 60. On Cold Mountain there was a mile or so stretch of open, grassy area. Yellow spring flowers were everywhere. I met a large group of college-age students out for the weekend who took my picture, and I took theirs with about four cameras. I also ran into the son again from the day before, followed after about 15 minutes by his mother. She and I talked a while. I think she was about ready to quit, as she looked and sounded exhausted.

I reached the Wayside at Route 60. It was very overgrown. With budget cuts, the state had not cut the grass. It was a nice spot, but the picnic areas were unusable. Three thru-hikers came up from the south as I was packing up. It was a father and son team that I had also met the day before, along with another young guy. Since I was headed home, I emptied my cooler and gave them each a beer, and what remaining snacks and fruit I had. You would have thought I was giving them gold. I drove back to the interstate and up I-81 which was becoming like an old friend.

Old friend as it was, the drives were getting incredibly long, with still trying to hike on the same day. Four weeks later, on Friday, June 26, I was waiting for Ken Wallace at the trailhead on the north side of the James River. It was about noon, and I had left at 5:00 A.M. I would leave my car at the parking lot there, and Ken would drive me south on the Blue Ridge Parkway to the trailhead right on the parkway at Petites Gap. I would hike the 10 miles down through the James River Face Wilderness to the footbridge and my car. I came to learn that designated wilderness areas have fewer blazes to mark the trail. The idea is to try to give people a "wilderness experience," with as few references to the outside world as possible.

The book described the section as a strenuous challenge. I did not find it so, but I was hiking north, and was starting at 2,400 feet and would end at the river at 600 feet elevation. Out of the gap there was a 700-foot climb up to High Cock Knob. It was a wide, good footpath, but not so steep as to be a problem. I had picked up my training at the gym, lost weight and it was paying off. Near the top it got steeper and rougher. *Don't get too cocky,* I thought.

Before descending, I could get a glimpse of the mountains on the other side of the James River. The mountains on each side formed an eight-mile gorge, very steep in spots, with lookouts along US 501. The descent was hard at first, and then became easier on the way down to Marble Spring. There was not much elevation over the next two miles. I came upon a thru-hiker, Slim, from North Carolina. He had started later than most, so it seemed doubtful to me that he could get to Katahdin by October, but he did not seem discouraged. He and I hiked and talked for several miles.

As we hiked around the shoulder of an open area, we came upon another couple of thru-hikers. They were gorging themselves on the wild blueberries that were growing in abundance along the trail. They were a married couple in their 30s. Greta had long, thin legs in between her boots and short hiking shorts, and a braided ponytail. Her husband was Heinz, a good-looking, athletic guy. Together they were the "Hiking Poles". They did not use poles, but were originally from Poland. They were now living in Palm Springs, California. Heinz had thru-hiked the AT two years before, so this time he brought Greta along. The previous year they had hiked the Pacific Crest Trail from Mexico to Canada.

Heinz worked as a Jeep tour driver in Joshua Tree National Park near Palm Springs in the winter season, and tended bar. Virginia, Ben, Michelle and I had just been to Palm Springs in January. Penn State was in the Rose Bowl, and we took a day trip to Palm Springs when we were out there for the game, so I knew of Joshua Tree, but we did not go there. I guess Heinz and Greta had organized their lives to take summers off to go on extended hikes. They traveled very light, and were fast hikers. I had no doubt they would make Katahdin.

Slim and I headed on and left the Poles to continue on with their berry lunch. There was a short, rocky climb up to the junction of the Belfast Trail, where we stopped for a break. The Poles came along, as well as Rufeo. Rufeo was a twenty-something from Pittsburgh, Pennsylvania. We chatted for a while, and they headed down. It was three miles down to the Matts Creek Shelter. Slim decided to tent camp about halfway down, so I was on my own. There were open views of the James River Gorge along the way down. The views were spectacular. There were switchbacks all the way down, which made the descent easier. It was almost 1,900 feet over three miles.

I reached the Matts Creek Shelter. The Poles, Rufeo and Sid were there. Sid was a fifty-something section-hiker from New Jersey. They were all purifying water from Matts Creek, and deciding on their plans for the rest of the day. We were two miles from the river and my car, so I offered to take any of them into town if they needed to go. They all jumped at it. It was about 4:30 P.M. The five of us headed along the flat trail along the river, and talked all the way.

We got to the southern bank of the James River at the James River Foot Bridge. The James River Foot Bridge was built in 2000. It was named for a president of the Natural Bridge Hiking Club by the name of Bill Foot. It was a pedestrian-only bridge. It seemed like a joke (foot...get it?). The bridge was about 20 feet above the water, and attracted a lot of people. On this sunny, warm day in June, young people were out in droves on the bridge. As a rite of passage in the local area, they would jump off the bridge or its concrete abutments into the river. This was a happening place. The bridge was needed because the AT hikers used to hike on the railroad bridge, which Ken told me was problematic if a train came along. Hikers would have to take off their packs and hold it and lean against the side so the train could pass. This sounds like urban legend stuff.

The Poles and Rufeo were all in, getting into the river. Greta threw on a long dress, took off her hiking clothes and donned a swim suit. Heinz and Rufeo got down to their hiking shorts and jumped off the concrete abutment where the bridge met the bank. Greta walked down to the river bank and swam out into the middle of the river. After watching the fun for a while, I told Rufeo that Sid and I would head across the bridge to my car. I would take Sid east to the campground in Big Island, where he wanted to go for a planned mail drop. It happened to be the place where Ken Wallace spent his summers. I would stop back and pick them up and take them west to Glasgow. Sid and I had a beer at the car, and I drove him the six miles along the river to the campground.

Rufeo and the Poles were waiting for me at the parking lot, and we headed along the gorge over the mountain on a winding road to Glasgow. It was about five miles. There was a small grocery. We all had a beer in the parking lot, and they went in to resupply. They were surprised to learn that Michael Jackson had died. They did not take long, and when they came out, they organized what they had bought into their packs, shedding most of the store packaging in favor of their large, Ziploc bags. This tends to be what thru-hikers do.

We headed back to the trailhead, but before we could get out of town, Greta spotted a greasy spoon hot dog joint. She got excited and asked that we turn around so that she could get some "fatty foods" which she was craving. We did, and all three of them chowed down on hot dogs, hamburgers, French fries and pierogies. It was almost 8:00 P.M. when I dropped them back at the James River trailhead. They had plenty of daylight to get to the Johns Hollow Shelter, less than two miles away. I gave them each a cold beer for the evening. They disappeared into the woods. I headed out to my motel, about 45 minutes away in Lexington, Virginia. Lexington is the home of two colleges, Washington and Lee, and Virginia Military Institute.

I had made arrangements to meet Ken Wallace the next morning at the Jennings Creek trailhead near Arcadia, Virginia. Although only about 6 miles from the interstate to Arcadia, and another 4 miles to Jennings Creek, it seemed remote. Arcadia had no services for the hiker. Ken would drive me up the rough dirt Virginia 618 to get to the Blue Ridge Parkway, and then 10 miles north on the parkway to Parkers Gap. Being an old guy, Ken was an early riser, but he did engage in late-night poker games at the campground. Ken had met Sid the night before.

The Parkers Gap trailhead is right on the Blue Ridge Parkway. Today's hike of 11.4 miles would be entirely in the Jefferson National Forest. Since I was hiking north to south, I was benefiting from a huge loss of elevation. It was not on purpose, it was just that the shuttle worked out better this way. It would be a relatively easy day. There were a few easy bumps down, up, down, up, down and up to Floyd Mountain. Walking around a blowdown, I took one of my few spills since hiking. I laughed when I landed on a bed of moss, a real soft landing.

At Black Rock Overlook, I met Jerry, a local guy whose truck was at Parkers Gap. He took my picture at the overlook. From the wooded summit of Floyd Mountain, it was a 2,300-foot downhill hike over four miles, so it was an easy, comfortable trail. At the bottom of the downhill, at Hamps Branch, there was the beautiful (built in 1992) Bryant Ridge Shelter.

The shelter had a partially enclosed, two-level sleeping area, and open-area covered decking on two sides of it, with a picnic table and benches. It was occupied by 20 Boy Scouts and leaders. They were on a practice hike for their upcoming trip to Philmont, the national Boy Scout camp in New Mexico. I talked to the leaders a while and laughed to myself that I had been to Philmont some 45 years (could it really be that long?) earlier. I think the Philmont experience has changed a lot in that time. They would fly out. I took a bus trip, four days each way. I had 10 days in the New Mexico wilderness. It was a great experience for me, and I'm sure it would be so for them. I had lunch at the shelter, enjoying their company.

There were switchbacks up to Fork Mountain, making the 800-foot climb over two miles easy, and then 1,000 feet down over a mile and a half to Jennings Creek. There were families and groups out for this nice weekend, camping along the creek. It was only about 3:00 P.M., but I headed back to Lexington.

Since it was early, I got cleaned up and headed down to Natural Bridge for dinner and the attraction. On the way I passed Foamhenge, a takeoff on Stonehenge. "It took 4-5 Mexicans and one crazy white man, six weeks to construct" the sign read. I had dinner at the quiet bar at the Natural Bridge Hotel, and then walked down to the attraction. Since our family had been there years before on our college trip to UVA, it did not seem necessary to pay the $20 to take the tour again.

The next morning, I checked out early, and drove out through Glasgow to the parkway and south to the Peaks of Otter Resort for breakfast. I stopped to take pictures at an overlook of the James River east of Glasgow. I also stopped at the trailhead at the James River Foot Bridge to take some pictures. It was 6:30 A.M. but the sun was up, and it was a beautiful morning, and the river was like glass.

I was the first one in the Peaks of Otter dining room at 7:00 A.M. It seemed quiet there this Sunday morning. The resort did not seem busy. It seemed to be another case of an underused recreation area. I headed north on the parkway to Petites Gap.

Ken was waiting for me at Petites Gap, which was not a long drive for him. I think we had an unspoken contest about who would be first at the trailheads. We both liked to be early. I asked Ken about his range for shuttling. He said he had no problem taking me all the way down towards Daleville and beyond. That was great, because Ken was very dependable, and available. Ken took me south to Parkers Gap to begin my 7.3-mile hike.

The hike started with an 800-foot climb over a mile and a half to Apple Orchard Mountain. At 4,225 feet, it is the highest point northbound until the White Mountains in New Hampshire. At the summit there was a radar dome of an air traffic control facility. Near the summit I came to the Guillotine, a suspended rock boulder in a narrow rock cleft. The AT passes right under it.

Except for a few 200-foot bumps, it would be downhill to Petites Gap. The trail crossed the parkway twice, and then moved away into the Thunder Ridge Wilderness on an old logging road, which made for easy walking. There were several great viewpoints along the way. I saw no one on this quiet Sunday morning. I was back at my car by noon, and began the 370-mile drive home. I did stop at a nice viewpoint on the parkway to take some pictures

I spent the summer hiking in Vermont and Massachusetts (13 days in 4 trips). I also entered two triathlons. One in July went well, and I finished 6th out of 11 in my age group. September was a different story.

I was in a race at New Jersey's Spruce Run Park, only a half an hour from our home. Virginia came with me, and Ben came to see it. I was a little worried about it, since it was a half-mile lake swim, and I found out the day before that the water temp was 65 degrees. I had not yet purchased a wet suit. I had tried the bike course (15 miles) a few weeks before, and I knew there was a climb up Jugtown Mountain that I could not pull. I decided to try anyway.

The race was a half an hour late getting started. When I went in the water, it took my breath away, it was so cold. I got off course and swam 50 yards past the final buoy before a lifeguard tapped me with a paddle. I was one of the last ones out of the water, since I was in the last wave to start. I headed out on the bike without eating anything or drinking much. People from the early waves were coming back from the bike as I was starting out. I got to Jugtown Mountain and tried, but I had to stop to walk my bike up at several spots. Not a confident bike rider, I was even slow on the descents. On the last hill, I had to stop for several emergency vehicles that were caring for a rider who had taken a spill. I may have been one of the last ones back to transition. I was not feeling well, but headed out on the run. I only got 10 yards and started to feel faint. I stopped and sat on the grass to recover, but it was not going to happen. I had to quit, which was disappointing to me. I just had not eaten enough to fuel my try. I would keep trying over the next few years, and always finished the events I entered.

Over the summer, Ben decided he wanted to try hang gliding. He talked Bethany, Kevin and me into accompanying him to the nearest school in upstate New York. Even though I do not like heights, I figured, on a training hill, I would not be that far off the ground. It turned out not to be much of a problem, since I hardly got off the ground anyway. The instructor was worried I might affect his liability insurance as the kite dragged me across the ground. He kept yelling that I was not following his instructions. He was right, so I gave up in the middle of the afternoon. The kids all did better, and Ben and Kevin went back for another day; but hang gliding is a long process to get even a beginner's license to fly.

It would be October 10 before I would get down to Virginia again. Ken was available, but was headed for Florida soon. I met Ken before noon at Jennings Creek, after the 375-mile drive down. He was early, but I was earlier. Ken drove me up Virginia 618 again to the parkway, and south this time, to the Bearwallow Gap trailhead on the parkway.

My guidebook described the trail as difficult in both directions, but I found it easy. I was losing elevation all day, heading north to Jennings Creek. It was only a 6.4-mile hike. There was a 500-foot climb on switchbacks to Cove Mountain. The leaves were all down at these higher elevations. The entire Cove Mountain Ridge consisted of knobs and sags up and down 10 times, but nothing long or tough. The footpath was not easy, but not hard either. There were some rocks and roots across the ridge.

I took a break at the Cove Mountain Shelter, exactly halfway. After the shelter there were some views across to Buchanan, and then another down towards Jennings Creek. The 2-mile, 1,000-foot downhill could not have been easier on a wide, graded path. With all the leaves down, I could spot the bridge at Jennings Creek a few hundred yards before I got there. I headed south to a cheap, flea-bag motel that I found in the Cloverdale/Daleville area. There was a Virginia Tech football game 50 miles to the south, so most of the rooms in a wide radius were booked this weekend.

Daleville is where the trail passes close to I-81. Ken was waiting the next morning at the hiker lot a half-mile from the interstate on US 220. He had driven 40 miles to get there, but still arrived well before our 8:00 A.M. meet time. It would be a 13.6-mile hike this day, so I wanted to get an early start. We headed south on Route 220, and then north on US 460. He then took a winding dirt road to pick up the Blue Ridge Parkway, right at Black Horse

Gap, my start point. I was hiking by 8:30 A.M.

The trail ran parallel to the parkway for the next six miles, but then moved away from it for good. The first two miles were very easy and downhill. Usually hikes out of gaps have a climb at the start; but this was downhill, on an easy grade. I was at the Wilson Creek Shelter at 9:30 A.M. There were three large southern men in their 40s there, who were just getting moving for the day. I felt uneasy about them, so I moved on. Over the next two miles there were some ups and downs, but easy trail. After crossing Curry Creek, it was a strong 700-foot climb, using switchbacks, in less than a mile. Even though I was in good shape, I was breathing heavily. I stopped at Salt Pond Road for a break, and it was another strong 200 feet up until it leveled out. There were wooden steps initially from the road. The trail followed the crest of a ridge for the next two miles.

The trail connected to an old fire road, which was a brief but steep climb up to the Fullhardt Knob Shelter. The shelter was deserted. I was over eight miles into the hike, and it was just noon. I was making very good time. I relaxed over lunch. I could tell from my maps that it was a gradual five-mile down all the way to Virginia 220.

Initially there were long, graded switchbacks to take me down the first two miles. Then I crossed some roads and hiked through open fields, where I could look back up to Fullhardt Knob. There was quite a little rise up through an open field that did not seem to show up on the elevation profile. I passed a section-hiker about my age who was coming down the hill. He did not seem to want to talk, and moved on.

I crossed busy US 11, which parallels I-81 all the way from Harrisburg, Pennsylvania. It was a populated area. I crossed under Interstate 81. Check. The trail corridor for the last mile ran right along I-81 for most of it, and some was on private property. Before I knew it, I popped out onto Route 220. I got an ice cream at the gas station, and had a short road walk on the busy highway to my car. My motel was two miles away. It was only 2:30 P.M., plenty of time for a nap and watching some football.

The next morning, I packed up early and met Ken Wallace at Bearwallow Gap. He drove me back to Black Horse Gap, where I had started my hike on the previous day. I would hike north back to my car. I had been looking ahead to the sections south of Daleville, and the first one was over 19 miles. It looked tough, and I thought undoable for a day hike. That *camping* word started to creep into my head, thinking that was the only way. Ken said if I got an early start, it could be completed in a long day. He would even stay in a motel in Daleville to give me an early shuttle. I thanked him for the thought. I have not seen Ken since.

The trail would directly parallel the parkway for the entire eight miles. It would cross the parkway three times, and bumped into it two other times. The viewpoints today would be the viewpoints on the parkway. It was a flat walk across the ridge, with no elevation bumps of more than a few hundred feet. The day looked on the map, and actually was, one of the easiest and nicest days ever on the trail.

It was a cloudy day, but the views of the Peaks of Otter and The James River Valley were terrific. There was still color in the hills and valleys. It was Columbus Day, but there were few cars on the parkway, and no hikers out. I completed the section in a little over three hours, and headed home.

Getting to Daleville seemed like a milestone, and a good stopping point. I'd made three trips to Virginia this year, and hiked 84 miles in 9 days.

For the year, north and south, I'd hiked 188 miles in 22 days, my most mileage in a year so far. Since 2002, I had now hiked a total of 976 miles, or about forty-five percent of the AT, in 101 days. I could almost think about setting a goal of finishing it someday. The goals were nice, but I was learning more about all the different people who were hiking the trail. Maybe it *wasn't* only about getting from point A to point B.

In November, Major Nidal Hasan killed 13 and wounded 43 at Fort Hood, Texas, the largest mass shooting ever at a US military base. Tiger Woods announced an indefinite leave from professional golf to focus on his marriage.

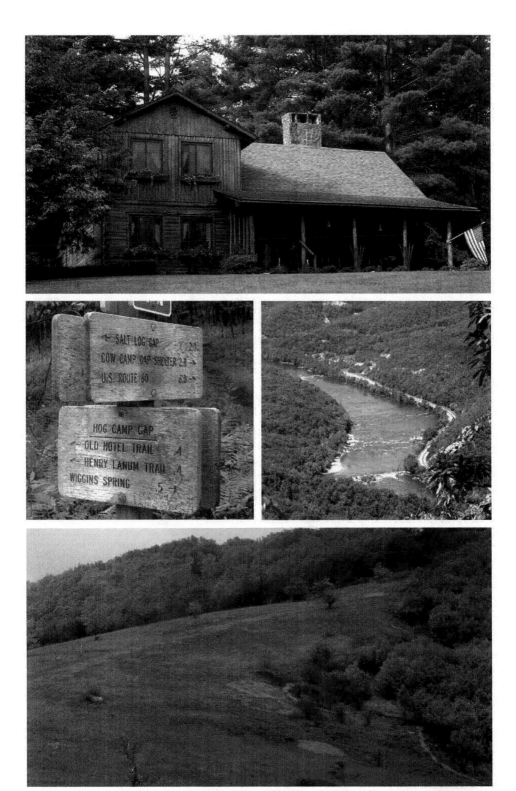

Top: Dutch House-Montebello VA. Middle: Trail at Hog Camp Gap; Above the James River. Bottom: Cold Mountain north of Route 60.

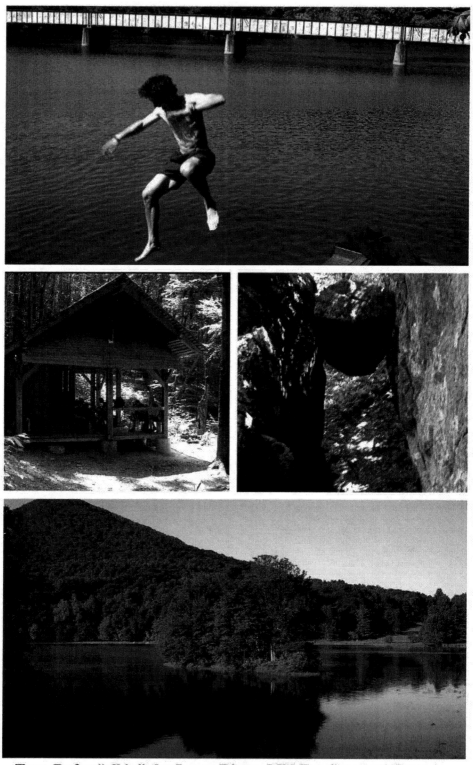

Top: Rufeo "all in" the James River. Middle: Scouts at Bryant Ridge Shelter; The Guillotine. Bottom: Peaks of Otter Resort.

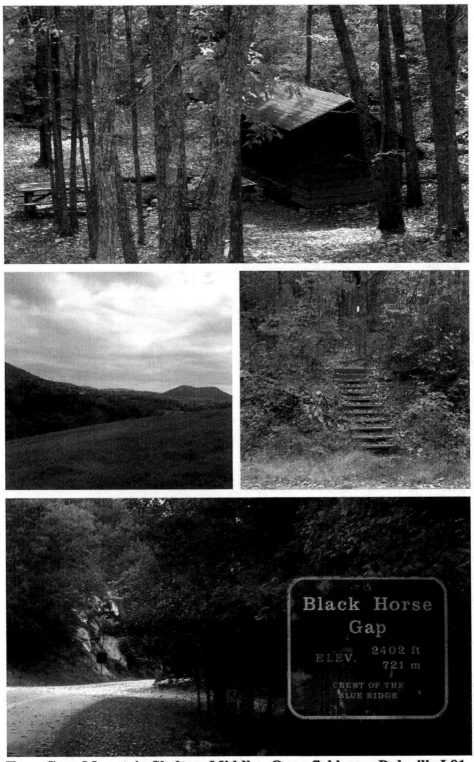

Top: Cove Mountain Shelter. Middle: Open field near Daleville I 81 crossing; Salt Pond Road. Bottom: Black Horse Gap.

2010 – North - Into the Whites

Over the winter, I spent time developing a plan for New Hampshire. This hut-to-hut thing looked great. There were eight huts in the Presidential Range of the White Mountains, which encompassed the northeastern part of the state. The southwestern part of the state looked remote, but had adequate road crossings, so it appeared doable. The White Mountains had two, thirty-mile sections with no road crossings, but the huts were each placed about a day's hike (only about 7 miles) apart, so you could do each of those sections in 4 hiking days and 3 nights in huts. I could finish the whole state (161 miles) this year. About 20 hiking days, I thought. Oops.

The huts were owned and operated by the Appalachian Mountain Club. The AMC operated not only in New Hampshire and Maine, but had chapters and operations all throughout the Northeast. I joined the AMC, which would pay for itself with discounts on hut stays. The huts were staffed by a crew of young people during the short summer season. They served breakfast and dinner, and sleeping was in open-bunk rooms. Although a stretch for me because of my poor sleeping habits, there was really no other way. Anyway, it seemed like fun.

It would be so much fun, I thought, I would recruit Ben, Bethany and Bethany's husband Kevin, to hike the section that included Mount Washington. Ben's wife Michelle was invited, but she decided it was not for her. Smart. What the heck, we would have the experience of climbing the highest mountain in the northeast. I knew some of it was above tree line and the weather was always an issue, but that would only add to the adventure. I did not have a clue that hiking in the Whites was taking this hiking thing to another level. If I had, I may not have even gotten them involved. In April, I got their commitment for the Fourth of July weekend, and booked our reservations. We would stay in the huts 2 nights, and hike 3 days, two up and one down, since down would be a lot "easier." I bought them each a headlamp for the trip.

As time went on, I started to have reservations about what I had gotten myself and them into. They say that when a northbound thru-hiker gets to New Hampshire, they have put in three-quarters of the miles, but only half the work. Although I had hiked some tougher sections, nothing had prepared me for the Whites.

To scope out what I had gotten my family into, I decided I'd better do a trial run on my own. I booked hut stays in the other, longer section in between Crawford Notch and Franconia Notch. Hiking for the section was described in my book as "extremely strenuous…and rewarding." I was nervous about it. I drove up early on Saturday, June 12, to a hiker's parking lot in Franconia Notch, just north of the Flume Visitor's Center. I was early for the afternoon shuttle which would take me to the Highland Center, AMC's flagship lodge.

The shuttle was about an hour, and I was the only one on the bus. We had about five stops at the various trailheads along the way. The driver told stories of moose and black flies. There were certain color shirts to wear and not wear. I never found it to be an issue. As we approached the Highland Center, the driver pointed out Mount Washington.

I bought a new "weekend" pack for all the things I needed for four days on the trail. My pack was about thirty pounds. I needed lunch and snacks for each day, plus a sleep sack. My local outfitter store told me I should get hiking boots, because my trail shoes would not cut it in the Whites. I carried my trail shoes too, for the hut stays, and in case the new boots did not work out, which they did. I bought some legit hiking pants with the zip off legs, and some synthetic shirts. It was now official.

The Highland Center was nice. I was looking around for a "cocktail" reception they have before dinner and ended up in a Dahlia (whatever that is) presentation, where I promptly excused myself. I met John from Concord. John was an AMC volunteer whose job it was to assist guests with their plans for their stay, kind of like a concierge. John was in the insurance business and we had a lot in common, since he was about my age. He had hiked in the Whites some when he was younger, and he seemed envious about my plan. He was quiet about the difficulty, giving me credit for all the miles I had already hiked on the AT.

Dinner was served family-style, and I ate with three younger guys from Boston, who had just finished the section I was embarking on. They did not paint an easy picture, talking about hiking down parts of the trail which was like a waterfall. It sounded tough. I did not sleep well in my nice bed and private room.

I was up early and packed my things, and was first in line for breakfast. I ate like it was my last meal. I had a second helping at a table with John and his wife, who were with the Dahlia presenter, who I apologized to. John offered to drive me down to the AT trailhead, which was about three miles away. That was great, since I did not have a shuttle reservation, and I could get an early start.

The trail starting out was something like I had not seen. It was very steep, and also rocky. Not small, pointy rocks like in Pennsylvania, but large ones, that you had to hop from one to another. Somewhere, my hopping and balance skills had become lost. Each step was a decision as you picked your way along the path. It was slow going. After about three hours I had only gone 2.5 miles, but had climbed 1,600 feet. I was tired already. I was encouraged though, since from the elevation profile, I was done climbing for the day.

The trail was still difficult over the next two miles, but I was not climbing any more. The trail was wet though, and there were many sections of puncheon (wood boards nailed to logs at each end) to protect the trail. I would see only a few people on today's hike.

The trail got easier on an old railroad bed for the next three miles. I took the side trail to Thoreau Falls and ate my packed lunch there. There were spectacular views to the east. Back on the trail, I came to the rock slides of Whitewall Mountain, and caught a glimpse of a white speck in the middle of a mountain quite a distance away. It could be nothing other than the Zealand Falls Hut, my destination. It looked so far away, but was less than three miles.

I continued to pick my way along the railroad bed, and was making a little better time. The last two-tenths of a mile was a steep boulder climb up to the hut. The hut crew (croo) were sitting on the porch. It seemed quiet, but it was before 3:00 P.M. I was instructed to just go in a find a bunk anywhere I would like.

Throughout the afternoon, more and more guests arrived. Groups of men, some families, some women with kids arrived. The hut is popular for families, since there were much shorter and easier trails to get there than the one that I had taken. The hut held about 40 people and there were at least 30 there that Sunday evening. Zealand Falls Hut was perched in the middle of a steep mountain next to Zealand Falls. The falls were right next to the hut, and the kids were running around and playing on the falls, which seemed dangerous to me. The moms seemed fine with this. There was little space around the hut because of the terrain. The views were terrific from the hut, and you could clearly see the railroad bed etched along the rock sides of Whitewall Mountain.

All the huts have limited electric generated by solar or wind power. Zealand had some hydro power because of the falls. Cooking was done with gas. It was interesting. Dinner was served family-style, and you were encouraged to only take what you would eat, since the food scraps would have to be carried out by the crew. The baked bread that night was horrible, since a crew member put in 10 times the amount of salt. The crew also carried in the perishable food supplies, which was no easy task. The huts had periodic helicopter drops of non-perishables and the gas tanks for cooking.

Hut stays are not cheap, about $70 to $100 a night, with the high end of the range on weekends. The rates are discounted for members of AMC and if you stay three or more nights in a row. People complain about the cost, but it included the dinner and breakfast, and helicopter flights do not come cheap.

After dinner, the croo put on a skit to make points about hut behavior and rules, and there was a nature talk of sorts. Of course, green thinking was encouraged.

One of the guests was Mike Conner. Mike was from Montreal, but spent up to 60 days a year volunteering in the Whites with AMC. He was a legend, and I read about awards he was given in subsequent AMC magazines. He had many experiences and tales of assisting hikers, and trail building and maintenance. He could pick out each mountain from the hut and tell what it was. He talked of bushwhacking across the top of Whitewall Mountain, since there was no trail up there.

Thinking about my upcoming family hike in July, I pulled out a map of the Mount Washington section, explained what my plan was, and asked about ways to make it less difficult. He had several recommendations. I asked about what appeared to be a shortcut trail on the first day and pointed to it. He took his finger and drew an X over the trail and said no. I remember it clearly now, but forgot a few weeks later.

I slept almost not at all, too pumped up and thinking about the next day. The weather seemed to be turning, which did not suit this fair-weather hiker. Breakfast was oatmeal and pancakes. I packed up and started out.

From the hut, it was a two-mile, 1,400-foot rock scramble up Zealand Mountain. It took me two hours. The trees were gone, replaced by scrub pines. The sky was gray, but it was still clear enough to see across the valley to Whitewall Mountain and the railroad bed. I walked on the well-defined trail through the scrub pines, still climbing towards Mount Guyot. It started to rain, and did not stop for the rest of the day. I pulled out my rain gear, opening the zipper at the bottom of my pack, where I had carefully packed it.

As I approached Mount Guyot, the scrub pines disappeared. I was above the tree line now, over 4,000 feet. I passed a northbound thru-hiker. Wow, he was early, and must have been a speed demon to be this far north in the middle of June. There was a short descent, and then a gradual up through some trees. I was hiking on the Twinway Trail. In the Whites, you should be aware of other-used trail names, since the AT seems to be de-emphasized.

I was soon above the tree line again, and it was another steep rock scramble up to the summit of South Twin Mountain. It was blowing hard and raining sideways. It was cold and stinging. The fog had rolled in. I crouched behind a rock and called Virginia, feeling lucky to have cell reception, and not knowing if there would be any at the hut, which was only eight-tenths of a mile away. She was glad to hear from me.

It was a very steep, tough, rocky 1,000-foot descent to the Galehead Hut, and took over an hour. I was being very careful, since it was very slippery, rain and water was pouring down the trail. I was glad to get to the hut.

I was one of only three paying guests at the Galehead Hut this quiet Monday night. Galehead is considered the most remote of the huts. I had a bunkroom to myself, and could spread out my wet clothes. More importantly, I could put on dry clothes and my warm wool shirt, since it was damp and chilly. As I used the bathroom, I noticed a bad smell.

I looked out the window, and a guy in a white hazmat suit was shoveling out the Clivus composting toilets into large, white drums a story below. At this high elevation, the facilities did not work so well, since they froze solid over the winter. They had planned to do the cleanout the previous fall, but the weather went against them. They would helicopter the barrels out over the next few days.

The other paying guests were John, a New York City Broadway actor, and Chuck, a thirty-something guy with a young family from Connecticut. Both were frequent visitors to the Whites and the huts. John did it because he loved the mountains and getting out of the city. Bob was a committed hiker and was on a mission, trying to bag all the 4,000-foot mountains in New Hampshire. A non-paying guest at the hut was Chris, who was a high-level staff member of AMC, who was in charge of all the huts and lodges. It was interesting at dinner to talk to all these guys and hear of their experiences.

The rain was picking up throughout the afternoon. Dale, a late-50s distance hiker came in. He inquired about "work for stay." Thru-hikers can come to the huts and stay for free if they do some assigned work, like wash dishes, clean the kitchen or bathrooms, and so forth. Dale was a chef from Pittsburgh, so he offered to cook, but dinner was mostly prepared. He was given other jobs. Dale was thru-hiking, but also had his car with him. He would get a shuttle and keep moving it north, 50 miles at a time, and then use it to get into town to resupply and stay in a motel once a week.

Three girls, drowned rats, from State College, Pennsylvania came in. They were not technically eligible for work for stay, since they were only out for a long weekend. With the heavy rain, the hut master and Chris would not send them out in the weather, so they were given jobs, too. The work for stay program allows only for eating after the paying guests had done so, and they had to sleep on the floor of the dining room. This seemed silly to me, since there were 30 empty bunks, but I guess the AMC can't be too generous with the program benefits, since the paying guests are paying large amounts, and the work for stay participants pay nothing. I would not have cared, but I understand what they have to do.

After dinner, with so few in the hut, the normal skits and nature talks were abandoned. Chuck was bird-dogging the State College girls, playing Pictionary. John could have cared less about the girls, and contented himself with back issues of *Appalachia* magazine. He liked to read about the "events" of the Whites. The events were mishaps and near mishaps of various people who come there to hike in the mountains, some of whom are totally unprepared for what they are getting into. I was beginning to understand. I did not want me and my family to be published in the next issue.

The rain and wind got heavier overnight. The wind-power device on the hut roof made a racket. I did not sleep much for the third night in a row, and at some point I decided to abandon my hike, since I was so exhausted. I had an out. I could hike the four miles down the Gale River Trail and catch a shuttle back to my car in Franconia Notch.

I was up early, packed up my still-wet clothes, and right after breakfast, I headed down the Gale River Trail. The Gale River Trail was very steep at first. Chris passed me like I was standing still. I had asked Chuck about a possible ride when we reached the bottom, but he was vague about whether or not he would wait, so I was trying to get down there before he did. I still had to be careful on the steep descent. After the first mile or so, the grade became easier, and the last two miles were fairly flat in the woods.

There had been an article in AMC's magazine I was remembering about a croo member of the Galehead Hut getting stuck while crossing the Gale River one of the several times that the trail crossed it. There was a sudden heavy rain storm, the river picked up suddenly, and she got stuck on a rock in the middle of the river and spent hours until she could be rescued. She had been transporting food up to this remote hut. Thank goodness her cell phone was working and she was able to call someone. Since then, the AMC has developed a plan to move the trail to the west side of the river to avoid the crossings. John had complained about that.

On the way down, I lost the trail, and thought I had to cross the river, which I did; but there was no trail on the other side. I crossed back and found the trail, but Chuck must have passed me while I was floundering.

I got to the trailhead parking lot and caught Chuck just as he was leaving in his Jeep, and convinced him it was not out of his way to drop me at Franconia Notch. He did, and it helped me, since I would have had to wait about four hours for the afternoon shuttle. Once I reached my car, I called Virginia to tell her I was safe, but that I was sure I could not drive all the way home. I crashed in a motel in Concord, the state capital, and drove home the next day.

I had quite a first encounter with the Whites. I continued to worry about what I had gotten my family into.

Nonetheless, Bethany and Kevin, Ben and I met at a commuter parking lot north, near Westchester, New York and began our drive up to the Highland Center near Mount Washington. Traffic was not great on the beginning of the holiday weekend, Friday, July 2.

We arrived about 5:00 P.M., and Bethany and Kevin immediately selected packs and poles from the LL Bean gear room in the basement of the Highland Center. Ben got a set of hiking poles too. We had dinner in the dining room, and then Ben and I went to a presentation by a blind hiker who planned to summit Mount Washington the next day, going up the "easiest" trail with his guide dog. I don't think he made it.

We had breakfast and waited for the shuttle, which was to take us around to Pinkham Notch, our starting point. We planned to hike the AT from Pinkham Notch to the Madison Springs Hut, stay there Saturday night, then summit Mount Washington the next day, and continue on to the Lakes of the Clouds Hut for Sunday night. Monday would be hiking 12 miles down to the Highland Center, and then drive home Tuesday. It was a good plan, I thought. Oops.

The 9:00 A.M. shuttle was over an hour late, and the drive around was about an hour. We did not start hiking until noon. Since we were hiking only about eight miles, I still figured we could make the hut by 5:00 P.M., or 6:00 P.M. at the latest. I led out in a sprint, which I could never maintain, but soon had a mutiny on my hands. Kevin took over at a reasonable pace, and I brought up the rear. We were not going slow, but not fast, either. Rocks and stream crossings slowed us down.

We passed the auto road at about the 2-mile mark. Shortly thereafter, we met a group of 50-somethings, two men and a woman, who was crawling on her hands and knees. She had apparently twisted her knee. Her companions were not helping her much, at her instruction. They had not called for help due to cell service. We tried ours and could get service, and then they could, too. They were not far from the auto road. Help would be on the way for them, so we felt okay about heading out.

A few minutes later, Kevin and Ben spotted a bear on the trail. It went around us on the trail, and headed toward the crawling woman. We all just yelled and we heard them yelling too, probably just to scare the bear away. There were quite a few people out on this holiday weekend. We leapfrogged a group of three women several times, who were also on their way to Madison Springs Hut. We finally stopped for a late lunch near the Suspension Bridge over the Peabody River. I pulled out and studied my map. I really wanted the hike to be fun and not a struggle, and was ready to abandon the AT if there was an easier way.

My map showed a more direct route to the hut, 3 miles instead of 4. We would also be avoiding about 500 feet of elevation of Mount Madison. I made the fateful decision to take the Madison Gulf Trail to the hut. It was about 2:45 P.M., and I figured we could hike the 3 miles to the hut and be there by at least 5:30 P.M. Kevin looked at the isobars on the map at the end of the trail and had an idea about the difficulty, but we headed out. Oops.

The first mile was a pleasant walk, and then the fun began. We had some rock scrambles up through some boulder fields. Then we came to a boulder field with a waterfall running down it. We thought we had lost the trail, but that was it. The blue blazes disappeared, replaced by rock cairns, since we were in a wilderness area. We arrived at a beautiful waterfall, where we paused for a minute. Two men came down the trail and gave us a warning about the difficulty of the trail ahead. I figured we were only about a mile and half away. It seemed pointless to turn around.

The next mile and a half took over two hours, with steep boulder climbs and a very difficult rock face. A few tears were shed, but we all made it. We had to climb up a chimney hand over hand. On another rock face, two young guys were flying down on their butts and took off. I almost called after them to help us, but they were gone.

Finally we started to come out above tree line and into the scrub pines. We reached the junction with the Parapet Trail, and I knew we were within a half-mile. We were through the hardest. We reached the hut at 7:00 P.M. and had missed dinner. The hut was full on this Saturday night of the holiday weekend. We found the four remaining bunks, none of which were together. Ben and Kevin took ones that were next to the ceiling. The bunks were 4-high in 2 large rooms. I took one on the floor. Bethany got a second-level one.

We got cleaned up in the filthy facilities, and the croo did feed us some cold turkey and mashed potatoes. The hut was in bad shape. There were actually flush toilets, but some were not working properly. This was the last season for Madison Springs Hut, as it would be torn down in September, and rebuilt and expanded. The hut was rowdy into the night. I slept very little, and I don't think Bethany did, either. Ben and Kevin did better. The hut stay was not very pleasant.

After breakfast, we got ready to head out. It was six miles to the summit of Mount Washington, and then another mile down to the hut. It was a nice day, but there was a strong wind blowing, which was intimidating to Bethany. She was not sure she wanted to continue. I told her we could take an easy route down off the mountain and find transportation. She decided to go on. The hike to the summit was all above tree line. There were some rock scrambles and steeper parts, but nothing like what we had encountered the day before.

After a few significant ups and downs, Mount Washington came into view. It looked far away. We kept on going. The wind started to die down, but there was a bit of a chill. We spied the Cog Railway. On the way, I started to think that maybe the group had had enough. Once we got to the summit, we could find a way down, and find transportation back to the Highland Center. The closer we got to the summit, the more Bethany's pace picked up, and she seemed to even be having fun. Ben was getting tired and was laying on his pack when we stopped. Kevin was solid.

We crossed the Cog Railway tracks, but still had the last bit to climb to get to the summit. We made it! We went into the summit cafeteria and had some lunch, mingling with the tourists in high heels. It was about 2:00 P.M. The group decided we'd had enough. I called the AMC and was able to get our reservations switched from the hut to the Highland Center. I was a blithering idiot on the phone when I spoke to Virginia.

We could have taken cars down the auto road, putting us on the wrong side of the mountain, but we were able to get seats on the floor of the Cog Railway to get off the mountain. I got a ride with a couple back to the Highland Center to get the car, and then came back to get the group.

There was a nice Fourth of July buffet at the Highland Center. We ate outside on the patio with a couple who seemed to be familiar with the trails, and they told us that the Madison Gulf Trail was probably one of the most difficult in the Whites. Bethany and Kevin googled it later and got a similar report. The White Mountain Guide said so, too.

I bought the book, *Not Without Peril*, a compilation of stories of deaths and near-death experiences on Mount Washington and the Whites. One hundred thirty-five people have died in those mountains.

We now had a free day on Monday, July 5. Ben decided to head home, so I took him down to Conway to catch a bus. Bethany and Kevin took a little hike up Mount Wiley. We had lunch at the Mount Washington Hotel, on the veranda. We all were recovering. Bethany, Kevin and I drove home the next day. On the road, Bethany was busy studying for her first classes in the MBA program at NYU.

I still had unfinished business in the Whites, trying to finish my hike to Franconia Notch that I had abandoned in June. The huts closed soon after Labor Day, so I did a do-over and drove to the Highland Center to stay on Wednesday, September 1. On Thursday morning after breakfast, I drove back over to Franconia Notch and caught the AMC shuttle to the Gale River trailhead. I was early, and explored Franconia Notch a little, including the Flume. I did not hike up the Flume trail, but looked around the visitor's center, which was near the trailhead parking lot.

My plan was to hike up to the Galehead Hut on Thursday, hike the AT from Galehead to the summit of Lafayette on Friday, and then hike the 1.1

mile down to the Greenleaf Hut to stay on Friday night. I would then hike back up to the Lafayette summit and across the ridge on the AT, and down the AT to my car at Franconia Notch. That was the plan.

At the trailhead parking lot, I met a father/son duo from Boston who were going to hike much of the same section I was, although they were going to camp, and not stay in the huts. We were the only ones on the shuttle, and we all got off at the Gale River trailhead. We were hiking up the Gale River Trail to the AT. I would back-track half a mile to get to the Galehead Hut for my second stay there.

I left before they did, and they did not catch up. It was that easy, three miles initially, along the Gale River, crossing it several times. I picked a nice spot to eat a sandwich I had purchased in Franconia. It was that same spot where previously I had lost the trail and tried to cross the river, and Chuck was able to get by me somehow. A couple on the way to the hut passed me. I started the difficult climb up the last mile of the Gale River trail to the AT. My weekend pack was close to 30 pounds with all the extra food Virginia had packed for me. I had eight (total) large apples and oranges.

I was breathing heavy and sweating, but soon overtook the couple. The guy was large and was having as much trouble as I was. We reached the AT together, and sat to rest. It was only half a mile to the hut, and it was still early afternoon. When we reached the hut it was quiet. I found a spot in the same bunk room I had been in back in June.

Eventually, about a dozen people would roll in. Three groups arrived from the south. There was a German mother-daughter combo who had stayed at the Greenleaf Hut (my destination for tomorrow) the night before. I would be doing their hike the next day, only reverse. They talked about the difficulty, and that it had taken about 8 hours to traverse the 7.7 miles. It turned out they were the strong ones, as another group of three men came in after them, who took 9 hours.

About 5:00 P.M. an exhausted group of another three men straggled in. They had not stayed at the hut, but came up the Flume Trail to get to the summit of Mount Lafayette. They had actually hiked about 11 miles. They were from Ohio, and the son of the hike leader was a college student at Ohio State. He was in bad shape, having had stomach reduction surgery in the past few months. He just laid on the porch bench until dinner.

John from Montreal arrived. He was an AMC volunteer who was a paying guest tonight, but was going on to Zealand Falls to volunteer the next night. He knew Mike Conner. He and I shared a bunk room. I have never met anyone from Canada that I did not like.

Bob from Rhode Island came in from the north. Bob was a great guy. He was doing all 8 AMC huts in 8 nights. His route would mostly follow the AT. He was in his 40s, and in good shape, and loved the Whites. This was about his sixth trip up here since he lost significant weight about five years earlier. His wife had come with him the first few times, but something happened he did not explain (involving a bear), that ended her participation. In addition to the eight huts, Bob was also peak bagging, climbing as many 4,000-foot mountains as he could find. Soon after he arrived he was off with just a bottle of water to bag North Twin. It was four miles round-trip, but he was back in a few hours.

Bob also had a story of a hike he organized with friends a few years earlier. About six guys hiked up the Ammonoosuc Ravine Trail, then the AT to the summit of Washington. They would continue on in one day to Madison Springs Hut. It was a long, 11-mile day. The group got separated, and the weather turned bad. One of the older, heavier and slower hikers, Curt, got lost. Bob was frantic throughout the day. With communication between Madison Springs and Mount Washington summit, it was learned that a thru-hiker was assisting Curt, and he was on the way. The weather got worse, but Curt and the thru-hiker straggled in at about 6:00 P.M. Curt was suffering from hypothermia. They stripped him of his clothes and put him in a bunk with blankets, and he recovered.

Curt owned a business, and ended up offering the thru-hiker a job that he still has today.

After dinner, Mount Garfield was pointed out. It looked so far away (it was only three miles), but it also looked very steep, and went over 4,500 feet. That was all I could think about during the night, not to mention that Mount Lafayette beyond and twice as far, was over 5,300 feet. Needless to say, I did not sleep well. I had learned to double up the thin hut mattresses when the hut was not full, so it was not the discomfort of the bunk. I was just anxious about the next day.

The next morning, Bob and I started out. I told him not to wait for me and that I would be fine, but for some reason, he took me under his wing. Bob was clearly a much stronger hiker than I was. He was also 15-20 years younger.

The first 2 ½ miles looked flat on my map's elevation profile, but it was anything but that. No long climbs, but difficult short ups and downs. Every now and again, Bob said he wanted to stretch his legs and would take off, but would wait for me every 45 minutes or so. The Garfield climb did not disappoint. It was straight up over 1,000 feet in seven-tenths of a mile. I was sweating and breathing heavily. Bob was long gone, needing to stretch his legs. I almost missed the spur trail to the summit of Garfield. Bob was waiting there, and he took an unflattering picture of me sucking wind.

We took a break for lunch, and I told Bob not to wait, but he sincerely seemed to want to hike with me. He said I was easily keeping up my end of the bargain. From Garfield you could easily see the ridge across the summit of Mount Lafayette. If only there was a bridge across the deep ravine.

It was a nice, sunny day, but there was a little chill in the air. We headed down the steep western side of Garfield over the next mile. Then we began the 2-mile climb up 1,800 feet. There were several false summits, which means to the hiker, it appeared that you had reached the top at several points, only to find that when you got there, you had more to go. About halfway up we were totally above tree line. The wind started to pick up, and the air got cooler. We rested about 300 feet (elevation) from the summit. I changed out of my soaked shirt, and opted for long sleeves.

The summit of Lafayette was busy, with about 10 people up there. It included a couple from Saratoga, New York. The guy was on his cell most of the time. It seemed his occupation was gambling of some sort. We spent some time on Lafayette enjoying the views and looking down at the Greenleaf Hut, 1.1 miles and 1,000 feet below. Eventually we headed down. The hut disappeared from view as we got into thick scrub pines below the tree line, but the trail emerged at the top of a low ridge at the hut.

Bob and I had a bowl of soup, which is offered by the croo when the hikers roll in. Bob and I found bunks in the same area of the hut. Cell reception was sketchy, but if I sat in a certain place on the back steps, I could let Virginia know that I had arrived. Bob could use my phone too, since his was out of battery from seven days out on the trail.

The hut was not full on this Friday night of Labor Day weekend. The dozen of us fit around one table for the family-style dinner. The group included some AMC volunteers in for the weekend, and Trish. Trish was an experienced hiker from Massachusetts. She had her two young daughters, about 8 and 10 years old, with her. Dad was not a hiker. The hut croo has programs for young kids to become young rangers if they complete an age-appropriate workbook. An awards ceremony is held at breakfast.

I did not sleep again for the second night in a row. All I could think about was the trail description for the next day's hike along Franconia Ridge. "It is exposed to the full force of storms which appear rapidly and violently, with hurricane force winds and freezing conditions even in summer." I had visions of walking across a razor's edge with precipitous drops on either side. After the three-mile walk there was a very steep 2,800-foot descent over three miles to my car in Franconia Notch. This was all after climbing the mile and 1,000 feet. back up to the summit of Lafayette from the hut.

The hut croo always gives a weather report each morning. Fog had rolled in, and Lafayette was not in view. The croo said bad weather was possible, and wind was picking up. Bob was going up, and after bagging the next two 5,000-foot mountains (Lincoln and Little Haystack), he would come down the Falling Waters Trail and continue on to Lonesome Lake Hut, about three miles west of Franconia Notch.

Wimp that I was, I decided to bail out. I could take the Bridal Path Trail down to the highway, and either catch a ride, or walk the three miles to my car. Bob tried to encourage me to go up with him, but I felt spent and intimidated, by the weather and the hike. My second attempt to complete this section was a dud.

The Bridal Path Trail going down from the hut was very steep and difficult. The fact that this was a path for horses to carry supplies to the hut and summit made little sense to me. I could not see horses climbing up through the steep boulders. I barely passed Trish and her two girls going down. Trish had the girls dressed with bright-orange vests so that they could easily be spotted should they get lost. The girls were gamers, climbing down the steep descent. I presumed they had come up this way the day before.

As I climbed down, the weather seemed to clear a bit. It was hard to know what it was like at the summit, although an email with Bob later indicated that the weather was not an issue at all. I was beginning to feel more and more like a wimp, but I also felt like I was a zombie from lack of sleep. I was okay with the decision. The pounding on my knees on the hike down took a toll. This was the first time I had experienced knee issues after a tough descent.

On the way down, I passed many people and groups headed up. There was a group of thirty or so headed to the summit of Lafayette for a wedding this Saturday of Labor Day weekend. Another group had a baby. Dad was carrying it in a front Snugli carrier. They did not seem to have packs or supplies, and therefore were totally unprepared, I thought, for what they were getting into. At the notch, a dad asked me about hiking up to the summit with his 3 and 5-year-old sons. Indignant, I advised him strongly against it. My wimpiness was coming through.

I reached the junction with the Falling Waters Trail and was almost to the highway. It had taken me 3 hours to hike down the 3 miles. I learned later via email that Bob saw Trish and her girls at the trailhead. I probably only missed him by about an hour or so.

I easily caught a ride back to my car. The father/son duo that I had met at the parking lot and shuttled with two days before were there. We had a beer together, telling of our adventures. I made it only to Concord, and crashed around noon in a motel, and slept all afternoon. I drove home the next day with my tail between my legs. Four days away from home netted me a whopping 6.6 miles on the AT. I was getting nowhere fast.

I was done with the Whites for the year; but a month later, on Saturday, October 2, I was waiting for a shuttle in Hanover, New Hampshire. I still had the easier (and it was) southwestern part of New Hampshire to work on. I had driven up that morning and had arranged for a 1:00 P.M. shuttle. I called Stray Cat of Apex Hiker Shuttle, and he wanted to come right away, which was fine. I had not purchased a sandwich yet, but I had plenty to eat, and my hike was only six miles. Stray Cat had thru-hiked the trail twice before, and was hoping to do it again in the next year or two. Having a limo business was just a gig in between hikes for him. He would help me for my planned hikes over the next few days. He was very dependable, and always right on time.

Stray Cat took me out to Hanover Center Road, and I would hike back to town. It was a very easy first mile or so. In a thick pine forest, I stopped for a snack, since I had not eaten. Soon after, I crossed a boardwalk bridge over a cattail marsh, where I took some pictures. About half a mile later, I lost the trail, walking right through some brush that had been placed to keep me from going the wrong way. When I turned around and went back, I was not paying close attention. I headed off back in the direction that I had just come. It was not until I got to the same cattail marsh and boardwalk that I realized it.

Back again I went, and was more careful, and saw my mistake of missing a turn up a switchback towards Velvet Rocks. The climb up, across and down Velvet Rocks was pretty, in a thick pine forest with soft, pine needle footing among rocks to be avoided. You had to pay attention. I reached the Velvet Rocks Shelter area, and seemed to lose the trail completely. I was less than a mile from town, but there were significant, uncleared blowdowns, and very poorly maintained trail. I was floundering, but about a hundred yards ahead was a trail runner from Hanover coming in the opposite direction. He was having trouble, too. We went toward each other and both found our way, but griped about the poor trail maintenance of the Dartmouth Outing Club. After all, we were only a mile from campus.

The last mile of the hike was on the streets of Hanover, passing the Hanover Food Co-op, which I went into. For the weekend, I stayed in a motel just south of Hanover, and enjoyed eating in sports bars in Hanover each night. Breakfast was always at Lou's. Lou's is always crowded, with a line on weekends.

The next day, I met Stray Cat at Hanover Center Road, and he would shuttle me out to the Dartmouth Skiway at Lyme-Dorchester Road. It was 12 miles today. Right from the steps at the road, it was steep climbing, about 1,200 feet over 1.7 miles to a viewpoint at Holts Ledge. Looking east to Lamberts Ridge and Smart Mountain, I saw where I would be hiking the next day. I had hiked around and to the top of the Dartmouth Skiway area, but did not see any evidence of the slopes on the trail.

It was a steep 1,200 feet down over 1.5 miles to a marshy area near Goose Pond Road. I was soon climbing again, 1,400 feet this time, to the North Peak of Moose Mountain. I had lunch at the Moose Mountain Shelter at a col between the North and South Peaks of Moose Mountain.

From the South Peak, it was a long, gradual, easy down over four miles to my car at Hanover Center Road. I drove back to my motel through Metropolitan Downtown Etna, as the sign read. It did have a general store and a volunteer fire company.

The next morning, Stray Cat met me at the Dartmouth Skiway. The section I was hiking was part of a 16-mile section that I did not want to tackle in its entirety at this time of year, with fading daylight. There did not seem to be any road crossings. As luck would have it, Virginia had bought me a book about day hiking the AT, written by Polly. Polly was a self-described slow and timid hiker, who had been working on the trail for years by hiking days. She was supported by her husband, who shuttled her to and from the trailheads. Her book consisted of a rudimentary log. She had split this section by accessing the AT near Quintown. Quintown was not really a town, but a cluster of about six houses that must have been summer places.

Stray Cat did not know of the trailhead but was game, so we headed back through Lyme Center and then to Route 25A, rather than a gravel road I had found that seemed like it would go direct to Quintown. The secondary unpaved road off Route 25A turned into a forest logging road that was not passable by Stray Cat's limo, so he had to stop, and I walked the remaining mile or so to access the trail. It was not hard to find, but was remote and deserted. The forest road followed Jacob's Brook. My hike would be about 10 miles.

A new bridge was under construction over Jacob's Brook. The base of the bridge was in place, but there was yellow tape across it, and a sign indicating it was not to be used. The trail was routed 50 feet upstream to a place to cross the brook on rocks.

From Jacob's Brook, it was a long, gradual, 1,700-foot climb, but over four miles, to Smart Mountain. At Smart Mountain, there was a Fire Warden's cabin. I'm not sure why, but I was kind of expecting it to be occupied, which of course it was not. I had lunch there. I opted not to try to climb the fire tower any further than the first flight of steps, so I could not get above the trees for any views. It had been a quiet day so far and I had not seen a soul. It was, after all, a Monday.

After a snack at the Ranger Cabin, I began the steep down Smart's Mountain to Lambert Ridge. In one spot there was a series of boulder steps, followed by log steps bolted into the rock face, which I navigated carefully. There were also steel rebar steps along some steeper rock faces.

Along level Lambert Ridge there were some great views to the south. It was a gray and cloudy day, but there was still good visibility. At one point, the slopes of the Dartmouth Skiway came into view. It seemed slightly past peak of the full fall colors, but still beautiful.

It was another tough two-mile and 1,400-foot descent from Lambert Ridge, and took a good hour and a half. I was weary from the long day, and the knees were taking a pounding. I saw about three people coming down from Smart's Mountain. Finally, I reached the Lyme Dorchester Road crossing, but still had two miles to go. The trail ran parallel to the road. I was tempted, but did not just road walk back to my car.

It was a rocky and not easy trail back to the Dartmouth Skiway parking lot and my car.

I got back to my motel and checked the weather, which was looking shaky for the next day. I was planning to do the remaining six miles from Quintown out to Route 25A, and then drive home. With the weather, my hurting knees and an intimidating-looking climb up Cube Mountain, I decided I'd had enough, cancelled Stray Cat, and drove home the next morning.

For the year, I did 62 miles in New Hampshire in 8 days on the trail, a far cry from my plan of completing the entire state (161 miles). I had spent about 12 days up there, some of it completing side trails to access or bail out on the AT. I was still thinking about those unfinished 40 miles in southern Vermont. Oh well, maybe next year.

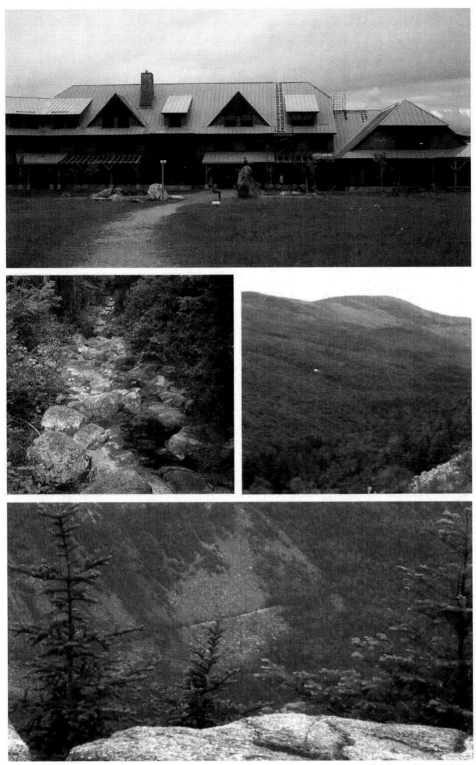

Top: Highland Center. Middle: New Hampshire trail; Speck of Zealand Falls Hut. Bottom: RR Bed (AT) on Whitewall Mountain.

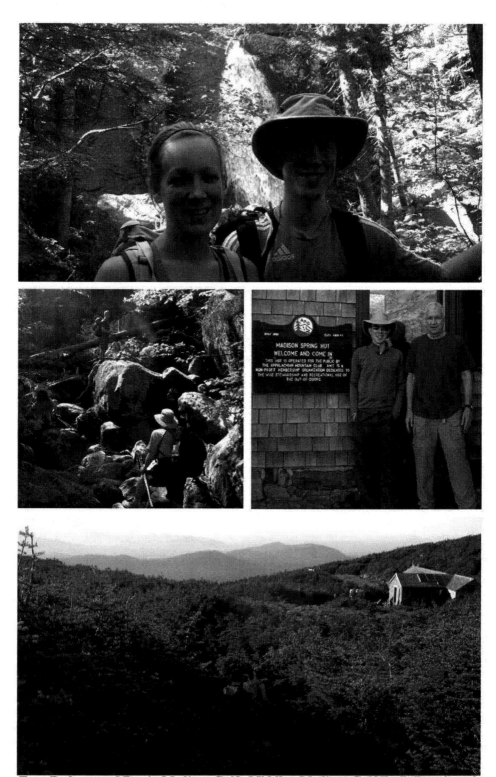

Top: Bethany and Ben in Madison Gulf. Middle: Madison Gulf Trail; Dennis and Ben at Madison Spring Hut. Bottom: Arriving at Madison Hut.

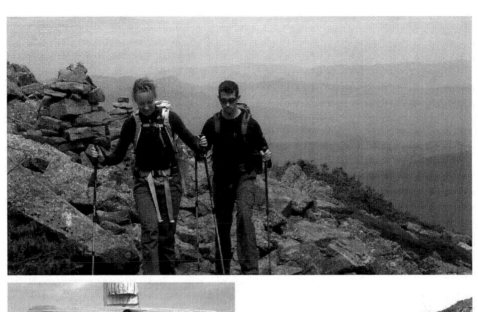

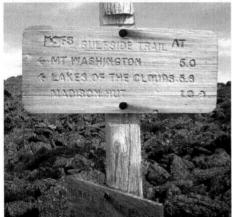

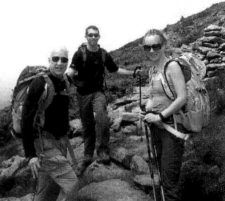

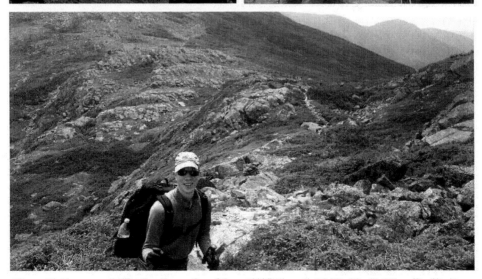

Top: Bethany and Kevin along the ridge. Middle: Gulfside Trail; Dennis, Kevin, and Bethany on the way to Mt Washington. Bottom: Ben above tree line.

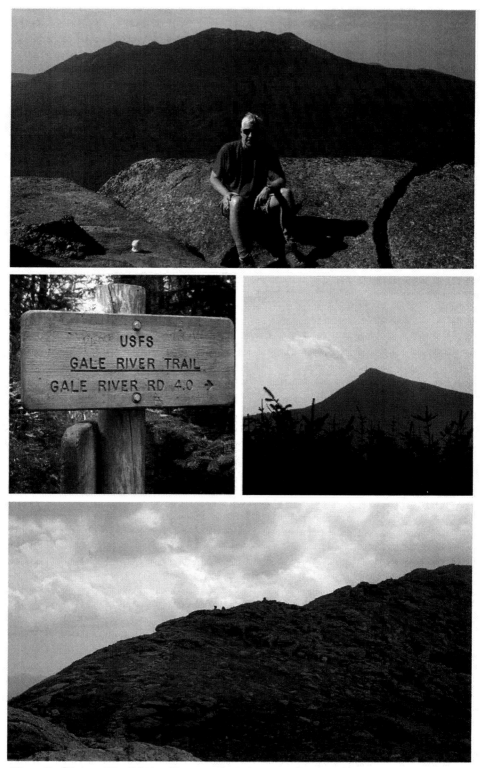

Top: Resting on Garfield on the way to Lafayette. Middle: Trail to Galehead Hut:
Mt Garfield from Galehead Hut. Bottom: False summits of Lafayette.

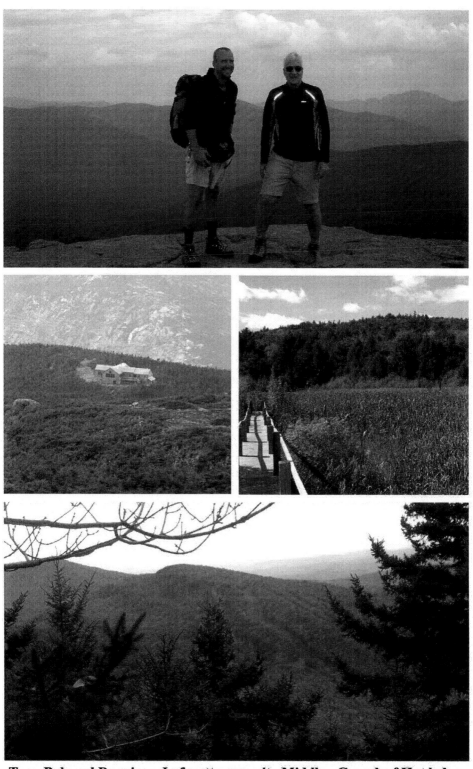

Top: Bob and Dennis on Lafayette summit. Middle: Greenleaf Hut below Lafayette; Cattail Marsh near Hanover. Bottom: Dartmouth Ski Area.

2010 – South - Remote Virginia

On January 12, a 7.0 magnitude earthquake devastated Haiti, killing 200,000 people. Tax season of 2010 had its challenges. Dallas, a retired partner and contemporary of mine (we actually became partners on the same date) came down with cancer, and he eventually passed away in July. Strange that he had moved into Tom's office. The office remains empty. Dallas did not have a large client list, but he did need help, and most of his clients had to be transferred during the height of tax season. Like Tom, he tried to work, but found it difficult.

In March, Congress passed and the president signed a new healthcare law, "Obamacare." In April, a BP oil rig off Louisiana exploded, killing 11, and thousands of gallons of oil poured into the gulf each hour until July. In May, a terrorist failed in an attempt to explode a bomb in Times Square.

I was very focused on hiking in New Hampshire this year, but wanted to continue to work on Virginia, too. Having completed all the sections to Daleville, the trail now was west of Interstate 81 for about 150 miles, into a remote part of southwest Virginia.

The first section south of Daleville was 19 miles and seemed difficult, so I skipped it and decided to look further to the south. I also needed a new shuttle driver, since in all fairness, I was out of Ken Wallace's range.

From the AT shuttle list, I was lucky to pick out Homer Witcher. Homer lived in Daleville, but some of the sections to the south would be quite a journey. I would also find out that cell reception really became an issue at most of the trailheads that I would use. Homer turned out to be dependable, but he did have other things on his plate.

I think Homer was about my age (10 years in either direction), but it was hard to tell. In 2002, Homer's wife (his younger than he, second wife) told him that she thought his job as a hospital lab director was killing him, and told him to quit. They and their two children (then a daughter, 12 and a son, 9) decided to hike the AT as a family. They became the "Walking Witchers" and completed their thru-hike. Homer had a book that was published on their adventure. Homer's wife Therese would get a job when they returned, but Homer did not.

Homer was interesting. He was a runner, and one day told me he would be late getting to me, depending on how fast he ran the 5K he was entered in. Several of his children (I think he had seven total) were in the race with him. He claimed his first and second wives were the best of friends. Homer was a hard-working guy in a lot of things, but did extensive trail maintenance, shuttling, and even relocated a section of the trail in the area. He told of making some "rescues" when he would get a call from someone on Tinker Mountain, just above his home.

For my first day, on May 14, Homer sent his now 19-year-old daughter, Taylor, to shuttle me. Taylor was in Community College, and actually hiked the AT a second time solo the year before as her high school senior class project. I was early, as usual, and was waiting at the Virginia 311 trailhead on the ridge of Catawba Mountain. I had driven the almost-400 miles down that morning. The large trailhead seemed active, and a few thru-hikers went by while I was waiting. They all seemed in a hurry to get to Daleville for a zero day (a rest day with zero miles logged). It was an easy drive out to Virginia 624 through Catawba (a town of only a few houses, but a post office and restaurant and a closed store). My hike would only be six miles, but it was early afternoon.

I had barely left Virginia 624 when I overtook Lab Rat on the switchbacks ascending towards Sandstone Ridge. Lab Rat was from Georgia, and had just retired from a state research lab, where he'd worked as a biologist. He was attempting a thru-hike, and seemed to be making good progress, though he was not, by his own admission, very fast. We hiked for a while together, and we swapped cameras. He sent a picture off to his wife to update his log and website. Eventually I went ahead, but told him I would wait for him at Route 311 with a beer, which I did.

It was a pretty hike, along some streams and through some meadows. It was only May, but a very hot day. The trail corridor was narrow, and we were not in a national or state forest that I had been accustomed to. We passed by some old, dilapidated farms.

The last three miles were across the aptly named Sawtooth Ridge, with some short but steep PUDs. At Virginia 311, I had a beer, and waited for Lab Rat, who rolled in about half an hour later. I had another beer with him, and he headed off to Tinker Mountain. He planned two more nights out in that inconvenient 19-mile section before reaching Daleville. I was still ignoring it. I was off to my Salem, Virginia motel.

The next day, I drove out to the remote trailhead at Virginia 621 in the Craig Creek Valley. Thank goodness for the accurate trail descriptions (exactly 6.5 miles west of Virginia 311). It was very remote, with no cell reception. All I could do was wait when Homer did not make his approximate meet time of 10:00 A.M. He had told me of the 5K run he was in that morning in Roanoke. He was doing less than 25 minutes for the 5K, which to me sounded great, since my 5K times in the triathlons were closer to 35 minutes.

As I waited at the trailhead, two thru-hikers came in and started drawing water from the creek there, using care to purify with their filters. Talking to them helped to pass the time. I gave them each an apple, which seemed like gold to them. Homer arrived about 10:30 A.M. I was antsy because of doing an 11-mile hike, and this was a late start for me. It was thirty miles and took forty-five minutes to drive west around Sinking Creek Mountain to get to the Route 42 trailhead, but it gave Homer a chance to tell me his story. He was on the road two hours to help me today, and was more than fair with the shuttle amount, so I was generous. I'm grateful to these AT shuttle drivers, and have been very lucky to find good ones.

From the trailhead at Route 42, the first mile or so was in and out of pasture and woods. Being out in the open, you could see the long ridge of Sinking Spring Mountain. After a mile or so, I began the long 2-mile climb up 1,400 feet to the top of the ridge. I was in decent shape and it was not that hot, but I was still breathing heavily when I reached the top. At the top, there were three thru-hikers resting from their climb. They were two late-50-something guys from the Midwest, and Sonia from Israel via Canada. This was Sonia's tenth year attempting a thru-hike. Sonia was in her late-30s, and was a big girl with a big pack. She was married, and living in Montreal. She had never made it to Katahdin, and rather than picking up where she left off the year before, she just started again at Springer. There is no one way to hike the trail.

I walked with the three of them for much of the five flat miles across the narrow ridge. The narrow ridge made for good views into the valleys, both to the east and the west. It was a partly cloudy and pleasant day. We were not always together, but seemed to leap frog each other. One of the guys said that he had started at Springer, decided to go home for a while due to a minor injury, and to rest for a while. His wife told him she had made plans while he was away, and encouraged him to get his butt back there. The guys were early retirees and hanging tough. They were over 500 miles into their thru-hike. I wonder if any of them made it to Katahdin. Only 1 in 4 does.

After the 5-mile walk on the rocky Sinking Creek Mountain Ridge, we began the 2,000-foot descent over the next 3 miles. It was a steep and rocky down, but about a mile short of the road, we reached the Niday Shelter, where all three planned to spend the night. About eight thru-hikers had accumulated there, and were beginning their evening chores of getting water from the nearby stream, unpacking their sleeping bags and pads, and spreading them out in the shelter and beginning the cooking of their evening meal. I did not usually observe any of this, since I was usually off the trail in midafternoon. Since I had gotten a late start today, it was nearing 6:00 P.M. I offered the services of transportation to a convenience store, but none took me up on it.

It was an easy last mile to my car. I was on my way back to Salem for a late dinner at the Applebee's.

The next morning, I met Homer at a general store on Route 311, which was about a half a mile from the nearby Route 624 trailhead that Taylor had dropped me at two days earlier. She had noted that there was no safe parking there. From the store you could see the ridge where I would be today. Had I known what to look for, I could have probably made out Dragon's Tooth.

I left my car at the store with permission. It was a 20-mile and 30-minute drive out to the remote dirt road (Virginia 620) with a ford crossing over a stream, and cows along the road.

Homer dropped me at the trailhead, and asked me to report any blow-downs I noticed. He had assumed responsibility for maintenance of this and other trail sections. He had even relocated the section immediately to the south, what sounded like single-handedly. What a guy.

My hike for today was only seven miles. The trail crossed Trout Creek on a wooden bridge, and then began a 1,000-foot climb over two miles to a ridge on Cove Mountain. There were actually two blowdowns to negotiate on the way up. I never called Homer. It was another nice day, although the sky was slightly gray. There were still good views at spots down to the Route 311 valley, and across to North Mountain. It was an easy footpath across the ridge. I snapped a picture of a turtle on the trail.

The trail became more difficult for the last mile before getting to Dragon's Tooth. It was rocky, and had little PUDs to negotiate and a not steep, but 500-foot climb up. Dragon's Tooth was a neat place. I had it all to myself on this early Sunday afternoon. It was a very well-maintained area, with good signage. Dragon's Tooth is a 30-foot tall monolith of a rock formation sitting right on top of the ridge on Cove Mountain. There is a trailhead lot on Route 311 just for those wanting to climb up to Dragon's Tooth.

The climb down from Dragon's Tooth was not for the faint of heart. Although trail builders had put a lot of effort into it, the grade was very steep for over half a mile, going down large, sharp, boulder steps. At one point there were some rebar titanium hand/foot holds to climb down/up with. A group of early-twenty-somethings, in sneakers, came charging up, think-ing they were close to the top, which they were not. The trail leveled off for another half-mile, and then began to descend less steeply on nicer trail. I made a wrong turn at a junction, and then backtracked, and was not sure I was going in the right direction. I knew if I was going down, I must be right.

I got to Virginia 624, and then had a half a mile road walk to my car at the general store. I went in to buy a burger and thank them for allowing me to park my car there. Then I was back to Salem.

I woke early the next morning, and it was pouring rain, unexpectedly.

The radar on the weather channel was socked in green. I decided to cancel my short hike and hit the road by 6:00 A.M. I called Homer on the way. He was expecting to hear from me.

When I got home, I realized I had now hiked over 1,000 miles on the trail.

After my June and July hikes in New Hampshire, I decided to bite the bullet and tackle that 19.6-mile section from Route 311 to Daleville. It would be my longest day ever to that point. There was no other way, since there were no road crossings and no access trails. Homer said it was very doable, but he was running 25 minute 5Ks, and was a self-described fast hiker. I wanted to do it before the days got too short. I figured I would be shot the day after, so decided on just hiking two days this time. I would also fill in the section I bailed on because of the rain. I had a continuing education conference in Hershey, Pennsylvania on Thursday, August 19, so I figured I would leave from there to head down to the HoJo in Daleville. Traffic was horrible, and I did not get to Daleville until after 11:00 P.M. It was getting tougher and tougher to hike on the same day that I was driving the full 400-mile distances.

On Friday, I did not have to get up that early, since I had a short 7.6-mile hike. I had not arranged for a shuttle with Homer, but instead loaded my bike into my SUV to shuttle myself. This was a first. The trailheads for the short hike were less than 10 miles apart. I had been to both trailheads in May, and I remembered it would be a flat ride. The area was remote, and would have meant Homer would be on the road two hours again.

I had a leisurely breakfast at the Waffle House, and then packed up to head to the Virginia 621 trailhead, with the creek nearby. I had my new weekend pack that I had purchased for the Whites. It could accommodate my bike helmet and lock. I decided I did not need to bother with the poles, since they would be a nuisance on the bike ride.

From the trailhead it was a nice, easy bike ride along Virginia 621, which had minimal traffic. After leaving the wooded area, I passed a few cow pastures, and then came to a street named Donkey Drive. I stopped, and six donkeys ran over to the fence to line up for a picture. I think they were expecting me to feed them, which I did not. I continued on to dirt Virginia

620 for a few short miles, fording that stream on my bike this time. When I got to the trailhead at Trout Creek, I hid my bike in the woods and locked it up.

I started off south on the trail up a big climb of 1,500 feet over two miles. The trail was very nice, but it was a little steep, even with the switchbacks. I think this was all Homer's work. I was glad to get to the top, because I was done climbing for the day. Once on top of the ridge on Brush Mountain, it was an easy old woods road hike another two miles, until a side trail for the Audie Murphy Monument.

Audie Murphy was the most-decorated WWII soldier, and after the war he became a movie star. My dad and father-in-law would always talk about Audie Murphy. The monument was the site of a plane crash that took his life in 1971 at the age of 47. In addition to a large granite marker that was decorated with flags and wreaths, people also built cairns in the area. It reminded me of White Rocks in Vermont, but nothing of that scale. There was a peaceful bench where I could have lunch.

It was a very easy, nicely graded and sloped trail down to the Craig Creek trailhead and my car. I had seen no one on this summer Friday. The northbound thru-hikers were long gone, and the southbounders would not have been down this far yet. I had to drive around to pick up my bike, which was no big deal. Shuttling myself had worked out very well in this situation. I took some pictures along the road back of the dilapidated farms and cow pastures. Virginia loves the pictures of any animals. She especially liked the donkeys. I had dinner at the Mexican restaurant, which was not that great. I was awake during the night thinking about my 19.6-mile hike the next day.

I was at the Waffle House at 5:00 A.M. the next morning, eating like it was my last meal. Homer was picking me up at the Daleville HoJo at 6:30 A.M. The trail crossed US 220 within a few hundred feet of the HoJo, so there was no reason to even move my car. I continued to eat at the HoJo breakfast bar as I waited for Homer.

My White Mountain pack was loaded. I was wearing my new boots, and had my trail shoes in my pack in case I got blisters. I had a gallon of water, and enough food for an army. I had extra clothes in case it got cold or rained. My pack was probably 25 pounds. It was not that long a drive out, one exit south on the interstate, and then up Route 311 to the trailhead on Catawba Mountain. I was hiking by 7:00 A.M. I said goodbye to Homer, and have not seen him since.

There was little elevation gain over the first two miles to the Catawba Mountain Shelter. I did not stop, and did not see any activity. On the way there were several wooden bridges (no streams) built along some steep sections. These bridges were needed to prevent erosion on the steep slopes as we wound around the mountain. After the shelter, I began the 1,000-foot ascent over two miles to McAfee Knob.

It was only 9:00 A.M., but there was a young couple there already who had hiked up from the road, too. They said they were just friends, but I think they were both hoping something would develop. She was visiting him for the weekend. We swapped cameras. They headed back down, and I continued north on the trail, and in a few yards entered Devil's Kitchen, an area of large block rocks with steps woven through the middle.

I descended down to Campbell's Shelter but passed on by, wanting to keep the focus of the day's mileage in mind. I continued on the easy descent towards Brickey's Gap, making good time. At about the 7-mile mark, I hiked down off the ridge into an open grassy field on a woods road with vehicle tracks, and followed them to another ridge and old road. I realized I was now on a blue-blazed trail, and had lost the AT. I arrived at the remnants of an old abandoned farm with what appeared to be pigsties, and got confused because there was a Pig Farm Campsite in the area that I was well beyond.

As I should, I turned around and tried to retrace my steps, coming back to the meadow and following it to the other end, but could not find the AT. I went back and forth several times. I thought I may have been on a cutoff trail that would have taken me to Lamberts Meadow Shelter, cutting off Tinker Cliffs, but I did not want to do that, and was not sure anyway. Great, on my longest hike ever, I was lost, and could not find the AT.

I called Homer. He and Therese were driving and told me to retrace my steps, which I had already done. A little panic was setting in. I pulled out my map and compass. I knew if I headed west, or even north, I would have to find the trail, since it looped around heading north, and then took a U-turn at Scorched Earth Gap and headed almost due south. I floundered, and finally just decided to bushwhack due east. Three minutes later, I was on the ridge and the AT. Whew! What a relief.

It seemed like an eternity, but I was probably only lost about 45 minutes. I actually found the AT at a spot that I had already been. As I continued north, I came to that same grassy field, and was much more careful this time. In the middle of the field at an overgrown spot, the AT left those tire tracks on the old woods road, took a sharp left, and went into the woods. The turn was very overgrown, and was not very obvious.

When I was floundering, I was actually in an adjacent field that was similar to the one where I'd made the wrong turn. I was retracing steps that I had not taken.

I tried to calm down, and called Homer and left a message that I had found my way, and called Virginia, but did not let on to her what had happened. I ate some lunch and drank plenty. I was still not halfway. I started the climb up to Tinker Cliffs.

For a half a mile, the AT runs right along the edge of Tinker Cliffs, not great for someone with a fear of heights. I know the views were great, but I spent little time there, and focused on getting past this hazardous place, wanting to keep moving. When I got to the end of the half-mile, I figured I was done most of the climbing for the day. I changed out of my boots for the trail shoes, and put on a dry shirt. I was still not halfway, and it was after noon.

The next mile was a steep down of 1,000 feet in a little over a mile. The steepness was mitigated some by switchbacks. I passed Scorched Earth Gap and went right on by Lambert's Meadow Shelter. I wanted to keep moving. I reached a low area, and sat down to rest and eat. I hadn't bought any decent sandwiches for this day's hike. I had opted for some convenience store wrapped white bread lunch meat things, which I could barely choke down with water. I forced myself to eat. A hiker has to keep himself fueled and watered. I remembered the mantra for the White Mountains, "Eat before you are hungry, and drink before you are thirsty." I was trying. The next six miles were not easy, following rocky Tinker Ridge. Although there was little overall elevation gain or loss, there were short little technical PUDs. I forced myself to stop and drink along the way.

I had not taken many pictures today, considering the good opportunities. I did get some nice shots looking west to the Carvins Cove Reservoir. It was getting to be late afternoon. The sky was gray, but it was August, and humid.

I finally reached a power line that had a view down into Daleville. I could see the orange roof of the HoJo. I still had two miles to go. The next mile was a very steep down. This section was unrelenting, and I thought it would never end. I reached the concrete bridge crossing Tinker Creek, and took one last break, even though I was within a half-mile. Finally, I emerged at US 220, and was done. It was 6:00 P.M. It had taken me 11 hours to do the 19.6 miles. Considering the difficulty and the fact that I was lost for a while, I did okay.

I stopped at a convenience store and bought a pint of much-deserved ice cream, and walked down to the HoJo. I called Virginia, and then Homer. I had a beer in the room, ate a few peanut butter crackers, and soaked in the tub for about an hour. I came out of the bathroom all wrinkled and stiff, ate the pint of ice cream, and went to bed. I was driving home before daylight the next morning.

The next 100 or more miles on the AT in the far southwest corner of Virginia looked very remote, except for the town of Pearisburg. The AT conference the next year would help me do the final 100 miles or so in the most southern part of Virginia. It seems like I have been working on Virginia forever. I started in 2004, had hiked about 300 miles in the state, and still had 200 miles to go. Virginia is by far, the biggest-mile state for the AT. Hikers get discouraged, and many people quit there, since it seems so endless.

I have been considering myself more and more lucky when it comes to solutions presenting themselves on the AT. It is that "trail magic." In yet another example, my *Journeys* magazine showed up earlier this year. It had an extensive article about a bed and breakfast/hostel in the remote mountains just south of Pearisburg.

The story of Woods Hole Hostel and Mountain Retreat was fascinating. You can read the story on their website, but here is the short version. In 1939, newlyweds Tillie and Roy Wood found a little cabin in the Sugar Run Valley, and purchased it for $300. Another $300 got them an adjacent 100 acres. For 40 years they rented it to hunters. In the early '80s, they began to go there in summers, from their home in Atlanta. They built a barn/bunk-house and began to open it to hikers, since they were only half a mile from the AT. This was Roy's idea, which Tillie was not sure about. Eventually, Tillie warmed to the idea, and began serving the hikers breakfast. They officially opened to hikers in 1986, and in 1987, Roy passed away.

Tillie continued to come back every spring for the next 22 years. Tillie gave the hikers a place to rest in the bunkhouse, and served them breakfast in her small cabin kitchen. Her granddaughter, Neville, started coming from time to time since she was four years old. At age 89, Tillie passed away from cancer in 2007. As she was dying, her main concern was what would happen to the hostel that she had come to love. Now grown, Neville promised her grandmother that she would take it over, not being sure that she really could. Neville had worked with her grandmother the previous two summers. She had met her now-husband Michael when he had done a thru-hike in 2005. They married at Woods Hole in 2009. During this period, they did a major renovation/expansion. They funded it by placing the property into a land conservancy. Neville and Michael have been running it since, and have taken Woods Hole to another level. They live there year-round, and from the B&B, hostel, and shuttling, they seem to be thriving. You can't make this stuff up.

I had enjoyed my experience at the Dutch House, so I emailed Woods Hole about a 4-day hiking plan for late October, and staying 3 nights at the B&B. It was a good time for them, since the hiking season was winding down. They still had guests and hikers, though. So there I was, on October 29, waiting at the Route 42 trailhead that Homer had dropped me at back in May when I had done the section to the north. I had driven the 400 miles that morning to get there, and it was about noon. Neville was right on time in her small, 10-year-old Toyota. She told me where to park in this remote area, with cow fields all around. It was a long drive to get to the end of dirt road Virginia 632 in the John's Creek Valley. I don't know that I would have ever found it on my own, since the route went off the edge of my AT map. Neville had no problem.

From the road, I crossed John's Creek and began the 1,700-foot climb over 2 ½ miles up John's Creek Mountain. The hike today was only 7.4 miles. It was up 2 miles, across the ridge, and 3 miles down. The climb up was steep and rocky in spots, and not too bad in others. In about an hour I reached Rocky Gap, and a dirt road crossing. There were a few rowdy hunters parked near the trailhead. I was a little unnerved, and moved quickly across the road. When I was out of sight, I ran a little. I heard them yelling, but I'm not sure what they might have been saying. It was another steep 500 feet in a half a mile to get to the junction with the John's Creek Mountain Trail, where I finally figured I could relax a little. I was on top of the ridge now, and was done climbing for the day.

I bypassed a few side trails on the ridge which would have gotten me to some better views. It was a gray day. The views between the trees showed that most of the fall color had faded, but the brown leaves were still on the trees. I began a very steep descent of 900 feet in less than a mile. The footing was good. I arrived at the Laurel Creek Shelter and ate my lunch. It was quiet.

Once I left the shelter, the grade was a very easy down across Piney Ridge over the next two miles to the road. I crossed a barbed-wire fence on a stile, and entered a pasture. The last mile was in open fields. There was a picturesque farm with bright green roofs along the route. The open hills all seemed to have cows grazing. I reached my car and headed to Woods Hole. My car's navigation system actually had the address, which belied the remoteness of the location.

Woods Hole was a magical, welcoming place.

The renovated and expanded main house had a great room, with a loft above the dining area, where Michael and Neville slept. In the back was a large country kitchen. Off a large foyer, which was part of the renovation, was a new personal/dressing area where they did massages, yoga and meditation sessions. It had futons, massage tables and a beautiful bathroom. The upstairs of the addition had two beautiful guest rooms, and a bathroom serving both bedrooms.

Neville is an artist, so the home is decorated with a lot of her work or accessories that she picked up along the way. There was no shortage of those. Neville is also an outstanding cook. She is a loving and welcoming person; that comes from her southern graciousness. It is hard to imagine how she can prepare a dinner each day, for anywhere from 2 to 20, and not really knowing at 4:00 P.M. exactly how many would show up. She is adept at getting everyone to pitch in for the meal preparations and cleaning up afterwards. She is a licensed massage therapist. She is a trained yoga instructor. She runs the inside of the house. Hiking boots had to come off on the porch. Sunrises could be seen from a swing on that porch.

Michael is a true Renaissance man. He grew up in western Pennsylvania, and is a Penn State graduate. A biology major, he worked in the pharmaceutical industry for a time, but seems to have found his calling. He is also a massage therapist. He has become a bee keeper and farmer, and takes care of everything outside of the house. Michael has to plow the remote dirt road in the winter, since the state only does it to a certain point. Michael is tech savvy. They have no TV, but do have satellite internet. Michael keeps up the website, and they get their news online. Winters can be long.

Michael and Neville's relationship is on display 24/7. Michael just teases that, out of the 2,000 hikers Neville must have met, she picked him. Neville is not a friend of alcohol, but I could sneak Michael a beer every now and then, just not in the house.

They both seem to be smart about business. Hikers can sometimes be on a budget, but Michael and Neville seem to be sensitive to people's needs and ability to pay, without being overly generous or allowing themselves to be taken advantage of. They offer "work for stay." While I was there, Pack Mule was staying in the bunkhouse for an indefinite period. He got a free bunk and meals, and maybe a minimum wage for working with Michael all day. Pack Mule was about 40, and seemed to be in some sort of transition stage in his life (as hikers often are). I don't think he had a home anymore, and clearly had limited resources. He was just hiking the AT continuously for now. He was homeless, or maybe just another version of a HOBO. Hikers who might be recovering from minor injury or foot problems (which happens often) might stay for a week on a "work for stay basis."

The bunk house slept about 12 on the enclosed second floor, accessed by a ladder. Mattresses were on the floor. The lower level had some storage, and a common area open to the elements. A shower with hot water was available except in the winter. They sold beverages, snacks and some supplies on an honor system. There was an outhouse 50 yards up the hill. A distinction was made between inside and outside guests when it came to using the facilities. All of it seemed logical and was working, as far as I could tell. Three dogs and two cats roamed the grounds.

There was a shed-sized woodstove out next to the driveway that provided heat and hot water to the compound. Large stacks of wood were ready for the long winter. Outside of the kitchen was a wood-fired pizza/bread baking oven. Large gardens were just off the front porch, protected with wire and mesh fencing to keep the critters at bay. The gardens were as organic as possible. Michael and Pack Mule were putting up posts for a fence to keep sheep that they would hope to get by next summer. Michael was also getting the back yard ready for a major berry bush planting and vineyard. Quality showed through in everything Michael was doing. Michael reminded me of Kevin, my son-in-law, and someday I thought they should meet, if I could work it out.

Neville showed me to my room. The room was large, and had three single beds, though I had reserved it for myself for the weekend. She said that there would be no dinner at Woods Hole tonight. There was a group of four hikers who were staying there, who Michael had shuttled that morning. They were doing a 19-mile section (I of course was skipping that this weekend) just north of Pearisburg, and we would meet them at a Mexican restaurant in town after dark, when they would expect to get off the trail. Friday night was often Neville's day off from cooking. It was usually slow on Fridays during the hiking season, since hikers would bypass Woods Hole to get to Pearisburg by Saturday morning, before the post office closes. Hikers often have mail drops in trail towns.

After showering (limited to five minutes), I loaded my car with Neville, Michael, Pack Mule, and Roger and Sandy. Roger and Sandy were staying in the other B&B room. They were a married couple from southern New Hampshire in their late-50s. Roger was hiking the trail, and Sandy was the shuttle. She would drop him each morning, and then do the antique store/ outlet mall thing and pick him up at the end of the day. He was working his way south, and had done the entire trail to this point. They were very nice and friendly, and tech savvy. They would google-map the AT trailheads to look at parking, etc. They also did a DVD about Woods Hole, which they sent me a copy of. It was terrific.

Dinner was fun as I got to know Michael, Neville and the other guests. It was determined that Keith and Margaret, a married late-50s couple from Charlottesville, Virginia, were planning the same section as I was the next day. We were going to get a shuttle south to Virginia 606 and hike the 14 miles back north to Woods Hole. Roger and Sandy were going that way, and could drop us off. This worked out great, and there was no cost for any shuttles. Even though shuttling was part of the Woods Hole business plan, Michael and Neville always tried to arrange the least-expensive way for their guests.

Mario was at dinner also. Mario was a late 60s section-hiker, and we had a lot in common when it came to the sections that we had each done. He was down here for about a week, but was headed home the next day. The 19-mile section that he had done this day had stretched his limits, he said, but he did it. I was encouraged. We also talked about some of the more rugged sections in New Hampshire that I had not yet completed. He had done most of them. He said they were all hard, but doable in a day. It was encouraging. He had camped those long sections in southern Vermont. *Darn.*

The next morning, there were 10 of us around the breakfast table. Neville asked everyone to introduce themselves, tell where they were from, and say what they were thankful for. I was thankful for finding Woods Hole. It was a common theme.

Roger and Sandy dropped Keith, Margaret and me at our trailhead. Keith and Margaret were completing a thru-hike this year. They had started at Springer in April, skipped 300 miles in Virginia, and then picked up at Front Royal and headed north and made it to Katahdin the month before. They actually had done that 300 miles in previous years, but were doing it again to complete the "thru-hike". A thru hike is considered hiking the entire trail in one calendar year. It does not matter what order. People often jump around due to weather, heat, bugs and foliage. There is no one way to hike the trail. Since they were from Charlottesville, Virginia, they could do some of this on weekends.

Margaret was a teacher, and had a deadline of sorts to get back to school by December. Keith was a retired banker who had worked quite a bit in international finance. They were terrific. Keith had lost about 40 pounds over the summer, and was much more adept now at getting up the hills than when he had started out. They were certainly both in better shape than I, having hiked 2,000 miles in the last six months.

The first seven miles of today's 14-mile hike were very easy and level along Dismal Creek. It gave an opportunity for good conversation. I fell in behind them. I enjoyed hearing of their thru-hike experiences. A dirt road also paralleled the trail. It was a Saturday, and we encountered a few hunters on the AT along the way. One had a deer in the back of a pickup truck as we crossed the dirt road. One hunter was particularly overweight, and was struggling a little. He radioed a friend for assistance, and insisted that we go on and he was fine. None of us wanted to take the side trail to the Falls of Dismal. It would be a long day anyway. In three hours we were at the Wapiti Shelter. We stopped for a break and to eat. Neville had packed a trail lunch for me, which she seemed to enjoy doing.

Right after lunch we started a 1 ½-mile, 1,400-foot climb up to Sugar Run Mountain. It was tough and relentless, and I was soon left behind as I gasped for air and had to stop. Margaret was the first up. They waited for me at the top of the ridge. Hikers seem to wait for each other once a climb is complete, but they all want to climb at their own pace and not stop and wait *during* the climb. It makes sense. My ego was a little bruised that I could not keep up. That was the only climbing for the day. I actually did not stop, not wanting to hold them up, although it was not necessary, since it was level from there to Sugar Run Road.

Along the ridge of Sugar Run Mountain there were some fantastic view-points across Wilburn Valley toward Pearis Mountain. It was a cool day. The color was gone for the year. I had changed out of my soaked shirt from the climb, but needed long sleeves on the mountain. I did wait at the view point so that we could swap cameras, and we finished together. With my bruised ego, I decided to lead out and set a quick pace. Margaret was on my heels, but Keith fell behind. I'm not sure what I was trying to prove. Along an old woods road part of the trail I stopped, as thousands of small birds seemed to be frantic in front of us. Margaret and I marveled at the scene.

We crossed dirt road Virginia 612, which would have taken us to Sugar

Run Road. I jokingly said we could do a road walk. Margaret just looked at me. I took the trail, which for that last mile and a half was very rocky, with a few small PUDs. At one point you had to climb down a 10-foot embankment in kind of a chimney. We reached Sugar Run Road. Michael had a sign posted about the location of the hostel, with an arrow pointing the way. It was a half-mile road walk to get there.

We all showered and cleaned up good. It was only the six of us for dinner that night, including Pack Mule. He and Michael wore ski hats at the table. Neville prepared a fantastic meal. After dinner, Michael had rented a video which we all watched in the small living room, trying to find a space to sit among the dogs that seemed to think they had priority.

The next morning, Keith and Margaret took me into Pearisburg and dropped me there at the trailhead. On the way out Sugar Run Road, a cow stood in the middle of the road. Keith had to honk to get it to move. I was hiking back to Woods Hole from the north this time. Keith and Margaret were doing another section and meeting Michael at their trailhead, and then they were headed home for a few days. I would be hiking the 10.5 miles alone today. We said our goodbyes, but did not swap contact info, which I regretted, and have not seen them since.

I started out on a back street in Pearisburg behind a Ford dealership. There was a short walk through an empty lot pine grove that was well maintained. Then the fun of a 2,000-foot climb over the next 2.5 miles began. After a mile, I crossed Virginia 634 and continued up. The climb included some very rocky spots that went around the side of mountains, circling small ravines. The leaves on the trail made it difficult to see the small rocks on the trail. I tripped a few times, but never went down. The climb continued up to Angels Rest. The views from Angels Rest and half a mile further along were spectacular, back toward Pearisburg and the New River. The trail began to level off, and at a power line, there were views to the east along Wilburn Valley Road, which was my route to drive to Woods Hole from Pearisburg.

The next three miles to Doc's Knob Shelter was unique. It was along an easy old woods road, walking inside a rhododendron tunnel. The blooms were all gone this time of year, but it was still interesting. I ate Neville's trail lunch at the shelter. There was a last view down toward Sugar Run, and then downhill over a rocky section to Sugar Run Road and back to Woods Hole.

Michael and Pack Mule were still working on those posts for the sheep pen. It was early afternoon. I shared the last of my beer with them when they quit for the day. Ed and Nancy arrived from North Carolina. It would only be the six of us for dinner. It seemed to be the end of the hiker season, and Michael and Neville were planning to leave for a family visit in Georgia. A friend and neighbor would stay at the hostel to accommodate anyone who showed up to use the bunkhouse, but no meals would be provided. Pack Mule would stay around too, although I would find out the next spring that he had left in mid-November. Neville felt badly, but his stay did not end well. Pack Mule was a smoker, and ran out of cigarettes. Neville did not see the need to get him to town for a few days, so he got mad and left.

Ed was a retired military officer and sometimes section-hiker of the trail. He had stayed at Woods Hole earlier in the year and brought Nancy back, since he wanted her to see the place. Ed was a precise engineer-type and a wood craftsman. He made pens, which he proudly showed off. They were marvelous. He spoke of building a garage on his property, using extreme care and precision. I think it took him four years, but I'm sure it was well-planned and thought out, and the pictures he had showed that it was beautiful. Nancy loved the finished product, but seemed to have a little trouble with the time it took. She was a lovely, gracious Southern Belle. Michael asked Ed to make a pizza shovel to use in the oven out back from a piece of wood Michael had. Ed was glad to say he would.

After breakfast the next morning, I packed up and followed Neville 15 miles past Pearisburg to a trailhead on Route 635, which ran along Stony Creek. It was very remote, and had no cell reception. I left my car at the trailhead and had an inkling it was not the one I wanted, but did not say anything. There were two trailheads at Route 635. One where I left my car actually crossed the road. There was another two miles south on the AT and closer to town, where the AT came within 100 yards of the road, with an access trail and a small parking lot. I noticed it on the way back toward town.

Rather than taking some back roads to get to my starting point, Neville drove all the way back to town, and then out the long road leading past

Mountain Lake. Mountain Lake Resort looked like a nice place. Its claim to fame was that it was the film location of the movie *Dirty Dancing*, starring Patrick Swayze and Jennifer Grey. Of course, the movie supposedly took place in the Catskills. Mountain Lake was a struggling resort because it had a major problem. The lake next to the resort and seen prominently in the film had naturally drained itself, so there was no lake anymore. The locals called it Mountain Lakeless.

We reached the top of the ridge on the Salt Sulphur Turnpike and the trailhead. I thanked Neville for everything, and she headed off. The trailhead had some tents in the area that were hunting camps, but I saw no sign of life. It was a Monday, and the calendar had flipped to November.

The hike along the ridge of Big Mountain was flat, but annoyingly rocky. It was a very gradual downhill, too. A few gunshots were a little unnerving, but I did not see any hunters or anyone. There were not any views. I arrived at Bailey's Gap and the shelter, and ate another of Neville's trail lunches. I had only hiked four miles, but only had a mile to go. My planned 7.3-mile hike had turned into 5.2 miles. There was nothing I could do about it. The last mile was very steep at first, but the trail was good, and the last half-mile was in a very pretty area. I crossed the road, and there was my car. I would make up the 2.1 miles sometime, I figured, but the next section was already over 19 miles. Oh well. That was a next-year problem. It was before noon, so I would drive home that day.

The scorecard for the year was 88 miles in Virginia over 9 days, and 62 miles in New Hampshire over 8 days, for a total of 150 miles in 17 days. After 9 years, I had now hiked 1,126 miles in 118 days and was over halfway, or 51.6% of the 2,181 total trail miles. Might it take me another 9 years to finish? I'd be over 70. I guess that was OK.

On Christmas Day, the husband of one of my partners passed away suddenly at the young age of 49.

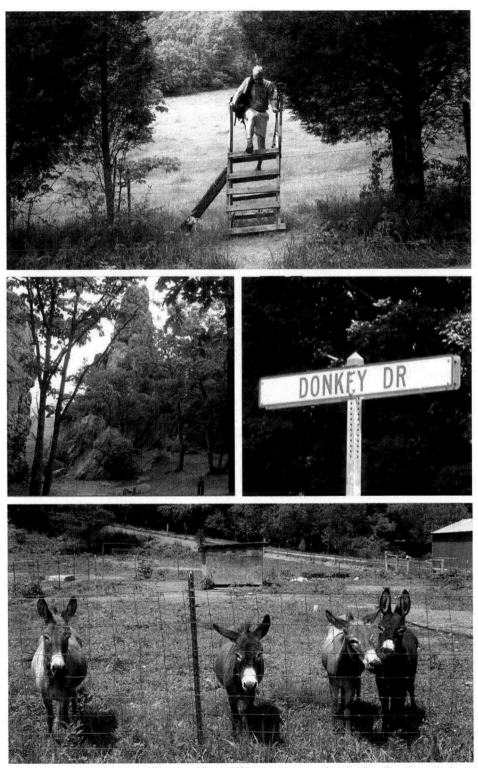

Top: Fence crossing using a stile. Middle: Dragon's Tooth; Donkey Drive along VA 621. Bottom: Friendly greeting in Craig Creek Valley.

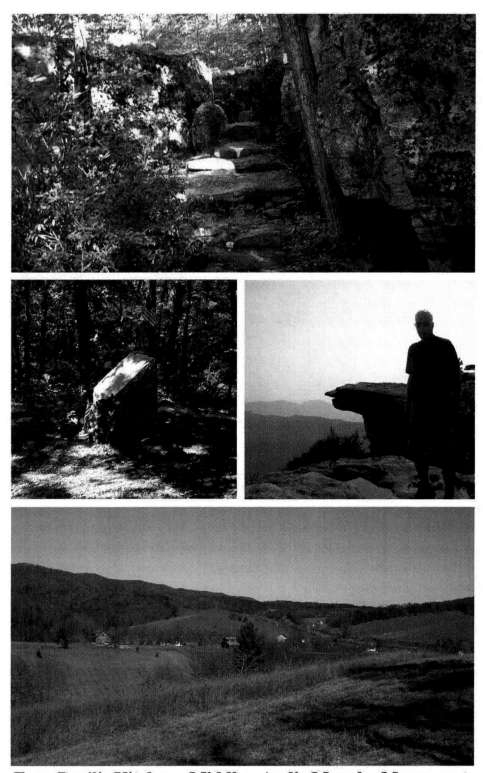

Top: Devil's Kitchen. Middle: Audie Murphy Monument;
McAfee Knob. Bottom: Remote Rt 42 Valley.

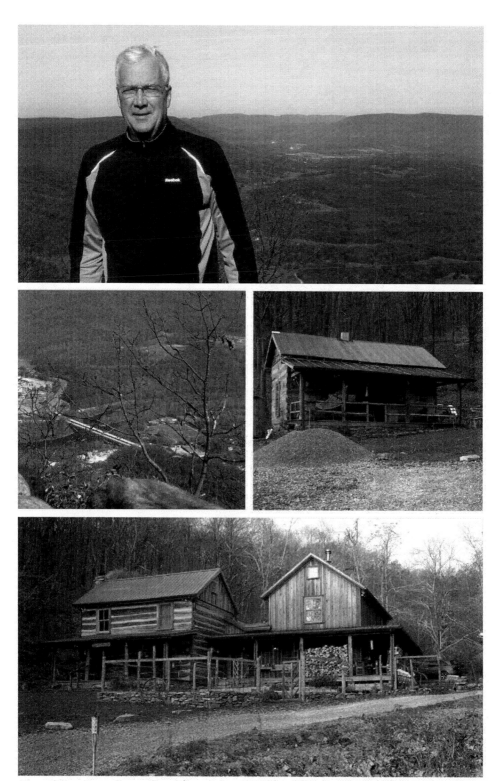

Top: View from Sugar Run Mountain. Middle: View from Angels Rest of Pearis-burg and New River; Woods Hole Bunkhouse. Bottom: Woods Hole B&B.

2011 – North - Finishing to Pinkham Notch

After my second trip to Woods Hole early this spring, I was ready to focus on the North. I had now hiked two 19-mile sections, which made the 17-mile section in southern Vermont seem doable. I would think about the 23-mile section later. The trail descriptions of two sections of the AT south of Franconia Notch in New Hampshire sounded very difficult. I had my new body working for me, having lost 25 pounds over the winter, and I felt like I was in the best shape of my life. Encouraged, I planned to check off a few sections over Memorial Day weekend.

After a partner's meeting on Thursday, May 26, I drove up to Manchester, Vermont, so that I could stay overnight, and get a very early start on the 17-mile section on Friday. Dot MacDonald agreed to meet me at the trailhead on Route 11 at 7:00 A.M. Dot knew the shortcuts up through Stratton Mountain Ski Area to get me to the Stratton-Arlington Road, which took about 40 minutes. It was good to see Dot again. I talked to her about the hike today. She did not think I would have a problem. She also was encouraging about the 23-mile section to the south toward Bennington, recommending that I hike it from north to south. Today's hike would be south to north. Memorial Day is the beginning of the hiking season in Vermont, because of the mud in the spring.

From the road it was a 1,700-foot climb, but over four miles. It really was not that tough. The trail was surprisingly good, and not that muddy.

I easily reached the Stratton Mountain Fire Tower in less than two hours. I was pumped. The summit of Stratton was pretty, with a little, well-kept ranger house that looked like it could have been occupied, but I'm sure it was not. The summit was dominated by hemlock and spruce. There is actually a short access trail to walk across to the north peak of Stratton's ski area which the gondola climbs to. Since I did not go up the fire tower, I could not see it. Dot said that when Stratton Ski Area was developed, care was taken so that it could not be seen from the trail at any point.

It was steep on the hike down over the next two miles and 1,500 feet. It was a little rocky, but not really very difficult technically. Over the last 11 miles there was little elevation gain or loss. Once down off Stratton, it was another mile to Stratton Pond and some campsites. It was quiet, and I would have thought that people would have been out to begin the Memorial Day weekend. My camera caught some images of some angels that were sent to protect me. I ate lunch at the Winhall River, but it was not even noon yet. I was making good time, and was halfway.

The William B. Douglas Shelter was about half a mile off the trail, so I did not go there, and left the Lye Brook Wilderness area. The next mile was on the old Rootville Road to Prospect Rock. The road almost seemed passable by vehicle, and eventually did go toward Manchester. Prospect Rock provided the only views of the day, down to the town of Manchester, where I was staying. It was a clear and nice day. It was a slight and easy climb up to Spruce Peak, and then across the ridge to the Spruce Peak Shelter. It was an enclosed cabin, and had a wood stove in it. The shelters on the Long Trail are set up to handle winter hiking. A sign said the shelter was built in 1984 by the Green Mountain Club, the US Forest Service and a Rutland Corrections Crew. I had three miles to go.

I was weary and fading, but the last three miles were not difficult. At a stream crossing, I forced myself to stop and enjoy a waterfall. I was glad to reach my car before 4:00 P.M. As much as I had agonized about this section and the one to the south, it did not seem that hard. I headed back to my Manchester motel.

The next morning, I tried to sleep in, and then had breakfast at a great "Upstairs" spot in Manchester. It was crowded, with the beginning of the holiday weekend. After breakfast, I packed up and headed cross-country to New Hampshire. I wanted to do that section north of Quintown that I had bailed on the previous fall. It was only 6.3 miles. I did not have an idea about a shuttle out in this remote area, but the roads around did not look long on my map. I had decided I could do it using my bike, which I'd brought.

I easily found the Route 25A trailhead. On my way there, I noticed a nice little hill or two, but it would not be a problem. It was a gray day. The bike ride was about 9 miles on Route 25A, and then a steady 4-mile climb up dirt Quintown Road, where Stray Cat had dropped me last fall. I left my bike chained to a gate, and walked the last half-mile to the trailhead.

From the logging road, I headed northeast up 500 feet to Eastman Ledges. It was pretty on the smooth rock summit. After a few pictures, I headed down. I did not take the three-tenths of a mile side trail to the Hexacuba Shelter. The signs at the trailhead confused me a little. The Dartmouth Outing Club signs seem to confuse me.

From the trail junction, I began the strong climb up Cube Mountain. It was 1,500 feet over a mile and a half. Parts were rock scrambles, and some parts were up some steep, but walkable smooth rock faces. Some of the spots were just roots and rocks on a tough grade. The forest turned into scrub pines when the elevation rose to near 3,500 feet. At the top, the nice day turned into a walk in the clouds, socked in, with no views. There was a chill in the air, so I stopped and put a heavy shirt on. I started down the steep descent.

There were some switchbacks and I began to hear voices, but it took some time for me to catch up to a group from the Dartmouth Outing Club. I called out hello as I approached them. I often call out when I encounter people on the trail, just so I don't startle them when we are on top of each other. The guys seemed protective of the girls until they realized I was not a threat. I hiked the remaining two miles with them and mostly spoke to Kate, a freshman from Connecticut. The group had parked their van at the Route 25A trailhead and hiked up to Cube Mountain, and were on their way down. I think I reminded Kate of her dad. She talked a lot, as girls can do. She slipped and fell at one point, and was shaken. She said that the Dartmouth Outing Club was mostly made up of freshmen and sophomores. The longer the kids were in school, they either lost interest, or had other things going on. I believe Dartmouth Juniors spend a semester abroad. I asked if they ever did any trail maintenance. She said none that she knew of. I suspected so.

We reached the full-flowing Bracket Brook, which had to be rock-hopped to get across. Rock hopping is no longer one of my strengths. There was a very pretty waterfall upstream. At the trailhead, the group packed up quickly, and started back to campus. I had to drive back to Quintown to get my bike before heading to my motel in Lincoln, and dinner at a sports bar.

The next morning, I drove back out the long and winding Route 118, and then Route 25 past Glencliff to the Route 25 trailhead. I had scouted it the day before. I called the Lincoln shuttle company before I left town. There was no cell service at the trailhead. I had tried to make arrangements in advance, but they said it was not necessary, which turned out to be correct. Still, I was pleasantly surprised when the driver showed up on time. We then had to make the long drive back down Route 118 to get to Kinsman Notch.

Today's hike was only 10 miles, but it was a difficult, steep climb to the summit of Mount Moosilauke and a difficult, steep climb down to Glencliff. For the northbound thru-hiker, this section is the first in the White Mountains and where the "fun" begins. I must have read the section description a hundred times. "This section ascends past cascades on rock steps, on wooden steps bolted into ledges, and over hand rungs of rebar (steel reinforcing bars) to the summit." It intimidated me, and I did not sleep well the night before.

The driver dropped me at the busy, large parking lot at Kinsman Notch. It was Sunday of Memorial Day weekend. After 100 yards, I was headed up 2,500 feet over two miles. This was the steepest section I had done to date, and the trail description fit to a tee. On the good side, I was in great shape, and had lost my pack weight over the winter. I could handle it. The hike was tough but beautiful for the entire climb next to the Beaver Brook Cascades. It was a good excuse to stop and view the wonderful waterfalls, one after another.

I was only a half-hour into the climb when I overtook two guys in their

20s. They were Max and Dan from Massachusetts. They were on a practice hike for something they planned in Colorado. Max was struggling. Dan was annoyed because Max had put 10 one-liter bottles of water in his pack to try to simulate his Colorado pack weight. He would not be doing a climb like this in Colorado. They were nice guys, and I just stayed behind for a while to talk. A family flew by. Finally, I got frustrated with the pace, and went around. There was still some ice and snow on the trail in spots. It was an incredibly steep, but wonderfully built trail. The rock steps were an engineering marvel. I don't know how they do it. Two northbound thru-hikers went by, skipping down the mountain at a brisk, and what I thought to be an unsafe, pace. They asked about getting a ride to Lincoln at Kinsman Notch. I said I did not think it would be a problem, since there seemed to be quite a few cars and a lot of activity at the big parking lot. The White Mountains are an easy hitch from locals or other hikers. Quite a few trails originate at Kinsman Notch.

At the summit of Mount Blue, the trail leveled off. Spruce trees started to dominate. It was getting foggy at the higher elevation. I reached the junction with the Benton Trail. A young family was just coming up. From my map, it was not clear where they had hiked up from. They took my picture at the trail signs, and I took one of the four of them. In the picture, I looked thin. *Wow.* The family sprinted off to the north peak of Moosilauke. It was four-tenths of a mile to the summit, at 4,802 feet. From the trail junction, I emerged totally above the tree line.

The summit was like Grand Central Station. There must have been 30 people. Many were huddled behind rock walls, trying to stay out of the chilly breeze. Most were prepared and had wind shirts, or even coats. I pulled out my wind shirt and put it on. The summit was totally socked in with fog, so there were no views down into the valley. Funny that it was a beautiful, sunny day when I started at Kinsman Notch, 3,000 feet below.

Many people at the summit had hiked up 3.5 miles from Ravine Lodge. Ravine Lodge is along that winding Route 118, and is run by the Dartmouth Outing Club. A girl I talked to had done so, and she was freezing in a T-shirt. The family took my picture next to the summit sign. I headed across the open ridge to the south peak of Moosilauke. On the way, I descended into the scrub pines with the well-defined rocky trail. If you google-map Moosilauke, you can see the trail clearly on the satellite view. I passed a family. Past the south peak, I started the difficult steep down. It was unrelenting. My poles were a nuisance. They do not help much on steep climbs or descents. It was easier to hang onto trees to keep my balance while climbing down the steep rock steps.

I passed a dad whose family was lagging behind. The family was out for a long weekend camping trip. They seemed not prepared for what they had gotten themselves into. I think the dad was a few hundred yards ahead to keep them moving, and so that he did not have to hear the whining. I passed three young teenagers with Mom struggling to bring up the rear. They asked how far to the summit. I lied and told them it was not much further. It was only about a mile, but it could take them over an hour to get there.

Finally, I reached the junction with the Hurricane Trail and was down. I still had a pleasant, level walk over the next two miles to the trailhead. I passed a young couple sprinting up the trail. They asked me how far it was. I said how far to what? They said to the top. They were in sneakers and T-shirts, and had a half-empty pint bottle of water. I said it was 3 hours up and 3 hours down. It was 2:00 P.M. They seemed crushed, and decided to go just a little further.

At the road, you had to ford Oliverian Brook. It was flowing strong. There were no rocks to hop, and no bridge. All I could do was wade in. That was a first. The dad had mentioned something about climbing out a tree branch to get across, but I was on the wrong side of the brook. It seemed hard to do, anyway. I made it to my car, and drove back that long Route 118 for the third time that day, to my Lincoln motel. The girl at the sports bar was getting to know me.

Bad weather moved in. My boots were wet, and my knees were killing me from my climb down Moosilauke. I bailed on my next day's easy hike south of Glencliff, and drove home on Memorial Day.

June came, and I decided to bite the bullet and attempt the 22.6-mile hike in southern Vermont. I would drive up to Bennington on Friday evening of Father's Day weekend, hike Saturday, and drive home Sunday. I was in good shape. Now was the time. Since it was June, I would have the most daylight of the year. I avoided the summer solstice. I have been told that people hike in the nude that day.

I arrived in Bennington in the middle of the afternoon and checked into my motel. I drove over to the Bennington Tower Monument, which dominated the skyline in the area. I took the elevator to the top and took some pictures out toward Bennington College. It is one of the most expensive colleges in the country.

I showered before dinner, and across the street from my motel, crowds were gathering. The high school band was there. They were waiting for the participants of "The Great Race" to arrive. The Great Race was an antique car rally of some sort. The group had started in Tennessee, and they were finishing today in Bennington. In a few minutes they arrived. There could have been 50 or 60 antique cars and trucks. They stopped traffic in town. It was fun. At dinner I ate like it would be my last meal, and splurged and ate my first dessert since the previous December. The brownie sundae sat in my stomach like a lump for most of the night.

I was up at 4:30 A.M. and ate the breakfast that Virginia had packed for me. I did not expect any diners to be open at that hour. I was at the Route 9 trailhead by 5:45 A.M., and Dot McDonald was right on time at 6:00 A.M. It took us an hour to drive the 40 miles around the Green Mountains to the east. Planning ahead, I talked to Dot about Maine. Dot loved Maine because of the remoteness and the beauty. I ignored the one-tenth mile road walk. Dot dropped me off right where I would enter the woods. I had plenty of food and water, and was off on my longest day to date. It was 7:00 A.M. Once Dot drove away, I really had little choice but to get to my car, 22.6 miles away. What the heck; that is not even a marathon, which normal runners can do in less than five hours.

The hike had no major climbs, and was a net elevation gain of only 1,500 feet over 12 miles to the summit of Glastenbury Mountain. There were a few 500-foot PUDs in between, but nothing that steep or difficult. I started out on nice trail, but it did not take long for the rocks to show up. It took less time for the black flies to show up. I was swatting all day when hiking and when I stopped, they were unbearable. That was the way it would be. There was nothing I could do about it except wear a hat, which made me hot, so I had it on and off. The trail had a lot of muddy spots, too.

I took a short break at Story Spring Shelter, and kept on moving. There were a lot of ferns in the area. I was moving well, and almost felt light on my feet as I skipped around the mud. Almost. Today's hike was entirely in the Green Mountain National Forest. It was a very cloudy day, and at times there was some fog and drizzle, but no significant rain. On the way to Kid Gore Shelter, I heard some major rustling to my right. A large, antlerless moose appeared from the brush, and just as quickly disappeared. I only saw it for a few seconds, and there was no way to get my camera out in time. *Darn.*

At the 8-mile mark, I reached the Kid Gore Shelter and took another break. I was making good time. By 12:30 P.M., I had climbed up to the base of the Glastenbury Fire Tower, the 12-mile mark and over halfway. I decided to eat my lunch there. The black flies made it very unpleasant, so I ate quickly and headed out.

Just 500 yards below the summit, I reached the Goddard Shelter. It was busy, and the first people I'd met today. There were four thru-hikers breaking for lunch. They did not seem bothered by the flies. I guess they smelled too bad. I also met Dana Brown. Dana was from Lancaster, Pennsylvania, and we figured out that he and I had both graduated from Penn State in the class of 1969. He was hiking the 40-mile section up to Manchester over four days with his two grown sons for Father's Day weekend. He was impressed that I would be hiking that distance in two day hikes. It was great to talk to him, but the flies made it not worthwhile to stick around, so I continued down and entered the Glastenbury Wilderness. I had 10 miles to go.

On the way down there were some lookouts, but the fog mitigated the views. I just kept my head down, and kept moving. I met two older guys who had just started today at Bennington. I don't know when they began their day, but they had only covered about 5 miles, and were planning to get to the Goddard Shelter, 5 more miles. It was late afternoon. They did not look like they would make it. They were section-hikers, and had met each other online and decided to hike the AT in Vermont together. One was trying to be patient with the slower one, who was struggling. I didn't think they would last more than a day or so together.

I have seen ads in trail magazines about people looking for hiking partners to slack pack parts of the trail, especially in the north. I think I'm glad I have never responded. I'm not always sure I can take care of myself, let alone someone else.

I started to fade at about the 17-mile mark, and reached a viewpoint that I thought I should have been well past. I almost cried. I got to Hell Hollow Brook and forced myself to eat an apple, a pack of crackers and a bag of trail mix. I still had three miles to go, so I needed to make sure I had the fuel I needed.

From the elevation profile, I was a little leery of the last mile and a half, because I thought it would be a very steep down. I was remembering the very steep climb up on the south side of Route 9 a few years earlier. It was not as bad as I expected. Finally, I reached the MacArthur Memorial Bridge over City Stream, and I was at my car.

I cracked a beer and called Virginia. It was quiet at the trailhead. No high school band was waiting to celebrate my triumph. It was 5:45 P.M. but seemed later, since it was a dark day. I had hiked 22.6 miles in under 11 hours. I had another beer to celebrate completing Vermont. I stopped to buy a pint of ice cream for dinner on the short ride back to Bennington. I showered and went to bed by 8:00 P.M. I was on the road at first light, and had breakfast in Albany.

After attending the AT conference in southwest Virginia in July, I wanted to get back to New Hampshire. I did not actually think I could finish the state, but I wanted to complete everything to Pinkham Notch. That would mean some more tough hiking.

I drove up to Lincoln, New Hampshire on Saturday, August 6. I had a plan for the next few days, but the weather was working against me. Sunday's weather looked bleak, so I switched my days at the Highland Center and the huts I planned to later in the week. There was an easier section to the southwest that I could fill in on Sunday, even if it was raining some.

I got up Sunday morning and checked the weather. It had poured overnight, but was not raining as hard now. I went out and had breakfast, and checked the forecast again. It seemed like it might be clearing a bit. I decided to go for it, and drove out that long Route 118 again to Route 25 to Glencliff, where I had dunked my boots in the Oliverian Brook. I had my bike with me, so I was planning to shuttle myself to Route 25A. It would be a 10-mile hike that did not look particularly tough from the elevation profile, and about an 18-mile bike ride. As I approached, it seemed to be raining a little harder. I had alerted Virginia that it would be late when I called her. There was no cell reception out here.

I arrived at the trailhead, and a car was there with its door open. I noticed a woman in the bushes quickly pulling her pants up. I moved my car back and forth a few times to give her some space. When she came out of the bushes, I parked and said hello. She said she and her friend had just arrived, and were getting ready for their hike. "Me too," I said. There was another woman in the car who started to speak, and I thought I recognized her voice. "Karen?" I said. She got out and came over and it was Karen, the hike leader from the Vermont conference two years earlier! She remembered me since I was a driver, and she was navigating in my car.

Karen and her friend Sharon had driven all night from Harrisburg, Pennsylvania to hike in the Whites for a few days. They had just arrived. They would be hiking the same section I was. They would do a key swap. Sharon would drive out to Route 25A and start to hike north. Karen would start to hike from Route 25 and hike south. When they met on the trail, Sharon would give Karen the car key, and when Karen got to it, she would drive back around to pick up Sharon. Hikers do this all the time. They would not get to hike together, but I guess they did not want to, because Karen is an extremely fast hiker. It was their thing. I offered the use of my car, but they were set. They said that I was more than welcome to join Sharon and hike back with her. Wow, this was trail magic. I just avoided an 18-mile bike ride, plus having to drive out and back to pick up my bike. It was fantastic.

Sharon and I headed out in their car to the Route 25A trailhead where I had ended with the Dartmouth Outing Club people. She led out. Sharon was about my age, but an experienced hiker. She and Karen had been to the Virginia conference this year, but I did not hike with them. I had seen Karen at the hike gathering place when she was leading hikes, but they did not stay on campus. Instead they stayed in town with other people from the Harrisburg Hiking Club. Sharon talked all the way, as women can do. She was very pleasant. She was married, but her husband did not share her passion for hiking, but had no problem with her leaving to hike.

Somehow she knew Graham Cracker from Florida, whom I had met at the Dutch House a few years earlier. Graham Cracker completed the trail, but not the year I met her.

The hike started out on an easy footpath, but climbed 1,000 feet over 2.5 miles, so not too steep. I could keep up with her, but not easily. She was supposed to be the slow one. We were less than four miles into the hike when Karen came flying by. We of course had driven around, and she had started hiking first. Sharon gave the car key to Karen. We continued to Ore Hill, and then down to Route 25C, crossed the road, and Sharon kept on moving. We were halfway up Mount Mist when I told Sharon I needed a break to eat something. She waited patiently for the ten minutes or so it took me to eat an apple, but I put my pack on (she never took hers off) and stood up, and she was off. On the steep climb down toward Wachinpauka Pond, she did stop for a minute to talk to an Asian couple who seemed to be looking for the pond, which they had passed. They did not believe us, and continued on.

Sharon really moved the last two easy miles to the car. She did stop once to take pictures of some bright-yellow fungus on a dead, fallen tree. Karen was waiting for us when we arrived at the trailhead. She had driven around, gotten gas for the car, stopped at the hostel in Glencliff to check it out, and still beat us back. I would have been dead hiking with Karen. Sharon and I had done the 10 miles in just over 4 hours, a blistering pace for me, but routine for her.

Karen and Sharon were planning to climb Mount Washington the next day, and then were driving all the way up to Katahdin to meet someone who was completing a section-hike of the entire AT. They planned a celebration with him. Tonight they were staying in a hostel in Gorham. I offered my motel room for a shower, but they declined, and were off. Once I had cell reception on Route 118, I called Virginia. She was surprised to hear from me so early, and was as amazed about my trail magic as I was. She said she had goose bumps. I have had a lot of luck on the trail with logistics.

I stopped at Franconia Notch at the hiker's parking lot to hide my bike in the woods. I thought I might need it there two days from then to retrieve my car.

The next morning, I was at an early-morning breakfast spot at 6:00 A.M. I drove out to Kinsman Notch, and was ready to start by 7:00 A.M. The guide's trail description for today's hike gave me nightmares. "Hiking here is extremely strenuous due to the change in elevation from both ends and the often wet and rugged footway." It did not disappoint. The section was 16.3 miles. I was only planning to hike 13.4 of it today, to the Lonesome Lake Hut, and then the other 2.9 miles tomorrow back to Franconia Notch, and the hiker lot where I'd left my bike.

The Lincoln Shuttle Company dropped off two thru-hikers just as I arrived. They were doing the full 16 miles today as a slack pack. They had stayed in Lincoln the night before, and would also tonight. The guy's trail name was Lost and Found. The girl's was Pony. I would leap frog them for the day, and we actually would get to Lonesome Lake within minutes of each other. Lost and Found would wait for Pony throughout the day, since she was slower.

They left the parking lot before me. From Route 112 heading north, there was an immediate steep 800-foot ascent in half a mile on rough trail. About halfway up, I passed Pony in her yellow rain jacket, who was setting up her music in her headphones. She did not seem to be having fun, and was never very talkative. I seem to have met many thru-hikers in the Mid-Atlantic States who did not seem that happy. They had hiked a long time, and were not yet in view of the end. Thru-hikers seem more happy at the beginning and end of their journey.

The next two miles were not steep, but still, the trail was very difficult, with rocks and roots. Every step had to be planned. The trail ran along Olesons Brook, which was loud and full-flowing with the rain of the previous few days. It was misting this morning again. At about 9:00 A.M. and only having gone about three miles, I took a break to eat something. Pony came by, and barely said a word. I continued to pick my way along the difficult trail, with short but steep ups and downs.

At the East Peak of Mount Wolf, I did not take the 60-yard side trail to the view because it was a straight-up rock scramble. The next three miles were downhill, but the rugged trail continued. I reached the Eliza Brook Shelter, but did not stop, since I had just taken a break. I could hear voices at the shelter. I was at the 7.5-mile mark, but it was after noon already. I figured I should just keep going.

I began a long, tough climb along some beautiful cascades. The rocks and roots on the trail were incredible. After an hour and only about a mile of steep climbing, I emerged into an open area on puncheon at Harrington Pond. I stopped and looked at the cliffs and ridge of the Kinsman Mountains right in front of me. I was exhausted, and almost cried. Just then, Lost and Found came up behind me. I said, "I think we have to go up there." He said, "Sweet!" He was having a ball. He and Pony had taken a break at the Eliza Brook Shelter with a few other thru-hikers. Lost and Found stopped for a minute, but then headed out. I followed for a while, but he just disappeared.

The next mile was a straight-up climb up to the summit of South Kinsman, and took over an hour. It was difficult, and was on the outside of the mountain. There were precipitous drops. Someone told me later that they were afraid they would fall to their death. At one point I took my pack off to take a drink, but had to make sure it did not fall, because it would not have been retrievable. I overtook a retired couple heading up. They were from Indiana, and had decided on a White Mountain adventure. They had started the day before at Kinsman Notch, where I had started today. They were clearly in over their heads, and the wife kept saying they would have to go back to Indiana and reconsider their plan. I felt like I should help them, but really did not know how. I went by and did not see them again. They were not planning to get to the Lonesome Lake Hut, but a camping area about two miles away.

I met a family from Pittsburgh, Pennsylvania who were coming down the mountain. The dad was in front, and a 13-year-old son was with Mom, 50 yards behind. Mom was terrified of the steep, open descent, and was very slow going down. They had started in Franconia Notch the day before, and had stayed at Lonesome Lake last night. It was about 2:30 P.M., and they had started at 8:00 A.M. It had taken them over six hours to go four miles. They found the climb up to North Kinsman very difficult, which was not what I wanted to hear, since I had to go down it.

I finally reached the summit of South Kinsman. The weather was breaking, and the sun was peeking through some clouds. I was above tree line, and the views were spectacular. You could see Interstate 93 running down through Franconia Notch. Harrington Pond below looked far away, but was actually about a mile, but 1,000 feet down. I took a break, but not for long, since I still had over three miles to go. It was the nicest walk of the day down, and then up the col between South and North Kinsman, all above tree line. I bypassed the spur trail to the summit of North Kinsman. I just wanted off the mountain. Be careful what you wish for.

The next mile and a half was a very steep down of 1,500 feet from North Kinsman. Many of the drops were on unwalkable (for me) steep rock faces. About 20 times, I threw my poles down ahead and slid down on my butt. I was exhausted, and this was the safest way. The down was unrelenting, and seemed to take forever. Finally, I reached the bottom, and the last mile was on level, but still rough, rocky and root-filled trail. I reached Lonesome Lake Hut, tired but happy. Lost and Found was there, still shirtless. Guys who thru-hike often do so without shirts. Pony came in about 10 minutes behind me, followed by three or four other thru-hikers. It was 5:00 P.M. It had taken me 10 hours to hike the 13.4 miles. I was encouraged that I could keep pace with a 20-something thru-hiker (Pony). I considered this my toughest day on the trail so far. I don't know how I would have made it without the weight loss and being in good shape. I told the kids that I thought it might have been as hard as hiking the two days up Mount Washington, but doing it in one day. I still believe it to be true.

Lost and Found wanted to hang around at the hut for a while, but Pony was impatient to head out. They had another three miles to get to the interstate at Franconia Notch. Pony did not want to hike in the dark. I was happy to be staying at the hut. I don't think I could have gone another 100 yards.

The hut croo told me where my bunk room was. Lonesome Lake had two separate bunk houses, and small bunk rooms of four bunks each. I had a bunkroom to myself, which was nice. I got cleaned up and changed clothes for dinner. My hiking pants were filthy from sliding down Kinsman on my butt. I started to feel good, and was recovering already.

The hut was half-full with about 20 guests. Dinner was at 6:00 P.M. I had dinner at a table with Roger, who worked for the Relief Division of the United Nations in New York City. He was from the Netherlands, and his brother and cousin were visiting him during his vacation. They were up from the city for a long weekend of hiking. Charlie and Donna from New Hampshire were also at the table, with their two grandsons, who were 7 and 9. All had hiked up the three miles from Franconia Notch. They would hike back to Franconia the next day. The Lonesome Lake Hut is popular among families, since it is a relatively easy hike to get there, and a nice place.

After dinner and the croo skits, Grace from Maine, an AMC volunteer, took the 20 of us on a nature walk down to Lonesome Lake. I don't know that I would have gone, except they said there might be a chance to see Bullwinkle, the resident moose of the area. He did not appear.

I crashed in my room, but did not sleep so well. It was well before the 9:00 P.M. lights-out. 9:00 P.M. is considered hiker's midnight. I was too excited about completing the tough day. I was up at the crack of dawn, and walked down all the way around Lonesome Lake, hoping to see Bullwinkle in the early morning, but he must have been shy. I was beginning to think he did not exist. I was back at the hut for coffee. The thru-hikers on the work-for-stay program, sleeping in the dining room, were just getting up. I went back to my room to pack up. Breakfast was the standard oatmeal and pancakes.

In the morning, I found out that I had missed Cimmeron by a day. Cimmeron is an 88-year-old man attempting to "thru-hike" the AT this year. He had thru-hiked several times, years earlier. He had stayed at Lonesome Lake Hut the night before. I have "thru-hike" in quotes because from reading his trail journal that others were posting for him, he ended up hiking about 1,100 miles of the AT. He got as far as Pinkham Notch, and was stymied by Hurricane Irene and some injuries. He must have skipped some other sections as he fell behind schedule. He did drive to Katahdin in September, but for a variety of reasons, was not able to summit. From his trail journal postings and comments from others, he was a feisty old guy, who wanted to hike his own hike, and was not at ease accepting help. He mostly hiked alone. It took him three days to hike from Kinsman Notch to the Lonesome Lake Hut. He could not find a place to pitch his tent, so he just sat up and slept against rocks for the two nights.

The first mile down from the hut had more roots on it than I had ever seen. It was not steep, and not even that tough. It was a welcome respite from the tough day before. In about a mile I crossed Cascade Brook, and the trail became very easy, and ended up in some meadows. There were some good views straight ahead to Mount Lafayette. That was where I planned to go the next day, for my third attempt at completing the section between Crawford Notch and Franconia Notch. About halfway, one of the female thru-hikers who had stayed at the hut passed me. Her pack seemed small for a thru-hiker, but she was not slack packing. She was a nice kid and after a brief conversation, she headed on. I tried to keep up with her, but boy was she fast. In about three minutes, she disappeared. The trail followed Cascade Brook under Interstate 93 to the junction of the Whitehouse Trail, which was a mile to the parking lot where I had left my bike. There is actually no AT trailhead at the interstate. I arrived at the lot. I decided I was not up for the bike ride back to Kinsman Notch, so I called the Lincoln Shuttle Company. While waiting, I met two guys from Massachusetts who were hiking up Lafayette. They were only going to a campsite near to the top of the mountain today.

The shuttle arrived and took me back to Kinsman Notch and my car. On my way back, I passed four thru-hikers hitching out of Woodstock on their way back to the trail. I turned around to get them and take them back, which they appreciated very much. I went back to the hiker lot to retrieve my bike. I had a reservation back in Crawford Notch at the Highland Center for tonight. It was a 45-minute drive to get there. I decided to stay there because I got a discount for staying in AMC facilities three nights in a row. Plus, I really liked it there. Since it was too early to check in, I lingered at the trailhead a little to see if there was any thru-hiker who might pop out of the woods who needed a ride.

A van pulled up, and two gorgeous 20-something girls jumped out. They had just come into Lincoln from Vancouver, Canada, and were going to hike the Whites. They had stayed at a hostel in Lincoln, and the hostel owner had dropped them off. They had big packs loaded with a lot of food. I think they were experienced hikers, but did not seem to be exactly sure where they were headed and where they would stay tonight. It would be a long hike to get to the Greenleaf Hut, and I don't think they could afford to stay there. They did not have a decent map. I gave them one of mine that I could spare. I left them there as they tried to develop a plan. I had helped them all I could.

I checked in early at the Highland Center, and my room was ready. New at the Highland Center was a massive kids' playground that was under construction. I really needed a nap. At dinner I ate with Maury and his son Sasha from Pittsburgh, who were here for a White Mountain adventure. They were planning to hike up Mount Washington over two days, not on the AT, but the easier Crawford Path, and stay at the Mizpah Spring Hut. Sasha was a scratch golfer, and was hoping for college scholarships. Also at the table were three 40-something guys from Maine who where planning on hiking from Crawford Notch to Franconia, the hike I had started the year earlier and hoped to finish tomorrow. I described a little of it, but did not try to encourage or discourage them. It is hard to tell how experienced people are, or their abilities, when you are sitting across the dinner table. I just figure people know what they are doing, although I have learned that people don't when it comes to the Whites. One hundred thirty-five people and counting have died in the Whites because of not being prepared, or lack of judgment.

After breakfast the next morning, I bagged a trail lunch, and drove back around to that same hiker lot. My plan was to hike up the AT 6.4 miles, to the summit of Mount Lafayette, to complete the section. I would then hike the mile down to the Greenleaf Hut and stay the night. The next morning, I would hike down and hitch a ride, or call for a shuttle back to my car. It would be a steep three miles at first, but I was finding that it was easier on my knees to hike up than to take the pounding coming down. Of course, it is hard as I gasp for air on the climbs.

I left the parking lot and hiked over the Whitehouse Trail about a mile to get to the AT. The AT climbed a three hundred foot up toward the junction with the Flume Slide Trail. It was a foggy and misty, humid morning. My glasses got fogged up. My shirt was drenched from the beginning. It was not cool, so I did not need a heavy shirt. From that junction, it was a relentless 2,500-foot rock scramble straight up over the next two miles, until the top of the ridge. I actually enjoyed it. I was rested from the short hike on the previous day and a good night's sleep. I felt like I was getting some benefit from being in shape. As I approached each boulder climb as it appeared in my view, I even found myself taunting the trail a little. "Is that all you got?" "Is that the best you can do?"

Almost at the top of the climb I reached the Liberty Springs Tentsite. Tentsites in the Whites consist of wood platforms on which hikers put their tents. This is done to protect the fragile environments. There is usually a caretaker there during hiking season to collect a fee. The fee collections in the Whites annoy the thru-hikers to no end. They often ignore the rules, and stealth-camp in prohibited areas. The tentsite was very quiet, and I did not see any activity at all. It seemed like it was early, as dark as it was in the mist, but it was after 10:00 A.M.

Once on top of the Franconia Ridge, it was a pretty walk through spruce and hemlock on level trail that was surprisingly easy. Though there were rocks, they were well-worn on this old trail. Once I reached the ridge, I only had three miles to get to the summit of Lafayette. After the first easy mile, I was climbing again up 600 feet to Little Haystack Mountain. I was emerging into the scrub pine zone. It was foggy, and I could not see far. When I reached the summit of Little Haystack, I was halfway across the ridge. I continued up another half-mile and another few hundred feet to the summit of Mount Lincoln. I was totally above tree line now.

On the way I met those two guys who I had seen at the parking lot the day before. They had camped at the Liberty Springs Tentsite the night before, and had slack packed to the summit of Lafayette, and were on their way back to the tentsite. I asked them if they had seen the girls. They had, but the girls had continued on up the mountain, and seemed to be doing fine.

On top of Mount Lincoln, I encountered a group of about eight guys in their 40s and 50s. They acted like an army squad playing soldier. It was comical. They had hiked up to the Greenleaf Hut the day before, and were hiking back down to Franconia Notch today. The fog continued, and I could not see beyond a few hundred feet. I continued on toward Lafayette with a few short but not difficult ups and downs. I had visions of hiking on this ridge of precipitous drops on either side. That was not the case. It was a nice hike up there. I only wish I could have seen something. I was making good time, and climbed up the next rise, and a voice said to me, "Congratulations, you made it!" I said, "I made it where?" The guy said, "The summit of Lafayette." I had not realized that I was that far along. There were a few people up there, and one took my picture at the sign boards. There was not much to see with the fog, so I headed down the trail to the Greenleaf Hut. About halfway down, the hut came into view through the fog.

I arrived at the hut and had a bowl of soup, which the hut croo always has available for guest arrival. It was only 2:30 P.M. I had changed my reservation dates a few times because of the weather, and they had me on the list for tonight, but then crossed off. I'm sure it would not have been a problem, because the hut would not be full.

I talked to a thru-hiker who had come down to the hut for the evening. Thru-hikers don't often stay at Greenleaf, since it is a long mile down, and then up in the morning from the trail. It is also only six miles from Franconia, and younger thru-hikers would consider it a short day, especially if they had stayed in Lincoln for a zero day. I told him how I had been hiking the trail, and that I had done the middle of it. His comment was, "Oh, you have not done the best parts yet." He also said that since I only hiked three or so days at a time, that I never really got my trail legs. Thru-hikers will tell you it takes about a week for your body to get used to long hiking days. I guess that is true.

I was feeling pretty good, so I decided I would hike down this afternoon rather than the next day. I talked to the hut croo, and they said that even though the Greenleaf Trail was a little longer than the Bridal Path Trail (that I had taken the previous year) it was easier. The Greenleaf Trail would put me further from my car, but I would have to get a ride in either case. I put on a dry shirt and headed down the Greenleaf Trail. It would be three miles down to the Canon Mountain Ski Area at the interstate. It was not exactly easy, and there were several steep descents, and my knees were feeling it. I took my time. I circled around the base of Eagle Cliff, which was spectacular. I saw no one on the trail at all, and I felt small and insignificant and alone in the wilderness. I guess I was. I made sure to take a break and eat from my pack on the way down.

I finally reached the road, and was tired from the 11.3-mile day in the Whites. I walked over to the cloverleaf to hitch a ride. A few cars came by. People were coming from the ski area, which runs a tramway in the summer, but most of the cars were full, or were going the wrong way. A hiker who had come down behind me on the Greenleaf Trail arrived. He was thinking about going to the store at the ski area to resupply, but was concerned about the prices there. He wandered in that direction. At that point, I decided I would call the Lincoln Shuttle Company, since I was having no luck getting a ride. I told him he could go with me to my car, but he seemed uncertain.

About half an hour later, the shuttle van arrived. I saw the guy, whose trail name was Treadmill, sitting in the grass near the ski area entrance. I told him he could ride the shuttle with me, and with my car I would take him where he wanted to go to resupply, and then bring him back. After thinking for a while, he agreed. We got to the hiker lot and my car, and I paid the driver for both of us. Treadmill was not talkative, but he was thru-hiking, I guess. By coming down the Greenleaf Trail, he was not on the AT anymore. He said he was purposely hiking as many extra trails in the Whites as he could. His boots were completely worn out and the soles were flapping, and you could see his worn socks.

He wanted to go to a grocery store, so I took him. I offered to wait and take him back to the trail or to the hostel in town. He declined. He seemed broke, so I offered to help him, but he declined. There was nothing more I could do. I left him in the grocery store lot where he just sat down. I did my best to help my fellow hiker.

I was starved, since it was now close to 7:00 P.M., so I bought a burger in town and hit the road. I thought I would just get to Concord and crash in the motel I had been used to crashing in. I was exhausted. It had become a long day. I got to my motel in Concord and to my surprise, there were no rooms available, and the owner told me there would be no rooms for 100 miles to the south because NASCAR was in New Hampshire this week at the New Hampshire Motor Speedway in Loudon. The owner found me a room, but I would backtrack 10 miles on the interstate, and then drive another 3 miles to find it. Thank goodness for my navigation system. I finally got to crash at 10:00 P.M., well past hiker's midnight.

I drove home the next morning, encouraged that I had actually finished what I had planned to do that week. I now only had to finish the other half of the Mount Washington hike, and I would have completed everything to Pinkham Notch.

A few weeks later, Hurricane Irene came to the East Coast. It affected most of the Mid-Atlantic and New England. Flooding was widespread in Vermont and New Hampshire. The AT in the Green Mountains was closed for a month. The entire White Mountain National Forest area was shut down for three days. The huts closed, and all hikers got off the trail until the storm passed. When the storm passed, roadways had been washed away, and some trails were unusable. Route 302, where the Highland Center is located, was washed away at points south of the AT.

I had asked my family if they wanted to complete the Mount Washington hike that we had cut short the previous year. Ben's wife Michelle was eight months pregnant, so it did not work for Ben to be away. I'm not sure if I will ever get Bethany to hike with me again. However, Bethany's husband Kevin was up for it. I picked Kevin up in Hoboken on Friday, September 9, and we drove up to the Highland Center. Bethany had a weekend course for her MBA program at NYU, so it was a good time for him. I was glad to have the company.

The White Mountains were just reopened in time, but there was evidence of closed, washed-out roads as we drove through Franconia and around to Crawford Notch. We arrived in time for dinner. At dinner we sat with Marybeth and Mindy, 30-somethings from Richmond, Virginia. They were who was left of a group of about 20 young girls who had started section-hiking the AT 10 years before. Marybeth was a pilot, and they had flown her plane up to Gorham and gotten a ride back to Glencliff, where they had left off the previous year. They had hiked to the Highland Center, and did all the tough sections I had done over the last two years, including Moosilauke, Kinsman, and Lafayette. They had stayed at the huts, but camped a few days before they got to the Whites. They were planning to hike the AT to Mount Washington just like Kevin and I, so we decided to share a shuttle in the morning. We were both planning on staying at the Mizpah Hut the next night. Each day's hike would be about six miles on the way to the Washington summit.

In the morning, Kevin and I drove over to the Ammonoosuc Ravine Trail trailhead parking area. The trail is often used by day-hikers to summit Mount Washington from the east. The trailhead is an easy road walk to the Cog Railway Station. We planned to come down the Cog Railway the next day. Dan from Trail Angels in Gorham was late, but did finally arrive. We picked up Marybeth and Mindy at the Highland Center, and headed south and down to the trailhead. I say down, because heading south on Route 302, we lost about 1,000 feet of elevation, which we would have to make up. The road was closed, but we could get through to the AT trailhead.

Kevin and I headed out first. We crossed the Saco River on a beautiful bridge. I led at first, but as usual, was going at a pace I could not maintain. It was better if Kevin lead. From the road it would be a 2,000-foot climb over two miles to Webster Cliffs. It was steep and tough, and took two hours. I could handle it fine, but Kevin waited for me often. We passed a couple who was headed up only as far as Mount Webster. We got to Webster Cliffs, thinking it was the summit of Webster, which was another mile. All day, I was thinking we were further along than we actually were. As we were approaching Mount Jackson, people were coming down from there. I argued with them about where we were, but they were right.

The views from Webster Cliffs, Mount Webster, and Mount Jackson, as we hiked along and up the ridge, were spectacular. It was a beautiful, clear day, with views all the way to Mount Washington, ten miles away. It could be seen clearly, and could be identified by the towers and buildings on the top. The road, the railroad bed, and the visitor's center down in Crawford Notch were easily identified. The steep walls of Mount Willard on the other side of the notch made for a dramatic scene. Just to the south, the steep walls on the western side of the notch had caused the rain from Hurricane Irene to wash out the roadway a few weeks earlier.

Crawford Notch was the scene of a massive rockslide in 1825. The Willey family had built a house at the base of what is now Mount Willey. The entire Willey family was lost in the rockslide, because they all tried to outrun the slide. Had they stayed in their home, a ledge above split the slide, and the home was not touched. The bodies of the parents and two of the five children were found, but three children were not. The term "I've got the Willeys" comes from this event.

The climb up Jackson was above the tree line, and included an open rock scramble that was not for the faint of heart. I told Kevin that I thought we would have lost Bethany, had she been along. From the summit of Jackson we could see north all the way to the Mount Washington Hotel. The Mizpah Hut, our destination for tonight, looked like a spec on the side of a massive Mount Clinton. Helicopter flights were going on all afternoon. I'm not sure why, because this was the last weekend for most of the huts to be open with a full staff. They may have been bringing in supplies for the long winter. One croo member is at most of the huts all year and the hut is open, but provides no services. You can cook for yourself on the wood stove.

After climbing down from Mount Jackson, we reentered the woods. There were many people out on this beautiful Saturday. There is a relatively easy trail from the Highland Center up to Mizpah Hut, which is only 2.5 miles. We reached the Mizpah Hut in midafternoon. We were told where our bunkroom was. We were sharing it with five other people. Mindy and Marybeth rolled in a few minutes behind us. The hut would be full tonight, with about 40 guests. There were families and groups, including one large group of a dozen women who had carried quantities of wine along. They were huddled out of the wind on the sunny side of the hut having a great time.

Kevin and I had dinner with Marybeth and Mindy. Dinner was rowdy. I enjoy the huts more when they are only half-full, during the week. The croo had trouble getting their points across. After dinner, the talk about the infrastructure of the hut and its solar and wind power systems seemed to be of interest to Kevin. He and Bethany had just purchased a home to use on weekends near New Paltz, New York. They would spend the next few years gutting the house and renovating it themselves. I would help them a few times, and my first job was to clean out the two-level barn, the size of a 5-car garage. The property was on three acres, about six miles from the New York Thruway.

As usual, I did not sleep all that well. After breakfast, there was a ceremony outside because it was the tenth anniversary of 9/11/2001. It was a chilly Sunday morning, but would be another nice day, although more cloudy. We caught a nice break with the weather this weekend. Kevin and I packed up and headed up a steep rock scramble to the summit of Mount Clinton. From there we would be above the tree line all day. From Mount Clinton, the AT runs along the Crawford Path, which is the original and most often-used path to the Mount Washington summit.

There were gradual climbs and cols between each of the mountains. Hiking above the tree line is spectacular, and not that difficult on these well-used trails. We passed Mount Eisenhower, Mount Franklin, and Mount Monroe on the way to Lakes of the Clouds Hut. At each of the summits, groups had hiked up to post an American flag to honor 9/11. We overtook Marybeth and Mindy at the summit of Mount Franklin. There were a lot of people out this day. The White Mountain trails can actually be very busy on weekends, and this was a very popular trail.

We arrived at the Lakes of the Clouds Hut before noon. The croo was busy closing it down for the winter. This hut does not stay open, since it is above the tree line, and too cold and windy. It is only 1.4 miles and 1,200 feet below the summit of Mount Washington. It is the largest and most popular hut, and holds 100 guests. There could have been 100 people gathered around the outside taking a break from their hikes. The Ammonoosuc Ravine Trail terminates here, and day-hikers continue on the Crawford Path to the summit.

After a snack, we headed out to the summit, into the clouds which had developed. We could see the summit better the previous day from 10 miles away than we could now from less than half a mile. We reached the summit and took some pictures at the summit sign, got something to eat at the cafeteria among the tourists, and arranged for a ride on the Cog Railway down to our car. It turned downright cold, requiring the heaviest shirts we had. Marybeth and Mindy rolled in. They decided to end their hike here and take a car down the auto road, and then catch a ride to Gorham, where their plane was parked. While we waited for the next train, the clouds came in and out, but we did get a glimpse down to Pinkham Notch and across to the Wildcat Mountains. The Wildcats were on my agenda for next year.

We took the train down and actually had a seat this year, rather than having to sit on the floor. We road walked the half-mile to our car, and drove all the way home that evening. We got to Hoboken around midnight, and I was home about two hours later. I was tired, but happy.

A few days later, the Occupy Wall Street movement began in New York City.

I felt like I accomplished a lot in the north this year, completing everything to Pinkham Notch. The scorecard for the north in 2011 was 101 miles in 10 days of hiking, including 40 miles and two days in Vermont, with the rest in New Hampshire. I was encouraged that I would finish New Hampshire easily next year, and be well into Maine. Oops, don't get cocky and taunt the mountains. They can taunt back.

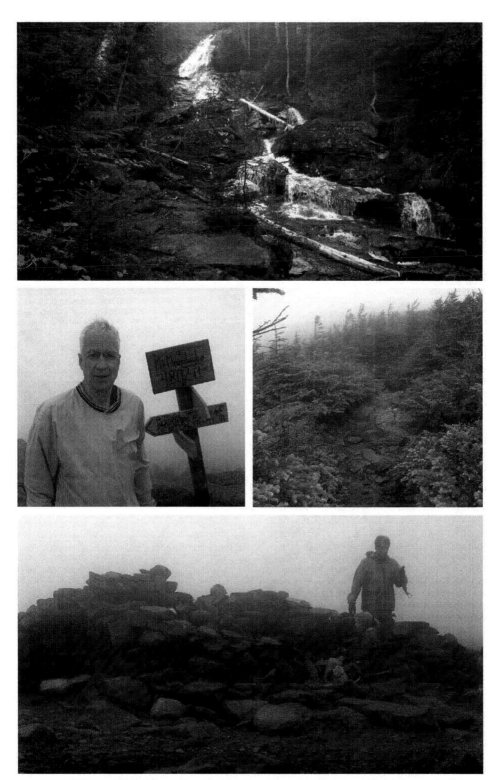

Top: Beaver Brook Cascades. Middle: Foggy on Mt Moosilauke; Trail through the scrub pines. Bottom: Keeping out of the chill on Moosilauke.

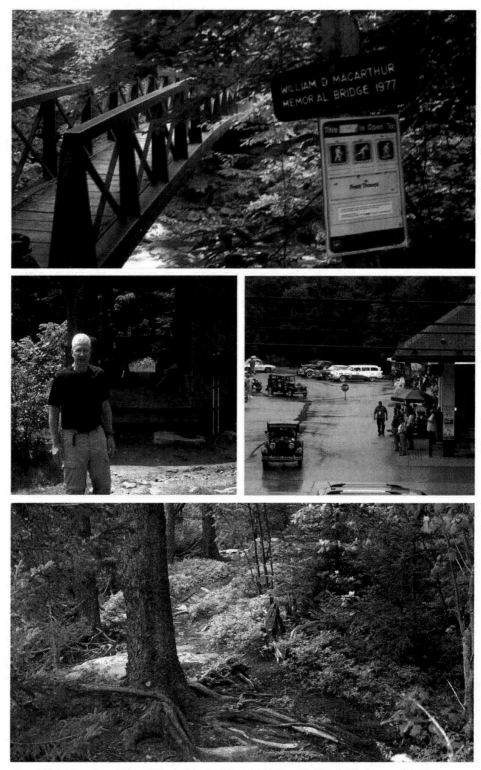

Top: Finishing Vermont at MacArthur Bridge. Middle: Goddard Shelter on Glastenberry Mountain; The Great Race finishing in Bennington. Bottom: Last day on Vermont trail.

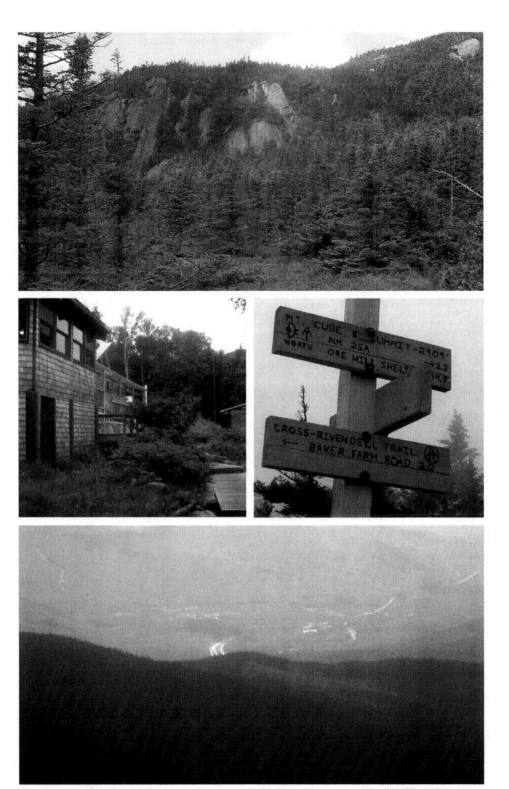

Top: Headwall of Kinsman Range. Middle: Lonesome Lake Hut; Mt. Cube summit in the fog. Bottom: Franconia Notch from South Kinsman.

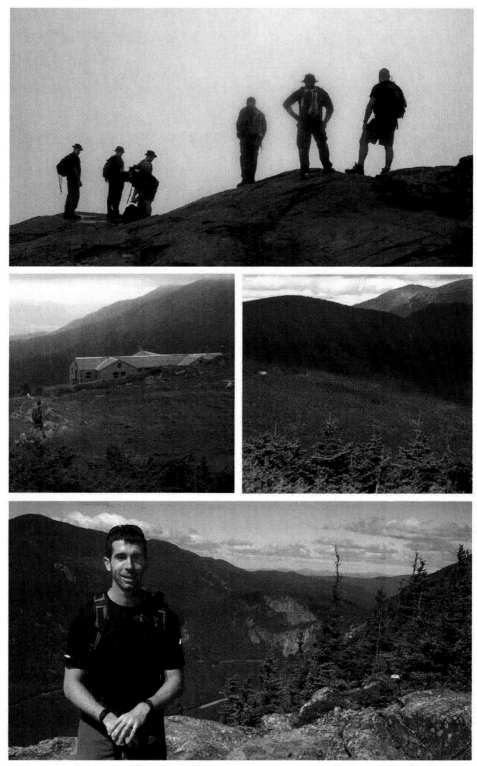

Top: Soldiering on Mt Lincoln. Middle: Kevin approaching Lakes of the Clouds Hut; Mizpah Spring Hut below the Presidentials. Bottom: Kevin on Webster Cliffs.

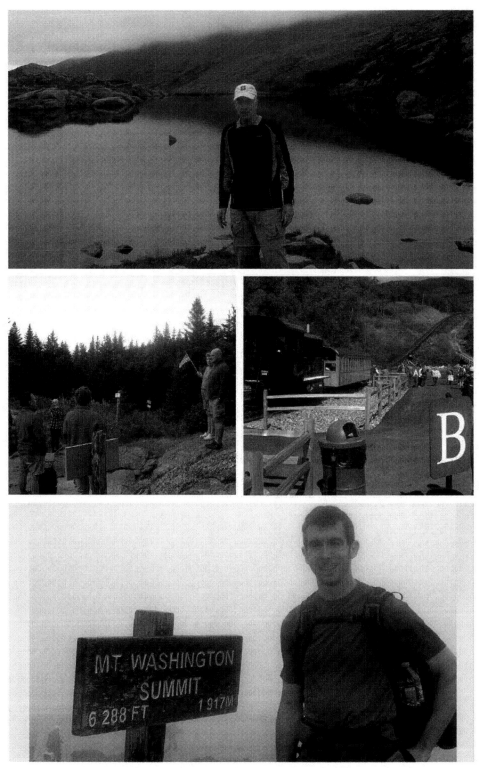

Top: Dennis at Lakes of the Clouds. Middle: 10th anniversary of 9/11 at Mizpah Spring Hut; Cog Railway. Bottom: Kevin at the Summit of Washington.

2011 – South - Virginia Conference

All I could think about in the winter of 2011 was getting back to the trail. Inexplicably, I would set my car's navigation system for Woods Hole on my way to work, and for Crawford Notch on my way home.

Beginning January 1, I became a disciplined eater, and stepped up my exercising. I was still doing triathlons, and was hoping to improve my times. I minimized pasta, potatoes and bread, but most importantly, ate nothing at the office that I did not bring. I did not eat one donut, bagel or goodie, which are plentiful during tax season. I gave up coffee, and started drinking green tea. "Treating yourself is going to the gym," a wise person told me. I politely avoided pizza nights that we have for the staff during tax season. I was at the gym five nights a week, and started going to a yoga class. I liked the yoga, mostly because it taught me how to stretch properly. I lost 25 pounds, and dropped down to less than when Virginia and I were married. Since I began hiking in 2002, I had lost 50 pounds. On the treadmill and track, I could break 29 minutes for a 5K. Could I keep the weight off? For the 2011 hiking season anyway, I became a lean, mean, mountain-hiking machine. I needed to be.

In January, Arizona congresswoman Gabrielle Giffords was one of 20 shot by an assassin. Six died. In March, an earthquake east of Japan triggered a tsunami, which in turn triggered a nuclear power plant meltdown, killing thousands. Prince William and Kate Middleton were married in April. Oprah aired her last show in May. NASA launched the final missions of three space shuttles, and ended the program in July.

In February, my aunt, the one whom Virginia and I had power of attorney for, passed away. She was 94. The last few years of her life were not easy for her. She had run out of money, but fortunately, she lived in a wonderful retirement home run by Mennonites, who accepted her limited income for her living there. She was in and out of hospice several times.

Over the winter, I was careful to sign up early for seven days of hiking at the AT trail conference in July. I wanted to make sure I got the hikes I wanted. The conference planners offered 200 miles of AT hikes from Interstate 77 near Bland, all the way down into Tennessee. I planned for about 70 miles, and chose sections that would help me find as many trailheads as possible, or that seemed remote, but not too far from the conference location in Emory, Virginia. I did not pick anything in Tennessee. I thought I could almost finish Virginia this year, which turned out to be correct.

I decided to head down to Woods Hole as soon as tax season was over, and planned four days with my new body. If I completed the planned sections, I would be all the way to Interstate 77. The logistics were working out perfectly.

I left home at 4:00 A.M. on April 29, and got down to Pearisburg around noon. Michael and Neville, from Woods Hole, arranged a shuttle for me, rather than doing it themselves. I met Don from Hoofers, his shuttle business. Don was a great guy and an early retiree from UPS. We met at an arranged intersection near town. Don said that there was a problem with the road out past Mountain Lake. It was washed out, and we could not get to my trailhead that way. Heavy thunderstorms a few days earlier had done a lot of damage in this area of Virginia, and there were seven confirmed tornados. The tornados were still evident a few months later on the way to the AT conference in Emory, Virginia, down near Abingdon and Damascus. Don said we could access the trailhead on the Salt Sulphur Turnpike from the back side of the mountain, but he did not know the roads.

It would be a long drive along Route 635 to get around, and then very poor dirt roads to get up the mountain to the top of the ridge. We both had SUVs. At one point, he asked me to go first, to make sure I wanted to do it. It was not easy, but we made it. It took another 45 minutes to drive back down and around to the John's Creek trailhead on the Forest Road 156, where Neville dropped me the year before to head south. Don would spend

2 ½ hours today to help me do a six-mile hike.

I was not hiking until 2:30 P.M. I crossed John's Creek on a 3-log bridge, and it was an easy hike to the War Spur Shelter. A few thru-hikers were there taking a break. I then began the strong climb up 2,000 feet to Lone Pine Peak. It was only another two miles, steep, but the trail was a nice footpath. I could handle it well, encouraging me that my weight loss had paid off. I did shed my heavy shirt, and was still sweating until I got to the top. A few more thru-hikers came by, but they don't usually want to stop. They just keep logging the miles. It was a nice, but cloudy day.

Once on top, it was an easy hike on a nice path across the ridge for three miles. Just short of my car, I came to Wind Rock. Beanpole, a 20-something good ol' boy, was there. He lamented that many of the thru-hikers he was with did not want to take the time to enjoy the views like this one. Looking down into the valley and across to Peter's Mountain, where I would be tomorrow, I could tell that the trees had only just begun to push their foliage. There was still a lot of brown.

I reached my car a few minutes after 5:00 P.M. The easy trail had made for a fast hike, despite the climb. I did not even take any breaks, except for water. It took me an hour to get to Woods Hole. I did not have time to shower before dinner, but I did not smell any worse than the other hikers.

It was busier at Woods Hole than the previous fall. Two tables were set up in the dining room. It was the middle of the thru-hiker season. Most all of the other guests tonight were thru-hikers. Book Smart was there. He was thru-hiking, but was staying a few days while his mother visited him. Sailor and Stretch were there for a few days. Both were recovering from injuries. I'm not sure what Sailor's issue was, but Stretch had blistered, infected feet. I helped him with some items from my first aid kit, and gave him a pair of my new wool socks, which he needed, since he had not been able to get to town. I gave him some cotton socks too, since he was always barefoot. It was nice to be at Woods Hole with some nice people with a common interest.

The next day, I planned to hike the 19.4-mile section north of Pearisburg. Michael agreed to get up early and be ready to leave at 6:00 A.M. Orange was appearing in the sky to the east, but the sun had not risen yet. I hated to not have Neville's breakfast, but I needed to get an early start. Michael and Neville were used to this. I dropped my car in Pearisburg, and Michael and I headed to McDonalds for breakfast; but then he knew of a diner that he wanted to patronize. That was fine with me, and I bought him breakfast there. He dropped me out at the nearer Route 635 trailhead at 7:45 A.M. I now had a gap of 2.1 miles that I would have to make up some time.

The long hike would be a climb up to the Peter's Mountain Ridge, and then 12 miles along the gentle ridgeline along the Virginia/West Virginia border, and then down to the New River in Pearisburg. Within the first mile, I reached the Pine Swamp Branch Shelter. Diehard was at the shelter, putting out the fire in the pit. It was chilly, and I was still wearing a wind shirt. Diehard said there were a few other hikers there, but they were long gone. He was older and said he moved much slower in the morning than the young bucks and does. The 1,300-foot climb up to Pine Swamp Ridge was not hard, since there was an easy path and many switchbacks. Once I was up on the ridge, it was nice to know I was done climbing for the day.

It was easy trail, alternating between some rocks and a cushioned pine needle path for the next five miles. The trail passed the junctions with the Allegheny and then Groundhog Trails. The Allegheny ran down to Route 635, followed by the Groundhog, which went north into West Virginia. I reached Symms Gap, and thru-hikers Nick and Kyle were there. They were from Indiana, and had just graduated from IU, as had Bethany and Kevin. They were even music majors. They were thru-hiking, since they were having difficulty finding jobs. There were open views into West Virginia, and winter views down into Stony Creek. The leaves had not pushed. It was bright, with a cloudy sky. I could still be in short sleeves.

There was more easy hiking on old roads along the crest to a power line, where there are always good views. At a stile over a fence into Rice Fields, I met three college kids out for a weekend class. They were part of a larger group that I would meet near the Rice Fields Shelter. The remainder of the local college kids, who all seemed very inexperienced, were struggling with their huge packs. This included the teacher, who was carrying a satellite phone. He could hardly walk. They were gathered on the north side of the ridge. They did not seem to want to go near the shelter across a stile in the woods. I believe they were spooked by the two bearded locals who seemed to be drinking. The group headed north after swapping cameras with me. I decided to move along, and left Rice Fields on another stile. It was well past 1:00 P.M., and I still had seven miles to go. I did not have my trail legs yet. The next four miles seemed long in the woods, though the trail continued to be easy. I was dreading the descent.

With 2 ½ miles to go, the descent came, and did not disappoint. It was steep, and my knees took a pounding. About two-thirds of the way down, two dads, who were part of another college group I would meet later, came by. One was having a hard time with a big pack. He wanted to know how far they had to go to Rice Fields, where this college group planned to camp. It was late afternoon now. I told them it was six miles. They had a big climb in front of them, and the one looked like a heart attack waiting to happen. This blowhard seemed like he would rather talk a good hike with me than actually work his way up the mountain. I wished them luck. Fifteen minutes later, the 15 college kids were resting with their teacher. They had not started climbing yet. This operation had not been well-planned.

The last two miles on rocky trail seemed to circle and take a very indirect route to the river. I was tired and annoyed. I think the purpose of this route was to avoid any contact or view of a large industrial site near the river. There were countless PUDs in between road and street crossings. I finally emerged from the woods and road walked to the bridge, climbed up the steps, and across the New River. The River was fast-moving, and very muddy from all the rain. It seemed like a long walk across the bridge and up a little hill on the road to my car in a parking lot of a closed home improvement store.

Exhausted, I drove back to Woods Hole. Neville was conducting a yoga session in the grass, which I joined to be a good sport. I was so stiff, I could not do anything. Neville had shifted me to another room. I showered, and then began to meet the large group that was there for this Saturday night. Neville would have dinner on the lawn and serve buffet-style to accommodate the 25 guests. The bunk house and the B&B were over-capacity. Several tented on the grounds.

There was a loud, boisterous group of 50-something AT section-hikers. Clair and Jenny, a mother-daughter team from Pearisburg, had taken my room. They were doing a 2-day hike from Pearisburg down to Dismal

Creek. I had done both those sections the previous fall. Clair's husband, who was in the US Foreign Service, would pick them up at Dismal Creek the next day. Jenny was a sweet girl. The family had lived all over the world, but had now settled. Why they picked Pearisburg seemed strange. Maybe they were hiding from something.

Not Far was there. She was an AT section-hiker from North Carolina. She was backpacking for about three weeks to recharge her batteries, she said. She thought I was a wimp for not camping, and was not shy to tell me so. She thought I should stretch myself more. She said there were some good and bad things that would happen on the trail, but they all made you a better person. I'm still not sure what I thought about her.

Gail was section-hiking north to south with her dog. Pickle was there with her dog, too, although her husband had arrived today to pick up her dog and to see Pickle. They slept in Pickle's tent. There was no room elsewhere. Pickle was a corporate attorney and at age 40, decided to leave her working career for a while to thru-hike the AT, which she did complete. Her husband took a picture of her, Book Smart, Stretch, Sailor, Gingersnap, Michael and Neville, which was on the cover of the AT magazine the following spring. Gingersnap was a 20-something, red-haired, outdoor dynamo, who was thru-hiking the AT, which was the tamest thing she had done.

The next morning, only about a dozen of us had breakfast in the B&B. I was heading south to meet Don. I parked my car at a small lot next to Kimberling Creek at Route 606. Don was right on time. It was a short drive along Route 42 to gravel Route 611 where the trail crossed. This would have been an easily biked shuttle, but I did not have it with me. At Route 42, there was a horrible dump at the trailhead, with smelly deer carcasses. I left quickly. The trail could not have been easier down 400 feet, and then 400 feet back up to Brushy Mountain.

A flat walk across the ridge got me to Jenny Knob Shelter. Three thru-hikers were just leaving, but I walked over. Smoke was there, sitting in his hammock, which was covered by a tarp. Smoke was hiking the trail in an unusual way. He was a weathered man in his 50s. He had worked as a welder. He only hiked every other day, and hung out at the shelters on his off days. He was not in a hurry, because he was essentially homeless.

He said he had an income that his sister would deposit for him as a credit at Walmart. Every month he would resupply. He was hiking up and down the trail, making sure to be in the south for the winter. This had been going on for four years now. Smoke had gotten his name because he smelled like smoke from the fire he always had going next to his hammock. He was pleasant, and very grateful for the apple and pack of crackers that I gave him.

I crossed Route 608 in Lickskillet Hollow after climbing down into the gap, and then back up to another ridge of Brushy Mountain. I ended the day by hiking a beautiful footbridge, crossing Kimberling Creek to my car. I completed the 9.6 miles in about 4 hours. It was pleasant and peaceful.

I drove over to a convenience store a mile away from the trailhead to get gas. I realized I could drive over to Dismal Creek Falls, which was close by. It was a beautiful spot. A man, who I presumed to be Clair's husband, was fly fishing below the falls. Clair had said this was his pastime. I drove back to Woods Hole.

Neville decided that she needed Sunday night off. Woods Hole had quieted down from the busy Saturday night. Neville liked the fact that I had a large vehicle and could transport a lot of people to a restaurant that she loved. About 10 of us traveled to the Palisades in Eggleston, Virginia, about half an hour away. The group included Book Smart, his mother, Pickle, Gingersnap, Michael, Neville and Melissa and David.

Melissa and David had just come in today. They were a couple who had met on the trail in Maine the previous summer. Both were attempting southbound thru-hikes. Melissa started with an enormous 70 pound pack. They hiked a brief time together, and a spark ignited. She was slow, and having great difficulty with her pack. David went on ahead, but after a few text messages, came back for her. David even carried her pack for a while. Eventually they got her pack pared down, and they continued together. An injury forced her to abandon her attempt, but David finished. They became a couple over the winter, and now David was back on the trail with Melissa, so that she could finish her hike to Springer. What love does...

Melissa was a psychologist. She said that research shows that a driver with a bumper sticker is 10 times more likely to be involved in a road rage incident. It does not matter what the bumper sticker says. Two bumper stickers means 100 times more likely. Etc.

We had a blast at Palisades. It was a quiet night there except for our group and a bluegrass band. Neville danced in between courses, and after dinner, we all square danced. Even me.

The next morning, we woke to the news that Osama Bin Laden had been killed by US Special Forces.

I packed up and headed south again. Don met me at that dump on Route 611 where I left my car. We traveled along Route 42, then up US 52, along Interstate 77, to the trailhead, and then over the interstate on Route 612. There did not seem to be any need to road walk half a mile down the hill to the trailhead. I entered the woods, crossed Kimberling Creek, and started climbing a steep 400-foot bump up to the trail junction for Helvey's Mill Shelter. I was breathing heavy and was a little lightheaded. I guess I'd had too much wine the night before.

Ron, a late-50s northbound thru-hiker came by. He was from Indiana. He said he hiked from sun up to sun down on his 25-mile days. He was no-nonsense. He did not have a map, and asked about the convenience store at Route 606. I told him it was a mile to the left of the trail. I said I would give him my map if he wanted to wait at the 611 trailhead. He was fast, and I was keeping up as we talked. I was feeling lightheaded again, and stopped to take a drink and that quickly, he was out of sight.

The rest of the hike was easy. Gail and her dog, whom I had met at Woods Hole, came by. Gail held her German shepherd close, almost like a blind person would. We chatted for a while. She planned to get to Damascus, Virginia. Damascus is a destination of choice for section-hikers. It is considered the best "trail town." I actually took no pictures this day. The trail was that unremarkable. I finished the 9 miles in less than 4 hours. As I relaxed at my car, Karen and Jessica popped out of the woods behind me. They were tall, lean, 50-something thru-hikers. Karen said, "Are you Dennis?" I said I was. They knew who I was because Don had picked them up as they hiked up the hill out of Bland. He delivered them to the trailhead. They split a beer I offered, and were off to the shelter. I wondered if Smoke was still there. Their plan included staying at Woods Hole a few days later.

I had completed my goal of getting all the way to Interstate 77. I was packed and ready to head home, but Michael had asked me that morning if I would give Sailor a ride north. I said, "No problem," and headed back to Woods Hole. It was early afternoon. Most of the hikers had moved on. Stretch was still there doing a project for Michael's new vineyard. His feet had still not healed.

Sailor and I headed out through Blacksburg to Interstate 81. Sailor was shy, and said very little on the trip. At the morning breakfasts, when Neville asked everyone to tell where they were from, Sailor would say "here and there." Sailor was in his 30s, and seemed to be in one of those transition stages in his life, and clearly did not like to talk about himself. He had multiple tattoos and ear, lip and nose rings. He texted his trail friends for most of the time he was in my car. They were at the HoJo in Daleville where I dropped him. He thanked me, and I was off.

After I dropped Sailor, I thought about all the people I had met, and my experiences on the trail. I was now in my tenth year. I really felt like I needed to start to write it all down. That would not happen until the following year, when it just started to come out. I made it to Staunton, where I crashed in a Super 8, and drove home the next morning.

In June, Kevin took charge of planning an outdoor adventure activity. He scheduled it for a weekend day, to introduce us to whitewater kayaking. Ben, Bethany, Kevin and I participated. Michelle was pregnant at the time, which eliminated her. It was a two-day course, but we only did the first day, due to a schedule conflict. We want to go back and finish, but have not done so. We learned the basics, which starts with how to exit the kayak when you flip over. It was fun.

I had been looking forward to the AT conference in July ever since I left the last one in Vermont two years earlier. July 1 finally came. I left at 5:00 A.M. for the 500-mile drive to Emory and Henry College in Emory, Virginia. I arrived in the late afternoon after a few needed naps on the road. Emory and Henry College had a beautiful campus in remote, southwest Virginia. The college had about 1,000 students. This conference had over 500 attendees, about twice the number that had been in Vermont. Emory and Henry College is a liberal arts college affiliated with the Methodist Church. They are the home of the WASPs (their athletic mascot) which seemed funny.

I registered and checked into my single room in a beautiful new dorm across the railroad tracks which divided campus. It took time to unload my car, and it was soon time for dinner in the campus dining hall. I met and got reacquainted with Julian, and we would often eat together, but would not be on any of the same hikes. My hikes were all set this time, and I planned to stay all seven days.

The next morning, the hike gathering place was a well-organized mob scene. Signs were posted with hike numbers where the hike leaders met their groups. Our hike had 20 people, and we divided into two groups. Our half would hike from Elk Garden to Massie Gap, and the other half would drive around to Massie Gap and hike to Elk Garden. It was only seven miles (plus another mile to get to the cars in Grayson Highlands), but there was a lot of driving. We would do a key swap, and I would drive someone else's car home. Paul and his wife Amanda were the hike leaders for our half of the group.

Our group included Rick from Lancaster, Pennsylvania. Rick and I hiked most of the day together. He was a great guy, and we were about the same age. He had recently retired and was at the conference with his wife, who did not hike. About five of the people were from North Carolina and all knew each other, but they were still friendly.

From Elk Garden at Virginia 600, the trail climbed up through a meadow, and paralleled the Virginia Highlands Horse Trail, which we abutted several times during the day. It was Saturday, July 2, so there were many riders out with their horses in the beautiful area. The pace was easy, but it was still hot and sticky. It was nice to talk to each person in turn throughout the day. Paul, the leader had thru-hiked the trail, but most of the others were section-hikers, mostly in their local area. All seemed to be members of their local hiking clubs. I had still not joined mine, and was beginning to feel bad about not having done so. There are 11 hiking clubs along the AT in Virginia, and they are very active in hiking and trail maintenance.

We reached the Mount Rodgers spur trail, which led half a mile to the treed summit. We all hiked up the easy climb to say we had been on top of the tallest mountain in Virginia. Since there was no view at the top, we just turned around and came down and had lunch at the Thomas Knob Shelter. A grandfather was there with his grandson. They were out for a long weekend. The grandfather was in his glory, teaching the teenager about hiking and camping. They were carefully looking at their maps to plan their next stop.

Soon after the shelter, we came to a grove of trees, where there were 30 or so wild ponies. It was the neatest thing to walk among and pet the animals, which included about four colts. They were very friendly, and tolerated us and ate apple pieces from our hands. We left the Lewis Fork Wilderness Area and were now in the Grayson Highlands. The rest of the day would be out in the open, in grassy meadows and rocky ridges. We climbed from Rhododendron Gap to Wilburn Ridge. We went through "Fatman Squeeze," a narrow tunnel in the rocks, and headed down a rocky section. A trail crew was there building rock steps to ultimately make the descent easier. We thanked them for the work that they do.

We continued on through the meadows of Grayson Highlands, where we turned off onto a side trail to get to the crowded parking lot. We met a Scout leader who seemed lost. It was a good thing she was on a practice hike for one she had planned for the next week with her group. We had a little trouble finding the car I was supposed to be driving back. I had not paid close enough attention to the make and model. Fortunately, Rick was on top of it. We had to pass Elk Garden to get back to campus, and our other group was still there, so I could drive my own car to campus.

I was always one of the first in the dining room for breakfast. Other early risers seemed to congregate at a counter, where we ate together for the rest of the week. The group included Ed from York and Rick from Lancaster. Ed was recently retired, and wanted badly to section-hike the trail. He had day-hiked all of Pennsylvania, but seemed overwhelmed by the logistics of day-hiking other sections. I considered myself lucky, being able to pay for shuttles and inexpensive motels. This can be an obstacle for many. I told Ed that using a bike to shuttle himself was a possibility in many places. I could have done more of this, had I owned a bike at the time.

Sunday's hike on July 3 was called moderate. It was actually a very easy one. There were only 7 of us, and I was one of only 2 men. The other man was John, a teacher, a 50-something hike leader from Lynchburg, Virginia. John was a double of a client of mine named John. I asked if he had any cousins in

Pennsylvania. He did not. Lynchburg is the largest city in the US without an interstate highway, he said. The rest of the group was older women, including the one who Karen, the hike leader, had "cut" from the 12-mile hike in Vermont two years earlier. The group also included Carolyn, the transplant recipient whom I had hiked with in Vermont. John and I hiked slowly out in front, but the rest of the group quickly fell behind, and we waited all day. I was surprisingly patient with this. John's wife Virginia (aka Jinx), was the sweep, usually the co-leader, who brings up the rear. She needed a lot of patience.

We started from Virginia 16 at the Mount Rodgers Headquarters and Visitors Center, where we waited as John and Carolyn shuttled a car. I did not drive today, since Carolyn preferred to, so I went with her. The visitor's center was interesting, and had a panorama of the area. A hundred yards from the visitor's center parking area, we arrived at the Partnership Shelter. It was a beautiful, new place, with running water and cold showers. Thru-hikers can call for pizza deliveries, which they can walk out to the road to get. It is rare that shelters are this close to the road. The shelter was apparently built so that thru-hikers would not stealth-camp at the headquarters building or use the rest rooms to wash up.

It was a long, slow day, but the older women were pleasant. They included Barb from Westfield, New Jersey, Virginia's home town, and Mary, a retired nutritionist who once was in charge of the food service for all the public schools in Chicago. At the end of the day, we again waited for John and Carolyn to retrieve her car, at the bridge over the South Fork of the Holston River. The slow hiker who Karen had "cut" from the hike said that she had enjoyed today's hike, and that she often had "trouble" with hike leaders.

Back on campus, I showered for dinner, and then after dinner, the evening's entertainment program was in Abingdon, 10 miles south on the interstate. The program was bluegrass, with apparently famous Wayne Henderson picking his guitar, and Jeff Little, a honky-tonk piano player. They were great. This small area of southwest Virginia is the home of bluegrass, and many bluegrass stars come from here and along US 58, the "Crooked Road."

Monday morning, I was signed up for a short (6.5 mile) but tough little hike up north. There would be 10 of us. We had four cars, so the leaders decided to hike together. We dropped two cars at the Route 42 trailhead in Rich Valley. The area also included Poor Valley. The distinction was the quality of the soil on different sides of the mountain range caused by some geological feature.

The group included Sheryl from Tennessee. I had hiked with Sheryl in Vermont. She loved the conferences and the trail, and got away whenever she could. She was, however, frank to say that her husband and three young adult sons did not give her a lot of support with her passion. The group also included Wayne and Shirley and their one-year-old son Bryce, from the Poconos in Pennsylvania. Wayne grew up near Allentown, and had thru-hiked the AT and was a Boy Scout in his youth. His boyhood friend Joe, who now lived in North Carolina was on the hike, too. Shirley carried Bryce on her back, and Wayne carried all the gear. Wayne and Shirley were experienced in all facets of hiking and camping, so bringing their son along was no big deal. They were actually tenting at the conference, and preparing all their meals. Their van had blown an engine about 100 miles from Emory. Undaunted, they left it at a garage, and some good Samaritans drove them the rest of the way with all their gear. They would get a new engine during the conference.

The hike leader was Steve, a soft-spoken guy from Virginia. The co-leader was more outgoing. She had a huge pack, perhaps to carry the emergency supplies for the group. The group also included Richard, a 67-year-old former military man, who also taught scuba diving as an adjunct professor at Old Dominion. Richard was struggling with knee problems. Kim, a member of the ATC staff from Harpers Ferry, was along as well.

We shuttled out to remote Forest Service Road 222, in Poor Valley. After an easy first mile to Lick Creek, we climbed a tough 800 feet on switchbacks to the summit of Lynn Camp Mountain. It was just as steep going down the other side. Shirley had no difficulty with Bryce on her back. He was good, and never seemed to cry throughout the day. I was amazed he could sleep in the pack. From Lynn Camp Creek we were climbing again, on an easier grade this time. We had lunch at the Knot Maul Shelter. We still had a little climbing to do until a somewhat steep descent to the picnic area at the trailhead at Route 42.

The next day, I was on a hike that would be contiguous to the north.

Our group of 8 drove in 2 cars to the Forest Service Road 222 trailhead. The hike leaders were a family from Winchester, Virginia, near Front Royal. The family included Lee, who acted as sweep, his self-described high-maintenance wife Terri, and their 19-year-old son, Cody. Lee said Cody would lead out and hike as fast as the group could. I needed to stretch my legs after some slower hiking days, and it sounded like a challenge.

Cody took off up the trail, followed by his mother. He set a blistering pace uphill, and his mother soon fell by the wayside. I was determined, and with my new body, kept up with Cody for the first mile. I was gasping. We had buried the rest of the group, and Cody did slow down some, just so I could stay with him. He was a geology major, having just finished his freshman year at James Madison U. He would humor the rest of us by putting rocks that he found interesting in his pack. He was a nice kid.

The two of us hiked for over an hour or so together, then he stopped to wait for the others as we emerged out of the woods to the open, grassy crest of Chestnut Ridge. I felt good, but was glad to stop. It was fifteen minutes before the next person emerged. It was Heidi, aka, Twig. Heidi said, "Wow, you guys really booked it!" Heidi was a 50-something runner and horse woman, who loved the outdoors. Her husband, a podiatrist, did not share her passion. She was originally from the Pittsburgh area, but they had settled near Washington, DC. They had compromised as to where to live, since he liked the city and she liked the more rural areas. They settled in horse country, and she rode her horse every day. She had become part of the early breakfast group at the counter. Fifteen more minutes went by until Richard, who was still having knee issues, and Lee, came out of the woods.

The steepest climbing was over, but it would be up another 4-mile gradual up to the Chestnut Knob Shelter. I decided I had proved my point about what a fast hiker I could be, and fell into the middle of the group. With Cody out front and Richard and Lee bringing up the rear, we did spread out during the day. It took another two hours to get to the shelter, where we had lunch.

We had lunch inside the enclosed stone shelter, since it had a table in it, along with some wide bunks. Terri was a show describing herself, and how she used to hate hiking, but was into it now. She wanted to keep moving all the time. She was the business person and bookkeeper for a construction business that Lee had. She and Twig both owned horses, so they had a common interest. I had lunch with Walt, a recently retired neurologist from Philadelphia. He said I was crazy to be doing triathlons at my age. He said I should do much more moderate exercise.

After lunch, we started the mile and a half descent to Walker Gap. About halfway down we met some in the group from the conference who we planned to key swap with. A couple said, "Who has the Acura?" I said me, and I swapped my key for their Suburban's key. Both our groups were spread out. We arrived at Walker Gap and waited for Richard and Lee, who did not show up for a long time. When they finally did get there half an hour later, Lee said that the hike leader for the other group would not let him leave the area until she was sure that our key swaps had occurred. It had, but she wanted to be sure. She had passed me after the swap, and I should have told her. I was too casual about it. Of course, she was right. If it had not occurred, there would have been problems, and a lot of driving and confusion to fix the problem.

While waiting at Walker Gap, we met an AT section-hiker who was hiking all the sections by doing in and outs, retracing his steps in every section. Wow, that would not be me.

The last five miles were a slow, gradual climb to Virginia 623. It was rocky and difficult. Our group spread out, but Cody would wait every hour or so for everyone to catch up. Twig and I solved some of the problems of the world. She did medical billing for her husband, which is a challenge to get paid for the services that are provided. Insurance companies are quick to reject claims, but she sounded like a bull dog to make sure they always got paid. I think it is hard to be a medical service provider, always having to persist with governments and insurance companies to get paid for what you do. I was familiar with some of this, having taken care of my aunt's affairs. It was shocking to me to see how little some medical professionals received for the services they provided to her.

I spent some time talking to Maryann from Georgia. She was a delightful woman in her 60s, and in marvelous shape. The day was getting long, and our group had lost track of how far along we were. We stopped at a lookout to the north towards Burke's Garden. Burke's Garden got its name when James Burke, a member of a survey crew in 1748, discarded some potato peels. A year later, the crew returned to find potatoes growing. As a joke, it became Burke's Garden, and the name stuck.

Burke's Garden was a beautiful valley, about 9 miles long, and 4 miles wide. It is surrounded by mountains on all four sides. In the late 19th Century, agents for the Vanderbilt family contacted local farmers about selling land so the family could build a large estate there. Nobody wanted to sell, and the Vanderbilts instead constructed the Biltmore Estate near Asheville, North Carolina.

As we waited for Lee and Richard, we pondered how far we had to go, and figured it could be another hour or so. As it turned out, we were only five minutes to the cars. I had a little trouble operating the Suburban, and it was a 30-minute drive along dirt and winding Virginia 623 just to get back to Route 42. We backtracked a little to Bland for ice cream, picked up I-77 to I-81, and back to campus. It was a long day.

That evening after dinner, I promised Richard I would take him to buy a knee brace. Virginia had purchased a simple one for me at a drug store, and it had helped. He seemed unsure, but humored me. Later in the week, he thanked me immensely.

The next day's hike would be my longest of the conference. Five of us would start at Interstate 81, and cross over to the north and hike 12 miles up to Route 42. Another five would hike in the opposite direction, and the leaders would do a key swap when we met on the trail. I did not have to drive. Our leader was Mark Wenger, one of my early morning breakfast buddies. Mark was planning to complete a section-hike of the AT later that summer. He had most of Maine to finish. He was the head of maintenance and construction at Colonial Williamsburg, and also had a construction business. He was an animal when it came to hiking and camping. Our co-leader was also Mark, a young 30-something, who worked for the Tennessee Department of Parks. The other two on the hike were "old guys." One just had sneakers. I thought to myself it would be a long day. Mark was careful to explain at the hike gathering place that there would be no possible outs on the hike. Once we got to the middle, it would be the point of no return.

Never judge a book by its cover.

George was 73, and a retired Methodist/Unitarian minister. But, he had hiked every day for most of his life, and even though he was a little slow up the hills (he said it happened at around 70), he was still strong and vibrant. Mark seemed to know him or of him, because George was a long-tenured trail maintainer and ATC volunteer in southwest Virginia along the crooked road. Mark showed him a lot of respect. Vance was in his late 60s, and his sneakers were well-worn from running half-marathons. He was never more than 10 feet behind young Mark for the entire day. Vance had retired a few months before from his job as a deputy sheriff in Kentucky. He became a sheriff at age 45, after 20 years as an accountant. Mark Wenger was the sweep, and hiked in the back with George. That put me in the middle.

We crossed Interstate 81 for the last of four times on the trail, and hiked through some open fields, where cows eyed us suspiciously. Watch out for those "meadow muffins," young Mark would say. We had a little 400-foot bump on easy trail to the site of the Davis Path Shelter, which had been taken down because of misuse by local teens. That is why shelters are not often near roads. The platform remained. Mark Wenger decided to take a long break, even though we were only an hour into the hike. He gave us a long narrative about the shelter, and what the ATC might do with it, and a general history of the area. It was interesting, but I thought we should be moving. The following spring, I would pick up my ATC magazine and learn that Mark Wenger was the new executive director of the ATC. His passion for the trail was right in front of me, but I was in too much of a hurry to absorb it.

We had two serious 400-foot climbs on our way to Crawfish Valley. George would fall behind, but quickly catch up. We met our opposite group, and all had lunch together while the leaders swapped car keys at the junction with the Crawfish-Channel Rock Trail. We still had another 800 feet climb over the next two miles to get to the wooded summit of Big Walker Mountain. When we got to Virginia 610, Mark thought his car should be there, but we actually had another two miles to go. The sky became threatening. I stopped to capture some pictures out in the open fields, and then had to hustle to catch up to the others, who were sprinting to the car. We made it to the picnic area at the Route 42 trailhead just as the clouds opened up.

The rain lasted half an hour, but during the storm, we made a wrong turn going by Hungry Mother State Park. The legend said that Native Americans destroyed several early settlements along the New River. Molly Marley and her small child were among the survivors taken to the raider's base. They eventually escaped, wandering through the wilderness, eating berries. Molly finally collapsed, and her child wandered down a creek until finding help. The only words the child could utter were "Hungry Mother." A search party found Molly dead at the base of what is now Molly's Knob.

That night after dinner, a rock band played in the campus auditorium. The band was OK, but the antics of the ATC conference attendees on the dance floor were the better entertainment. There must have been a wine reception I had not heard about.

Thursday morning, I was signed up for a hike back to the south, near Damascus. We would hike the 10 miles from Elk Garden to Creek Junction on US 58, the Crooked Road. I was learning why they call it that. Just check any map. There were 14 of us, and we decided to all hike together. We took four cars. I left my car at Creek Junction, and then the rest of us proceeded to Elk Garden, along Virginia 600.

Our leader was Jenni from Richmond, and our co-leader was Mary-ann from New Hampshire, who spoke with a heavy German accent. Other women were Karen, 62, a teacher from north of Baltimore, and Corina, 50, from Roanoke, but originally from the Dominican Republic, who came to this country as a college tennis player. Cindy from Texas was in her 40s, and said she had been a member of the ATC for 18 years, but had never hiked before this week.

The hike also included Ed from York, Andy from the DC area, Hank (50-something retired military) from Connecticut, and Ludwig, a 73-year-old retired New York Port Authority worker from Queens who had been retired 18 years, but hiked all year long. Rounding out the group were Bill from Scranton, who would soon celebrate his 50th wedding anniversary, another Bill from Allentown, Pennsylvania (the one person I would not get to talk to), Ed's friend Holt, a 50-something audit manager from Raleigh, North Carolina, and Craig from Rutherford, New Jersey, who would often bring up the rear with Cindy and the sweep, Jenni. Jenni and Maryann stayed near the back and told those of us who wanted to go ahead to do so, but to wait at designated places for the whole group to catch up.

The group was spread out over long areas. Hank was a rabbit, and Ed and Holt and others tried to keep up with him; but then would complain about how fast he was going. I just let them go, and hiked in the middle and talked to each person during the day to hear their life and hiking story. It was fun. From Elk Garden, we were climbing immediately, strong at first, and then more gradually up Whitetop Mountain. Whitetop Mountain was a completely open summit, with the distinctive feature of Buzzard Rock at 5,080 feet. We all waited there for the entire group to arrive, which took a while.

Hank was off like a racehorse, down a steep 1,900 feet over two miles to Virginia 601. There were a lot of switchbacks on nicely built trail, which did not make it difficult. We all had lunch at Virginia 601. It was getting to the point that Hank would want to leave as soon as the last of the group arrived at the designated stop point, which did not seem right, but the leaders did not seem to mind. They just continued at their own pace with Craig and Cindy. The whining continued about Hank's pace. The last designated stop was Lost Mountain Shelter. We had about three miles to go.

Ed and Holt asked Maryann and Jenni if four of us, including me, could go on ahead, so that I could shuttle them back to retrieve the cars. Ed had driven, but Holt and Hank could drive Jenni and Maryann's cars back. They liked the idea. Hank was off again, and I accepted the challenge of keeping up with him. Hank was single. He had hiked a lot of the trail, but never shuttled. He would always hike in and out, retracing his steps. He would "tag" a spot where he would turn around, and make sure that he would "tag" it on his next in and out from the opposite direction, so that he covered every inch of the trail. He also "baptized" himself at the rock spring areas to mentally thank those who had built it. He did some strange things. I rather enjoyed him, and could keep up with him, too.

We found Andy floundering around in the woods. He had missed the shelter, and had gotten ahead of everyone and left the trail to try to bushwhack across Whitetop Laurel Creek to get to the Virginia Creeper Trail, since he knew our cars were there. You should never leave the AT, even if you think you know where you are going. As we waited for Andy to climb up the embankment, Holt and Ed arrived, and I let Hank go ahead and finished with Ed and Holt across the 540-footlong Luther Hassinger Memorial Bridge. We were now on the Virginia Creeper Trail, which runs along the AT for about half a mile.

The Virginia Creeper Trail is an old railroad bed, now a well-used bike rail trail that runs 34 miles from the North Carolina border to Abingdon, Virginia through Damascus. People often shuttle bikes up to Whitetop Mountain to bike downhill on the Creeper to Damascus, and maybe on to Abingdon. We left the Creeper to get to our cars at the parking lot along Whitetop Laurel Creek under the bridge. We retrieved the cars, and were back about the time the last of our group finished the hike. We all stopped in Damascus for ice cream.

That night, I ran into Shirley and her baby Bryce outside of a Vermont trail talk I planned to attend. She and Wayne still did not know if their van would be ready. They had to get a new engine. I knew they were from the Poconos, and offered to help in any way I could. As it turned out, we decided we were going to be on the same hike the next day.

The dorms were closing on Friday, so we had to pack up before our hike. My hike today would be contiguous to the hike on Thursday, to the south from Creek Junction to Straight Branch. Both trailheads were on the crooked road, so it was an easy shuttle. In addition to Wayne, Shirley and Bryce and their friend Joe, the group included Ed from York and Jay from Ohio, who was 68 and retired military. Steve from Lynchburg, Virginia was the leader, and Mark from Tennessee Parks Department was the co-leader. Kathy from Connecticut rounded out the group.

I spent the first part of the day talking to Kathy from Connecticut. Kathy had section-hiked all of the trail in the north. She was still working on Virginia and south. She had started with a group of women who had a passion for it, but it became too intense for Kathy during her working years. She was getting back into it. Like me, she had done very little camping, and I was intrigued to know that she had hiked all of Maine without camping. She said even the 100-mile wilderness could be done by staying at places that would shuttle you in and out of logging roads. I asked about a 30-mile section north of Gorham, and she said there were side trails that you could go in and out on. I was beginning to wonder if I could hike the entire trail without sleeping on the ground. Few, if any, had done it. She gave me her email address to contact her with any questions.

Our group stayed together all day, which was nice. It was a chance to talk to everyone. We started out along the Virginia Creeper Trail, but soon left it for the woods. We would be hiking between the Creeper and the Crooked Road all day. At times, the Creeper Trail was visible through the trees, with the bikes speeding by. The first part, however, was more remote, and headed up to Straight Mountain, climbing gradually. The path had plenty of rocks and PUDs. Shirley was sure-footed with Bryce on her back.

At Bear Tree Gap there was a large group of teens from a church group. We had seen their van at the trailhead. They would be camping out this night. There were some easier sections too, with rhododendron tunnels with white blossoms everywhere. We had lunch at the summit of Straight Mountain when we knew we were done climbing. From the summit of Straight Mountain, there were a few steep descents. The last two miles were right next to the Creeper, and level along the Whitetop Laurel Creek. It was only eight miles, so it was a short day. We headed back to campus.

We could shower at the gym before beginning our drive home. Wayne found out that his van would be ready. I offered to take him the 100 miles north to get it because it was on my way. I felt bad that I had my bike, because I could not fit Shirley, Bryce and all their gear, too. Wayne would have to drive back for them, so they decided they would go visit Joe in North Carolina that night, and drive home the next day. It sounded like a lot of driving to me, but that is what they decided.

After dropping Wayne off and making sure his van was running properly, I started the drive home. I did not make it very far, as I was exhausted from the week. I was encouraged though, since I really felt like I was making good progress this year. At the conference, I was somewhat ahead (mileage wise) of many of the section-hikers, and many were envious of my day-hiking strategy. Ed, Holt, Hank and others wanted to know how I did certain areas and found shuttles. I could really see that finishing the trail without camping was possible.

During the week, they announced that the 2013 conference would be held in North Carolina, near the Smoky Mountains. Again it appeared that I would be lucky when it came to logistics, since I expected to be down in that area by then. As usual, though, I was studying the maps of the Smokys and there were daunting 30-mile sections with no road crossings. How could that section be hiked without sleeping on the ground? Oops, maybe I will be camping after all.

A few weeks later, I entered my seventh triathlon. It was the New Jersey State again. I came in 940th out of 1,366 in the race, and beat my previous year time by 4 minutes. Later in September I entered a race at the New Jersey shore, and did my first ocean swim in a triathlon.

After spending August and September in New Hampshire, I did one more trip south. I had sections to fill in on the way to Damascus. I could almost get there. I took the long drive down to Bland, Virginia. I arrived in the late afternoon of October 13, and checked into the Big Walker Motel. It was the only place within 20 miles of the trailheads I wanted to get to. I checked out the trailhead at the top of the hill from Bland on Route 52, near where the trail crosses Interstate 77.

I met Aqua there the next morning. I was lucky to find Aqua, and he would help me the next four days. I would be covering a wide area, so he did quite a bit of driving. Aqua was the current life partner of Ram Bunny, who ran a hostel on and off down near where the AT crosses Interstate 81 near Groseclose. He was very dependable.

I had planned to hike a 15.5-mile section. It rained quite a bit overnight, and I slept very little, thinking about the long day. It was very remote, and the trailhead at Virginia 623 was a long, winding road up to Garden Mountain, where I had hiked at the conference. I decided to cut the hike short. It was dark when I met Aqua, and it did not take too long to get to my revised trailhead. It was still dark, so he and I hung around a few minutes until daybreak. I was hiking at 7:30 A.M. I started on Virginia 615, which was not too far from Virginia 42. I told Aqua of my revised plan, and that I would meet him there the next morning at eight thirty.

I had shortened my hike to only seven miles. I realized it was still dark when I entered the woods. I got to a sign and put on my headlamp, which I had never actually used hiking before.

I would climb up almost 500 feet up to Brushy Mountain, but the trail was not difficult. The trail was thick with rhododendron. The white blossoms were gone. Daylight finally arrived, and it was actually turning into a nice day. There was a gradual down off the mountain, and then a slight bump up. The trail became very easy along some old woods roads. There were nice views down into the Bastian Valley on the north side of the mountain. The leaves were a bright, beautiful color. For the last three miles, the trail paralleled a forest service road, and I could hear a few cars above. At the end I was on a dirt and gravel road along a power line. On the way, the views were north along the I-77 corridor. It was only 10:30 A.M. when I reached my car. I felt silly when I called Virginia, and was mad at myself for being a wimp again. I ate an early lunch, and went back to the motel to take a nap.

There were slim pickings for restaurants around the Bland area. I had gone north to Bastian the night before for an okay Italian place in a strip mall. For dinner on Friday night, I drove down to Wytheville. Even though Bland is the county seat, it is a one-traffic-light town that does not seem to have much to offer to thru-hikers other than a slice of pizza and some supplies. It is a 3-mile road walk to get there down the hill to town. I believe a trail relocation is planned to avoid the road walk that I did not do. I drove it about three times.

The next morning, I checked out of the Big Walker and drove up to the Virginia 615 trailhead, where Aqua had dropped me the day before. We headed down Route 42, and took the very long, winding drive on dirt and rough Virginia 623. It was over Brushy Mountain, down over Hunting Camp Creek and up to the ridge of Garden Mountain. The 10 miles took 30 minutes. It was no problem in Aqua's truck. It would not be a bikeable road.

From the top of the ridge, it was downhill over four miles to Jenkins Shelter. The down of 1,500 feet was rocky, but with the elevation loss, not all that difficult. On the way, I met a local bow hunter. He was a large man, but pleasant. Even though he was on the trail, he said he often bushwhacked in the area because he was so familiar with it. Two southbound thru-hikers came by. About half a mile from the trail, I met two late-50-something guys. One was struggling. Both were nearing military retirement, and were out for a weekend camping trip. The struggling one had a recent hip replacement. His doctors had given him the OK to hike. He was a former Special Forces officer. The other was Evan from North Carolina. He actually had a cabin near the trail in North Carolina, and offered that I could use it when I was down there. The offer seemed genuine. We exchanged email addresses and corresponded once. Evan said I would see his son at the shelter. I would have continued with them, but they did not seem to want me to, since they were so slow. I went ahead.

Evan's son was at the shelter. He was a nice kid who had just graduated from college, and was leaving for the military within a few weeks. Evan and his friend struggled in. They cut their hike short. It was just too hard for the guy with the hip replacement.

There was an easy climb up to Brushy Mountain, and then down to my car. From the shelter, it was very easy. There was a beautiful, long bridge at the trailhead over Laurel Creek which had just been completed by the USFS in 2010. I was at my car early in the afternoon. I was still mad at myself for not doing both those sections in one day. I headed down to a new motel in Marian, Virginia. I was glad to be near civilization. Marion was not a metro area, but it offered more than Bland. At least they had a sports bar.

I had a long 15-mile hike planned for the next day, so I asked Aqua to meet me early at the trailhead at the bridge over the South Fork of the Holston River at Virginia 670 near Sugar Grove. He would drive me around to the Fox Creek trailhead on Virginia 603 past the Fairwood Livery. There were many horse trailers and horses in the corral. It was a busy Sunday. I was back in the area of the Virginia Highlands Horse Trail, which I would cross a few times today.

From Virginia 603 I would climb up 800 feet over two miles to Iron Mountain. There was a beautiful bridge over Fox Creek at first, and then a fence starting up the mountain to mark the trail. At the top of the mountain, there were a lot of leaves down. There is a distinctive *whoosh* of leaves as you hike along. Hiking down the mountain, the trail continued to be easy on well-maintained trail. The signs were some of the nicest that I had seen. They were frequent at all the trail junctions. After the 3-mile, 1,300-foot descent, the trail was level all the way to Dickey Gap. It was very pretty in the area around Comers Creek, and still above 3,000 feet. I passed two younger couples. One was out for a long weekend. The other couple was section-hiking.

At Dickey Gap at Virginia 650, the trailhead is within a hundred feet of Virginia 16. There were beautiful split-rail fences at the intersection. Elizabeth was there next to her small car. She was about my age, and a trail maintainer from Damascus. She was early, and waiting for a group of youth to assist her on a minor project to correct an erosion issue. I sat and had my lunch as she waited. She had been to the AT conference, and was very knowledgeable about the AT in the area. I had seven miles to go, so did not linger any longer. I hope the youth showed up for her.

I had a little more climbing, but less than 500 feet. On the way, I saw some orange flags where Elizabeth and the kids would do their work. It did not seem like there would be much to do. Virginia has the best trail maintenance. The trail continued to be very easy, and I crossed over High Point, and then down to the Trimpi Shelter.

I sat at the junction for a minute, trying to decide whether or not to hike down to the shelter, when Gerry came along with his two young sons. They were out for a brief hike, and headed to the shelter, so I decided to join them. Gerry's church near Sugar Grove held dinners on Saturday nights for thru-hikers at the height of the season. The boys loved playing in and around the stone shelter.

I left them at the shelter. It was more easy hiking for another mile, where the trail emerged into a pasture with cows. A bull was sitting right in the middle of the trail, so I gave him some space. I crossed a road where Gerry had parked, and then across the 120-foot bridge over the South Fork of the Holston to my car. Aqua said Ram Bunny was working at the sports bar again tonight, but I never met her.

The next morning, I checked out of the motel and took the short drive to a barn restaurant at Groseclose, where the trail crosses Interstate 81. Aqua was waiting. He would take me up to Mount Rodgers HQ, and I would hike the 11.5 miles back to the restaurant. From the road, there was easy hiking to the crest of Brushy Mountain. From there, I was up and down a few serious PUDs, which did not look that bad on the elevation profile, and down to a saddle between Brushy and Locust mountains. The climb up Locust was steep, but only about 400 feet, and then down to a dirt road crossing.

I had a snack at the road, and the first of two young couples came by. They were section-hiking, and headed to Damascus. I then started up to Glade Mountain. I was getting a little tired of all the ups and downs. Enough already. I had lunch at the Chatfield Memorial Shelter after descending off Glade Mountain. On the way, there were some views down into the Great Valley along Interstate 81.

From the shelter, it was downhill and level at the end. There were several road crossings, including one at the Settler's Museum, which was closed on Mondays. I talked to two southbound thru-hikers along the way. One had fishing poles sticking out of his pack. The other had a plastic whiffle ball bat. He claimed he would use it to ward off bears. He had carried it all the way from Katahdin. There were open areas down to the valley with plenty of views. I could start to hear the trucks on I-81. I met a woman from Lancaster, Pennsylvania, who often visited a family homestead in the area, and came out on the trail most days. I finally reached my car, tired but happy.

Inexplicably, I would gain weight on hiking weekends and when I got home, I was up 10 pounds since the start of the hiking season. By the end of the year, the 10 became 15. No problem, I thought, I would just lose it again over tax season, and maybe take it to another level. I figured I had the blueprint. *Oops.*

Nonetheless, I had kicked butt on the trail this year. I hiked 15 days in the south and totaled 149 miles. For the year, I had hiked 25 days, for a total of 250 miles. By 60 miles, this had been my biggest year.

I had now hiked 1,376 miles and was over 63%. I had not finished Virginia, but that was in sight. At the rate I was going, I could finish in three more years. *Oops.*

On October 4, I became Pop-Pop, when John Robert Heller was born to Ben and Michelle. In November, Virginia and I sold our house overlooking the Delaware River and bought a condo back in Allentown, six blocks from my office. It was a good move for us in all respects.

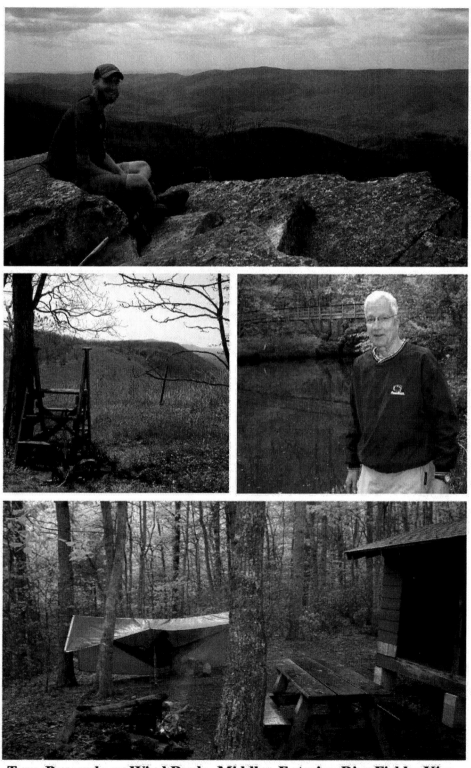

Top: Beanpole on Wind Rock. Middle: Entering Rice Fields; Kimberling Creek. Bottom: "Smoke" chillin' under his tarp.

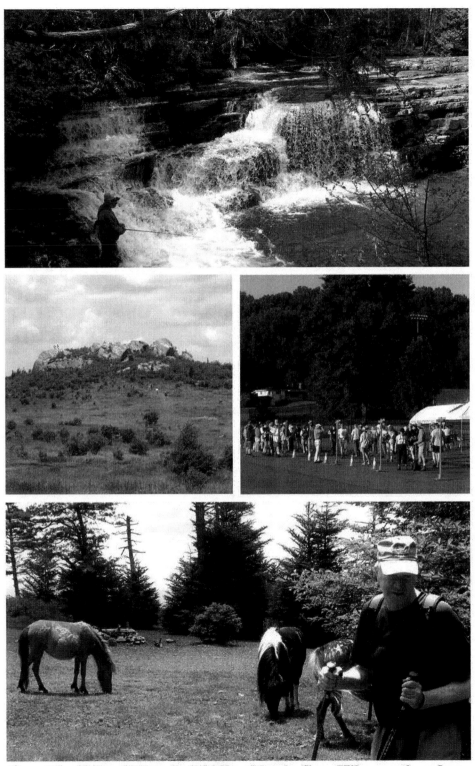

**Top: The Falls of Dismal. Middle: Massie Gap; Hike meeting place.
Bottom: Wild ponies in the Grayson Highlands.**

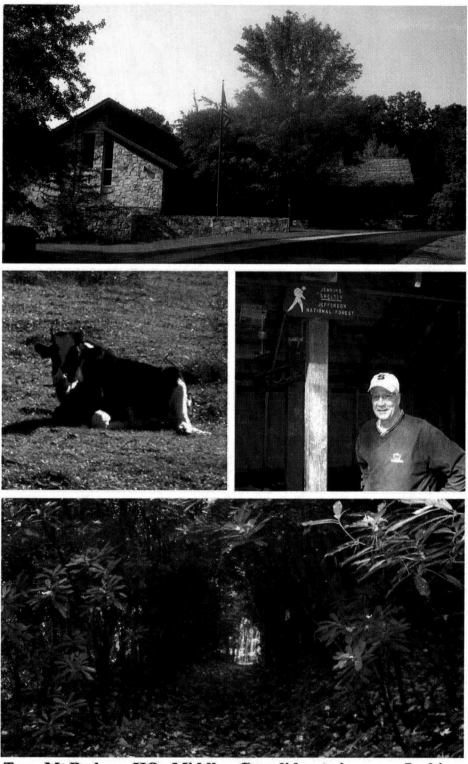

Top: Mt Rodgers HQ. Middle: Cow did not give way; Jenkins Shelter. Bottom: Rhododendron tunnel.

2012 – North - The Mahoosucs

On April 1, a well-known Boston biotech entrepreneur (67) fell on Mount Washington into Tuckerman's Ravine while hiking the Crawford Path with his son. His body was not recovered until late May. It was too dangerous to attempt a recovery. The White Mountains had claimed another.

I was psyched to get back to hiking in the North. I had completed everything to Pinkham Notch. From there, it was a tough 20-mile section to Gorham, and then a 30-mile section, without any road crossings, across the New Hampshire/Maine border to Grafton Notch. I studied the maps endlessly, and developed a plan. Six days, I figured. I made a reservation at the Highland Center for Wednesday, June 28. That would be my jumping-off point. Then I would hike up to the Carter Notch Hut on Thursday, and hike out to Gorham on Friday. I would hike the 30 miles north of Gorham over 4 days, using side trails to access the trail. Dan from Trail Angels would shuttle me. It was a good plan. *Oops.*

It was a long, tiring drive to the Highland Center. It was nice to be back there again. I had dinner with an early retired military pilot, Craig, who had started a southbound thru-hike in late May. A pilot friend of his was just joining him for four days of hiking from Crawford Notch to Franconia Notch to celebrate Craig's 50th birthday. Craig was hiking the AT barefoot, and his trail name was 2Go Barefoot. Craig and his buddy Jack were from Minnesota. Craig was working for the FAA now, but somehow could get the time off. Jack was a big guy, unlike Craig, who was trim and had been hiking for a month. Jack was a little nervous about what he had gotten himself into.

I did not say much. Who was I to give advice? It took me three attempts over two years to finish that section.

The next morning I got up early, but was not in a hurry. The hike was only six miles, and there was no reason to get to the Carter Notch Hut too early. I had a leisurely breakfast, but tried not to eat too much, trying to behave. I drove around to Gorham and found the Rattle River trailhead, where I would finish the next day. Dan drove me down to Pinkham Notch, my starting point. It was about 10:30 A.M. when I started out. Almost from the beginning, I was not feeling that great. The first mile was level and easy. About half a mile in, I was hungry, and felt weak. I stopped and ate an apple and some trail mix, and continued on. At Lost Pond, the trail started up the brutal climb of the Wildcat Mountains E, D, C, B and A. It would be over 2,000 feet in the first mile and a half. Steep. It did not matter.

I started the climb and only went 50 yards, and totally lost my breath and got dizzy. I stopped to rest, and tried to continue. I tried again. It was not happening. I sat for a moment, to try to compose myself. It would not be a good idea to get up there and get myself in trouble. It would not be responsible to myself or others who might have to help me. The mountain would be there another day. I turned around and climbed down. I sat at Lost Pond. I was very disappointed and discouraged. Two young people who I had seen sitting at Lost Pond came by. I told them I was not feeling well, and asked if they would hike back to Pinkham Notch with me. They actually were AMC interns who were doing some study at Lost Pond. I stopped a few times to rest, trying to be dramatic. I was starting to feel a little better.

Back at Pinkham Notch, I just sat for a while. I had all day to find a ride back to my car. A father and son team from northern Maine appeared nearby. They had just come down from Mount Washington. The dad went into Joe Dodge Lodge to call about a shuttle to get back to their car. My car was on their way, so I was able to tag along. Back at the trailhead, I could make myself useful by giving some thru-hikers from Tennessee a ride to town. I drove back to the Highland Center, switched my stay from the hut to the Highland Center, and crashed in my room. I was upset and not really sure what had happened. I really felt fine now.

The only thing I could imagine was that the 500-mile drive had taken something out of me. That, combined with the nervousness of the tough hike and not eating enough, caused my blood pressure to drop, causing the lightheadedness. It happened once at my gym. My blood pressure is low anyway. I would just rest the next day and see how I felt.

I drove back over to Gorham the next day and found my motel, but it was too early to check in. I decided to drive into Maine and scout out the trailhead at Grafton Notch. I thought there might be some sort of visitor's center in the state park. There was not. There was a slightly developed area at Screw Auger Falls, but no permanent ranger station. A box collected a $2 fee. There were a few rest rooms. The falls were neat, and there were a few young people wading in a pool under the falls. The parking area for the trailhead was a mile or so north of the falls. Sunshine from California was there, sitting in the middle of the large trailhead parking lot. A Maine state maintenance worker was talking to him.

Sunshine was in his third year of trying to complete the AT. He was in his 30s, and was a long-haired hippie-type guy. He was very pleasant. Two years earlier he started at Springer and quit after a few weeks, not understanding what he was getting himself into. The previous year he tried again and made it to Harpers Ferry, where he decided to abandon his hike that year and head back to California. This year, he started at Harpers Ferry, and was trying to finish and made it this far. He only had 250 miles to go to get to Katahdin.

Sunshine was exhausted from the hike of the previous few days in the Mahoosuc Mountains. I was starting to become intimidated by the difficulty and remoteness. I gave Sunshine an orange and some other snacks, which he devoured on the spot. He was waiting for a friend to come down off the mountain. The state worker seemed to have all day to chat. He told Sunshine that the remaining sections of Maine were not easy, but nothing like he had just finished. He also told Sunshine that a thru-hiker had drowned in a lake in Maine about a week before. Sunshine asked who, and when the state worker said his trail name, Sunshine became very upset, because he knew him well. The guy just went for a swim in the evening by himself and drowned.

I drove north to try to find Success Pond Road. Several of the access trails that I planned to use over the next few days were off of Success Pond Road.

I found it confusing, and did not get too far. I called Dan to cancel my shuttles for the rest of the week. I was getting more and more intimidated by the tough hiking up here.

I drove back into the little town of Bethel, Maine. I stopped at one outfitter to inquire about guides. They did not know of any. I stopped at another, and they did not offer any guides themselves, but trying to be helpful, they came up with a few people in town who they thought might be possibilities, and even looked up their phone numbers for me. One of the men was the head of the local rescue group. *Great, the town needed a rescue group.* It was just another reason to be intimidated.

I decided I would try to hike the next day on my own. I would not need a shuttle for my first day out of Gorham, because I had planned a loop hike up the AT, and then down a side trail on the same side of the mountain, with a road walk back to my car. I figured I could start out, and if I did not feel well or if it was too difficult, I could just turn around and go back. There would be a point of no return where I would have no choice but to go forward and finish. I would just start out and see how it went.

I had an early breakfast in Gorham, and had them make me a sandwich. I was at the Rattle River trailhead soon after 8:00 A.M. The trail road walks along US 2 and then on North Road across the Androscoggin River and up a little hill to gravel Hogan Road. After a few tenths on Hogan Road, I came to a small two-car parking lot where the trail turns into the woods.

At the trailhead, I met three guys from northern Maine who were going out for the weekend. They planned to hike up to Gentian Pond, camp there, and then hike down the Peabody Brook Trail the next day. I was doing the same thing, except they were going a little farther on the AT before coming back. The guys were in their early 50s, and had big packs. They were Mike (Speedy) who owned a construction company; John (Wolf) who was his lumber salesman; and Charlie (Chunker) who was Mike's financial advisor. I hiked with them for the first mile. Chunker fell behind, and when Speedy stopped to wait, I went on ahead.

The climb up to Mount Hayes was 1,500 feet, but over 2 ½ miles, so not terribly steep overall. It was still the Mahoosuc Mountains, so nothing is easy. My guidebook said "the range is wild and rugged. Be prepared for frequent climbs and descents and a rough and wet footway. Do not underestimate the time needed to traverse the range (three to five days (31 miles)).” I was planning four days, but adding 16 miles of side trails, to day-hike it. The Mahoosuc Mountains are considered some of the toughest hiking in the East. North on the AT toward Grafton Notch is Mahoosuc Notch, which is considered the single toughest one mile on the entire AT. That was for another day. The AMC publishes *The White Mountain Guide*. It is updated every year, and comes with a complete map set. I had the maps, and the AMC also has an online version of the guide, with extensive trail descriptions, which I had subscribed to. Some of the descriptions are frightening. *The White Mountain Guide* has over 4,000 miles of trails in it. My AMC magazine had said that three people had reported hiking all 4,000 miles. It is hard to imagine. None of those miles would be easy.

I was feeling fine and encouraged. I was hoping the disaster of two days earlier was just an aberration. I continued on to the summit of Mount Hayes. Every now and then there was a steep section. Soon I was at the summit, and continued on a level half-mile to the junction of the Mahoosuc Trail. Smooth rock surfaces dominated the pleasant summits. I met three southbound thru-hikers at the junction. They were nice but barely stopped, since they were psyched about getting to Gorham, only four miles away. They had finished Maine and were looking forward to the Whites, but mostly a zero day in Gorham.

I headed down into a pass, and then up to Cascade Mountain. It was 600 feet down, and then about the same up over the next two miles. I was still feeling good. I stopped for lunch and to enjoy the views. I could see Mount Madison and Mount Washington clearly. It was a nice day on the top of the mountains. I headed down to the Trident Col Tentsite Area. Once I reached Cascade Mountain, I was past the point of no return. The climb down to Trident Col was very steep, down about 500 feet in only three-tenths of a mile. The knees took a pounding. The sign there said only 2.7 miles to the Peabody Brook Trail, which was my exit point.

After another mile of easy climbing, but on still tough trail, I arrived at Page Pond. I knew I had to circle the pond a little, and soon found myself slogging through some mud. There were other footprints I was following, but I had lost the trail. I turned around and went back, spotted some blazes, and headed on. I was getting weary now. I knew I should still be climbing a little, but was not. I stopped to rest a while, and then continued. About 45 minutes from the pond, here came Speedy, hiking toward me. He said, "You are going the wrong way!" Indignant, and thinking he was pulling my leg, I said, "No I'm not." For a minute I thought they had somehow taken a different trail and gotten ahead of me. Of course they had not. From Page Pond, I had just hiked a mile in the wrong direction. I'm glad I met them, and would have figured it out at Trident Col because of the signs, but I was crushed.

There was nothing I could do but turn around. I hiked with them a while. I found my wrong turn at Page Pond. We continued on. Speedy was having some difficulty, and now Wolf was leading. Wolf and I climbed up the rock scramble to Wocket Ledge, where he took his pack off to wait. I decided to just stay with them for now. We waited 15 minutes for Chunker, and then Speedy to arrive. Speedy was still struggling. The guys were in good shape. They practice-hiked up a mountain near their home every Sunday morning. There were more good views back to Washington. Wolf took a picture of himself with my camera (a selfie), which was funny. I think he did it all the time. Wolf said he was energized by some Gatorade and some Emergen-C. I would buy both the next day. Emergen-C is high-dosage Vitamin C. Of course I ran it by my nutrition consultant, Virginia.

The guys were in no particular hurry. Speedy was wasted. They were camping at Gentian Pond. I was trying to get off the mountain. I stayed with them for a while longer. I was running low on water. They stopped for water often rather than carry it. At one of the stops, they let me use their filter to resupply. I would buy a filter the next day. After a little while, I found myself well in front of them again, and continued. Finally, I was at the junction of the Peabody Brook Trail, where I took my pack off to wait to say goodbye and thank them. Eventually I could hear them, but they had stopped at a stream crossing to get more water. I called out, told them I was at the junction, called goodbye, and started around Dream Lake.

I still had three miles to get down to the road, and it was past 4:00 P.M. now. The walk along Dream Lake was easy, much of it on puncheon, and then there were two relentless miles of steep downhill, about 2,000 feet. The knees were taking a pounding, and the going was slow. About halfway down, I passed a sign for Giant Falls, but really did not see any evidence of where they were. I passed a family coming up to the falls. It seemed late to be doing that, since it was 5:00 P.M. now. The tough down continued, but finally ended at the bottom of the mountain with a mile walk on an old grassy road. I had run out of water, a first for me. I finally had cell service, and called Virginia. It was close to 6:00 P.M. and she was getting a little worried.

I reached North Road, but still had a two-mile road walk to my car, back across the Androscoggin River to the Rattle River trailhead. I was there at 7:00 P.M., 11 hours after I started. I had hiked 9.6 miles on the AT, but with going backwards and down the Peabody Trail and the road walk, I had really hiked about 17 miles. It had become a long, tough day.

I was encouraged about what I had done, and decided to try some more. I figured I should take Sunday off, and then hike Monday. I called Dan to get back on his shuttle list. On Sunday, I took a drive up to the Berlin, New Hampshire area, and found Success Pond Road from the west. I stopped at the Northern Forest Heritage Park, which was a re-creation of an old logging camp. It was interesting. I napped and watched golf on Sunday afternoon. I was now a regular at the sports bar in Gorham.

On Monday morning after breakfast, I met Dan at the Rattle River trailhead again. He would drive me west to Berlin, and then out the long Success Pond Road to the Carlo Col Trail, which I would climb, then head south on the AT and back down the Peabody Brook Trail again. It was a good plan. Something did not feel right on the drive, and I was getting anxious. Dan was talking about someone he had picked up who had injured himself falling, breaking some teeth. About halfway out Success Pond Road, I told Dan to turn around and take me back. I just did not want to go.

I was not worried so much about myself getting hurt or lost. I would just feel terrible if someone had to come out to rescue me, not to mention the angst it might cause Virginia if she did not hear from me. I began to think it did not make much sense to be hiking in these remote areas alone. I was devastated, and not really sure what I was going to do. I was planning to come back in August, but did not want more of the same to happen. The definition of insanity is to do the same thing over and over, but expect a different result. I drove back to my motel, checked out, and drove home with my tail between my legs. I had just spent 5 days in New Hampshire to hike one day for a lousy 9 AT miles.

I thought about it a few weeks, and finally decided to call one of those names of licensed Maine guides that I had gotten from the outfitter in Bethel, Maine. One of the names was actually married teachers around 50, the women had said. I called the number and got Marie Keane. I told her who I was. She seemed to have at least some interest in helping me, so I emailed them the details of dates and times, and what I wanted to accomplish. They responded quickly. Marie and Steve's daughter, Katlyn, would be returning home from Chile soon. All three were licensed Maine Guides. They actually had a summer business (Wild River Adventures) of running canoe and camping trips in Maine and Canada, and all were very experienced. Steve and Marie had been doing this for 20 years, and their three kids grew up with it. There would be a daily fee, but they would do all the shuttles, and even made me lunches. Virginia was relieved. We closed the deal. I would go up in the middle of August.

I had unfinished business in Connecticut. There were two short sections that I missed when I was there in 2006 and 2007. Together they were less than a mile, but there is that pledge to pass every white blaze. Skipping those little pieces bothered me. I decided to take two days to drive to Maine. I would stop in Connecticut to make up those little sections.

On Saturday, August 10, I set my car's navigation system for Cornwall Bridge, Connecticut. As silly as it seemed, I realized I had skipped two-tenths of a mile by hiking down a side street (Sharon Road) instead of hiking all the way to Connecticut 4 from the north to get to my car at the parking area at US 7 and Connecticut 4 in town. I parked at the same parking area, and rather than walking up the road, I used the Breadloaf Mountain Trail to access the AT. It was easy trail, but a climb nonetheless, and I was sweating. I hadn't bothered to wear hiking clothes, and in the now heat of the day, my cotton T-shirt was wet when I got to the view at Breadloaf Mountain. It was a very hazy day, but I still could see across the valley to Silver Hill. I hiked down to the AT, and in a tenth of a mile I was at Sharon Road. Six years earlier, I turned left and hiked down the road. Now, I would hike down the AT, cross Guinea Brook, and then hike up to Connecticut 4. A mile down the road took me back to my car. I had just hiked two miles to fill in that two-tenths that I had skipped in June six years earlier.

Back on the road, I set my nav for Salisbury, Connecticut, about 20 miles to the north. The small hotel where I stayed on one of my first 2-day hikes now had a "For Sale" sign and was closed, a victim of the recession. I found the parking lot for the Undermountain Trail along Connecticut 41. I was making up a whopping seven-tenths of a mile this time. It would take me three hours to do it. In September of 2006, I missed a cutoff trail to get to Sages Ravine because of a bear. Then in August of 2007, I did not make it up because I was too tired. Oh well, the price we pay sometimes. I headed up the Undermountain Trail. At the parking lot, a van had pulled up with a mom, her teenage son and his girlfriend. We leapfrogged up the Undermountain Trail for the one mile to the junction of the Paradise Lane Trail. About that time, Mom sat down, feeling weak and lightheaded. I knew that feeling. I gave her my Gatorade and some Emergen-C.

After I was sure she was OK, I turned off onto the Paradise Lane trail to get to Sages Ravine. The trail was easy, but did not seem like it was used that much. From the valley I could spot Bear Mountain. I ate my lunch at Sages Ravine, where the AT intersected. I was in Massachusetts now. A family came down from Bear Mountain. It was Mom, Dad, 4 kids ages 6 to 12, and Granddad. Coming down from Bear Mountain was a serious hike, but none of them seemed the worse for wear. I was impressed. Granddad was probably a little older than me. He was enjoying himself with his family. Granddad had goals. He was trying to complete all the hiking trails in Connecticut, some 800 miles of them. After today, he will have finished all trails west of the Housatonic River.

I headed south on the AT and up Bear Mountain. It was only seven-tenths of a mile, but one tough climb. I got lightheaded (great) so had to take my time. I'm not sure how all those little kids made it down safely. At the summit of Bear Mountain, there was a rock pile tower to get above trees so as to have a 360-degree view. Either I never made it that far from the south in 2006, or it was new. Mom, the son and the girlfriend were just leaving when I got there. They had taken the shorter route. I was drenched. It was cloudy, but hot and humid.

I continued on to Riga Junction and down the Undermountain Trail. I was tired from the 6.7-mile hike, but the gap was filled in. No more thinking about that. I was off to my motel in Brattleboro, Vermont. I slept as long as I could the next morning, and headed up to Bethel, Maine, which would be my home base for the next week. The Keanes had recommended a motel. We planned to meet there later in the day. Bethel, Maine, population of about 2,000, is a cute little place. There is a nearby ski slope and Sunday River for recreation. I had lunch at Erin's Café.

I met Steve, Marie and Katlyn. They had been out scouting the trailheads on Success Pond Road to make sure they knew where they were. Steve and Marie had hiked most of the AT in the area, but years earlier. Katlyn had guided many hikes (mostly youth), but actually had not done the sections we would be doing this week. I had sent them a tentative itinerary, which they said was fine. Katlyn would be my guide for the first few days, and then Steve would take over. Marie would help with the shuttles, and might come along a day or so. They could not have been nicer. I knew I had made a good decision, and felt very comfortable.

For Monday, I planned a section north of Grafton Notch, avoiding the tougher Mahoosucs. It was kind of a warm-up for me, to see how it went. The Keanes had directed me to the only early morning breakfast spot in town. Like my diner at home, there was a group of older men all sitting together, solving the problems of the world. Steve, Marie and Katlyn all arrived at my motel, and I followed them to Grafton Notch. Katlyn and I would hike north from there, and Steve and Marie would shuttle my car up to East B Hill Road.

Katlyn and I started out on our 10-mile day. Katlyn is a beautiful young girl. In a week she would head back for her senior year at Saint Michaels College in Vermont. She was a Spanish Major, and had just gotten back from spending her junior year in Nicaragua and Chile. This was a good chance for her to make a few dollars for school, her Mom had said. Katlyn said she much preferred to be out hiking than going to a nearby resort to waitress. She really did seem to enjoy being out and hiking the AT near her home, where she had never actually been. I felt good about that. She was a member of her high school and college cross country ski teams, and would run cross country this fall to get in shape for ski season. The whole Keane family were cross country skiers.

Katlyn had guided overnight youth backpacking trips in the Whites. She had some stories about those adventures. When I would apologize for being slow, she would say it was nothing compared to the younger groups. She was extremely responsible, and always the most polite, and never made me feel like I was not keeping up my end of the bargain. I would tell her to go ahead if she wanted to, and that she could wait for me at the top of the climbs. She was trained to never leave her client.

Over the next few days, I would tell Katlyn of my hiking experiences. In the small world department, I mentioned Dot MacDonald, who had helped me in Vermont. The Keanes actually knew Dot, who was a close friend of a family member.

From the road, we were climbing immediately. The elevation profile was intimidating. The Maine maps had an extreme vertical exaggeration compared to the other states, which made it look worse than it was. We would go up 1,200 feet in a mile and a half. I had been on steeper, but the trail was not an easy footpath. There was a side trail to Table Rock, which Katlyn asked me if I wanted to take. She had been there many times with her dad, who hiked the difficult climb several times a week as his way of staying in shape. I decided just to stick to the AT.

After the initial climb, there was an easier mile. Easy is relative. Then we climbed another 1,000 feet in less than a mile to the scrub pine zone summit of West Baldpate. It was beautiful up there. My guidebook said Baldpate offered some of the best views of the Mountain and Lakes Region in all of Maine. True. There was a short, steep descent down West Baldpate into a col between the West and East Baldpate Peaks. There was a board and log ladder to climb down one of the rock faces. We stopped for a while in the col. It was great up there. The hiking in the col and the 350-foot climb up to East Baldpate did not seem that tough. Even though it was steep in spots, it was above tree line, and much of it was on rock faces. It was the nicest hiking of the day. Hiking above tree line is spectacular. Cairns marked the way.

On the summit of East Baldpate, we stopped for a snack at the signed junction with the Grafton Loop Trail. The view back down into the col and West Baldpate with Old Speck (tomorrow's hike) in the background were terrific. To the east along a ridge was a series of windmills. We still had six miles to go. We started down the very difficult 1-mile 1,200-foot descent of East Baldpate. I was slow.

Near the bottom, we passed a 60-something couple from North Carolina. They were day-hikers too, and were doing the same hike we were today. They'd started 90 minutes before us. A few days earlier, they did the section west of Grafton Notch, which includes the toughest one mile of the AT. This would be our hike tomorrow. Their description of it was incredible. They started at 6:00 A.M. and did not get off the mountain until 10:45 P.M., and had to hike down from Old Spec with their headlamps. A third member of their party quit and went home after that.

The trail became less steep on the way to the Frye Notch Lean-to where we had lunch. We had great wrap sandwiches Katlyn made that morning. We climbed 500 feet up Surplus Mountain. On the way, we passed five southbound thru-hikers, including some cousins, two shirtless guys from Connecticut and Massachusetts. They looked alike. From Surplus Mountain we had a three-mile descent on easier grade to Dunn Notch. At Dunn Notch, there was a challenging little crossing of the Ellis River, with a 15-foot bank on the other side. It was not as hard as it looked to get up. On the other side, we were at the top of a sixty-foot double water fall. By holding onto a tree and extending over a wooded cliff, we could get a glimpse of the falls. There were side trails to go down, but it was approaching 4:00 P.M. We did not even talk about going down. I think Katlyn had the idea; I was on an AT mission, and she left it at that.

It was another mile to the car. We arrived at four thirty, 8 ½ hours after the start of our 10.3-mile day. I did not get Katlyn home until almost 6:00 P.M. There were three great spots near my motel where I would have dinners.

The next morning, the Keanes arrived shortly after 7:00 A.M., and we drove out to Grafton Notch again. We left my car, and Steve drove us around to the Mahoosuc Notch trailhead on Success Pond Road. Both Katlyn and Marie would hike with me today. Marie was a strong hiker, but I could keep up. We would hike up the 2.1-mile access trail to the AT, and then 8.2 miles on the AT back to Grafton Notch. The hike up the Mahoosuc Notch Trail was surprisingly easy, belying what was to come. The access trail dumped us right into the south end of Mahoosuc Notch.

My guide book described Mahoosuc Notch as follows: "A deep cleft between Mahoosuc Arm and Fulling Mill Mountain. Giant boulders fallen from the notch's sheer walls have clogged the floor. Ice is found in caves here as late as July. As hikers follow the blazes, they must climb around and under house sized boulders and through caves and in some places, must remove their packs to do so. Traversing the notch is dangerous and difficult. Take care to avoid slipping on damp moss." It was all true. Some call it the most difficult on the AT. Some call it the most fun. I could see both points of view.

Marie had hiked the notch twenty years earlier with Steve. Katlyn had never been there. It was one mile of boulder scrambling that took close to two hours. There were quite a few people in the notch, and a large group from Outward Bound. It was clearly a destination hike for many. Marie was a shutterbug and between us, we took a lot of pictures, which we would swap. I looked a little frazzled at times. We made it out to the other side. I had banged my shin at one point, and Marie pointed out that I was bleed-ing. The left leg of my long pants and my sock and even boots were soaked in blood. I did not even know it. Somehow I had a puncture wound. Katlyn sprang into action with her first aid kit and patched me up.

We were through the notch, but the fun was just beginning. The climb up Mahoosuc Arm was the most brutal I can remember. It was as steep as some other climbs, 1,620 feet over 1.6 miles, but harder, and it took a lot out of me. It was another two hours. The views from the open summit of Mahoosuc Arm were great back down into the notch, which could be seen clearly. Old Spec to the east looked like a trapezoid, with its flat ridge. I did not think I had the climb up Old Spec in me, and started to think about a way to bail off the mountain, and mentioned it to the girls. They would have done what I wanted but in the end, there was no easier way off the mountain than the AT. Some of the nicest hiking of the day was in the alpine zone over the next mile to Speck Pond and the shelter. Katlyn spotted a grouse hiding behind a bush. There were views down to the north, and Success Pond and the road.

At the Speck Pond shelter we met a father-son team from Glassboro, New Jersey. The dad was in his 50s. It was their seventh year of section-hiking the AT. They had come through the notch and were wiped out, too. There was a mother, dad and 10-year-old son, section-hiking the Mahoosucs, who were planning to stay the night. I was recovering, and the next mile and a half up Old Spec was not as hard as I had imagined. There were a few challenging technical spots, but overall not nearly as tough as Mahoosuc Arm, except for it being later in the day. Five southbound thru-hikers, including the cousins we saw on the previous day, were coming down.

We reached the side trail leading to the wooded summit of Old Speck where we stopped to rest. Katlyn seemed slightly disappointed that I did not want to hike the six-tenths-of-a-mile round trip side trail for the summit views on a platform. We still had 3.5 miles to go, and it was now 4:00 P.M. I kept thinking about the couple from North Carolina who had to finish the hike with headlamps. I told them to go, and I would wait and rest, but they would not hear of it. We had planned to hike the next day, but I knew I needed a day off. Marie and Katlyn were able to use their phones to shift their appointments from Thursday to Wednesday, to accommodate me. The father-son team arrived and considered hiking the side trail, but they did not either, and they started down. We followed a few minutes later. In half a mile we came to a great viewpoint toward the east. We could clearly see East and West Baldpate, and the col in between. The father-son team was there, trying to figure if they were done for the day, or would try to make it to Grafton Notch.

The first two miles were not terribly steep, but still, my knees were taking a pounding. The last mile and a half was really tough and steep, 1,500 feet straight down. My knees were shot. We just kept moving. I was spent. Finally, we reached the beautiful area of the falls of Cascade Brook, and were down. We reached the car at 7:00 P.M. It had become an 11-hour day to hike 10.3 miles. I was not dropping the girls off in Bethel until after 8:00 P.M. Steve had dinner waiting and offered for me to stay, but I figured they should have the family time together.

I was glad to have the next day off, spending some time in the motel pool, but mostly napping all day. It was disappointing, but some bad weather moved in. It poured overnight, but the forecast indicated it might break in the morning. We decided we would wait an hour, and then make a decision. We went, but on the way out past Grafton Notch, Steve stopped to make sure I wanted to go. It would be foggy on the mountains, and Steve rightly pointed out that there would be no views. It would be Katlyn and me. She seemed to be sure it was fine with her if I wanted to go. I said yes.

We left my car at the Mahoosuc Notch trailhead, and then drove out further to the Carlo Col trailhead lot. The road got bad, and we had to road walk half a mile before entering the woods. On the road walk, a 20-something Asian guy was walking toward us. He was a southbounder, but had injured himself and took the side trail to get off the mountain. He would have at least a 10-mile road walk to the medical center in Berlin. Hopefully he could get a ride on Success Pond Road. The rain was letting up some, but the fog and mist would be with us all day. We would not shed our rain jackets until late. It rained much heavier in town, which was a minor concern for Steve and Marie, although generally they are not worriers.

Even though the rain was letting up, I had not counted on the streams that would be full-flowing down the mountain. The Carlo Col Trail was tougher than the Mahoosuc Notch Trail. We had to cross a stream four times just to get to the AT. Rock-hopping for me was not safe or possible. I had no choice but to wade across, with water over my boots and up to my shins. Hiking with water-logged boots was actually not as bad as I thought it might be.

Near the trailhead, we passed the Carlo Col Shelter, but did not visit. We got to the AT and headed north, climbing Mount Carlo. It was only 400 feet, but nothing was easy. We stopped to rest on the summit, in the alpine zone. As expected, it was fogged in. At times on the summits we could only see 50 yards. The next mile was down, and then up to the east peak of Goose Eye. On the way up there was a rock face climb on two sections of rebar bars, which looked intimidating, but were not a problem. We had to negotiate a few log and board ladders, which were very slippery. We had lunch on Goose Eye at the Goose Eye Trail junction. Katlyn even brought a mat for me to sit on. What a sweet girl.

There was nice hiking in the col up to the north peak of Goose Eye. Everything was wet. There was puncheon totally underwater, and many muddy areas to negotiate. At times it was not possible to stay on the trail. Water was running down any elevation gain or loss. Heading up, we passed those same five thru-hikers, including the cousins we had seen on our previous two days. This seemed curious, since we had taken a day off, and it was the next contiguous section. They responded that the Notch had "kicked their butt" and they only did four miles that day. We also met the family of three that we had seen two days earlier at the Speck Pond Shelter. They had huge packs, but were doing fine. At the summit of Goose Eye, we seemed to lose the trail for a minute. Katlyn soon found it, but the trail on the summit was starting to look the same to me. In the fog we could not get our bearings of the surrounding mountains. Having walked backwards on the trail two months earlier, I was concerned. Katlyn pulled out her map and compass, and assured me we were heading northeast as we should be.

She was proven right when we arrived at the Full Goose Shelter. It was dark, even though it was only around 5:00 P.M., and very foggy. There were four northbound thru-hikers in the shelter, but it was hard to even see in. We knew they were in there because they were talking to us. One was from Pittsburgh. They were all trying to dry out from the rain. They had stopped mid-day, hoping for better weather in the morning to go through the notch. The notch is a big deal, and on everyone's radar. Katlyn and I had a mile and a half to get to the Notch Trail, our exit point. It took another hour, and my knees took more pounding on the steep decline. The weather was finally breaking.

I knew when we got to the Mahoosuc Notch Trail it would only be another easy two miles to the car. Katlyn joked that if I wanted to go through the notch again, she was up for it. The Notch Trail provided three more full-stream crossings, soaking my boots again. We got to my car around 7:00 P.M., and I did not have Katlyn home until eight thirty. We had gotten a later start, but it was still a 9 ½-hour day to hike 11.5 miles (6.4 on the AT). I was spent, and my knees were killing me. I decided I needed another day off on Friday. I thanked Katlyn profusely for all her patience. She said she had fun, which I hope was true. She told her mother on the phone that she was glad that we went today, despite the bad weather. She seemed sincere. I would not see her again this week.

I had breakfast with Steve the next morning. I think he appreciated the business I was providing the family. Although they did mostly overnight canoe and backpacking trips (he had many stories), this was close to home for them. Hiking for them was at least, in part, recreation. The three of them could not have been nicer to me. I rested my body for the balance of the day.

On Saturday, we planned my last section of the Mahoosuc Range. I was able to arrange a shuttle with Dan for Steve and me, to save Marie a lot of driving. We dropped my car back in Gorham, right at the Peabody Brook trailhead, to save ourselves a road walk at the end of the day. Dan drove us around through Berlin and out Success Pond Road to the Carlo Col trailhead again.

The stream crossings along the Carlo Col Trail were not nearly the problem they had been two days earlier. Hiking with Steve would be different. Steve was not a big man, slim and in great shape. He is a physical education teacher and outdoorsman. When Steve was not teaching, running canoe trips, or spending time with his family, he was working on a "camp" property the family had up past Grafton Notch. It may have been in New Hampshire. Katlyn said that Steve liked Maine 26 because any time he was on it meant he was going to have fun that day, hiking or working on his camp.

This would be a very tough day. Although the elevation gain and loss was not that dramatic, the short climbs and descents were always steep and difficult. Steve would often get ahead of me and out of sight. I did not mind, and even preferred it. I felt awkward on the climbs up and down, and my knees were shot from the tough week. My balance was non-existent.

From Carlo Col, in half a mile we were at the sign for the New Hampshire/Maine border, which was a big deal to me. Moving on, there was a short but very difficult rock climb to a cramped, unnamed view point. A northbound thru-hiker from Germany was there, chatting with Steve. It was a nice day, and there were great views to the north and west. From there it was only a 600-foot net climb to Mount Success over two miles. It seemed, however, that we were always on a steep up or down. We had lunch at the Success trailhead. I was famished, and did not like the looks of the upcoming boulder scramble. Steve and I solved some of the problems with today's youth over a sandwich. We had both done some coaching.

The boulder scramble was as hard as it looked. I had to pull myself up through the difficult rocks. A hiker coming down seemed worried about me and said as much, telling me to take my time. He did not want the responsibility of helping to carry me off the mountain. We finished the climb through beautiful pine forests. The mile hike across the open summit of Mount Success was the nicest part of the day. There were great 360-degree views often. I could see Madison and Washington, and we could see down to the Androscoggin River. There was puncheon in many spots along the summit to protect the fragile environment. It had dried out a lot since two days earlier.

As we headed down, we met a couple who had just been to the wreckage of a 1954 plane crash. Two died, but five survived two cold December nights on the mountain before being rescued. The site is off the trail, and can only been seen if you know where to look. The hike down seemed very long. Over the next few miles we met two 70-something men a mile or so apart, who were ultra-light section-hikers. They were doing the 10 miles between Trident Col and Carlo Col today. I thought they might be a little old for this hike, but they seemed well-experienced and doing fine, so I did not worry about them.

Steve had hiked the entire Mahoosuc Range several times before. One time he was hired by a family (Mom, Dad, and two sons, 8 and 10) to backpack the entire 31 miles. After the first night, Mom and Dad decided they'd had enough.

The hike down to Gentian Pond was really getting long. The steep ups and downs just did not stop. At the Gentian Pond Shelter, we met a late-40s section-hiker who was staying for the evening. She admitted to being slow, and had only hiked the five miles from Trident Col today. She said she was hiking with two other women partners (60 and 40-something) who would be right behind her. It was another hour until we saw them. They were really slow, and seemed to be having great difficulty, and had not gotten to any of the really tough parts yet. They seemed to be in over their heads.

From a viewpoint near the shelter, we could see ahead to another mountain. Steve said that would be our last climb. From my memory of the elevation profile, I said no, that once we reached the shelter, we were done climbing for the day. Steve did not say anything, but of course he was right. There was more tough climbing, and then ups and downs to Gentian Pond, Moss Pond and finally Dream Lake. My knees were done. We finished off our snacks. Steve helped me pump some water because I was out.

We still had three miles to go down the Peabody Brook Trail, which I had been on back in June. It seemed a lot harder this time than I remembered. Steve asked me if I wanted to stop and rest again, but, "I can smell my car," I responded. We finally reached North Road. Beer never tasted so good to both Steve and me. It was another 13-mile, 11-hour day. It may have been my hardest day ever. Steve offered to hike with me for my planned fifth day, but I was done. I felt good that he could go along to take Katlyn back to college on Sunday. I dropped Steve back in town, and took two days to drive home.

Two weeks later, my puncture wound got infected when I was helping Bethany and Kevin with their New Paltz home. They ended up taking me to an emergency room. It took a few months for it to heal and for my knees to feel normal again. For both reasons, my gym visits were minimized, and I abandoned the idea of a fall triathlon. I visited an orthopedic doctor for my knees who advised, "No more running." I was not really upset about it. I planned to still do triathlons, just not run as part of my training. There were plenty of low-impact machines at my gym for training.

I was not really happy with my Maine/New Hampshire progress for the year. I spent two weeks up there and had covered only 41 AT miles. With side trails I hiked a total of 60 miles. It was what it was. On the good side, I was done with the tough Mahoosuc Range. Steve indicated they were more than willing to assist me as I headed north into Maine. That was comforting to me and Virginia. I'm sure Maine would offer many more challenging days. I was looking forward to it. I was not taunting the mountains anymore.

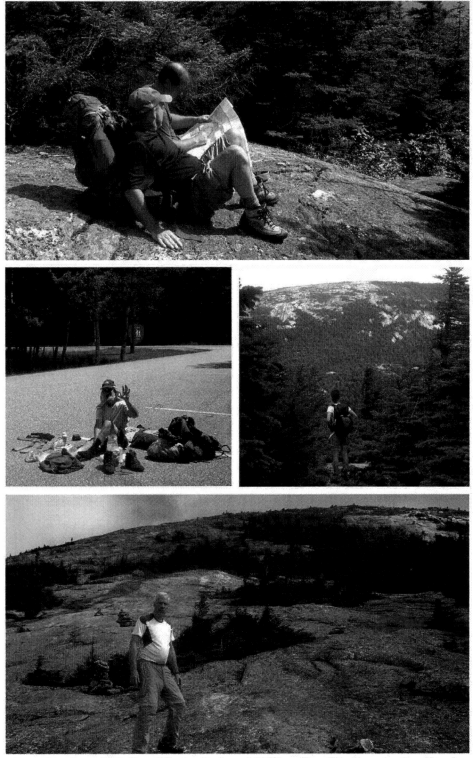

Top: Speedy and Wolf on Wocket Ledge. Middle: "Sunshine" at Grafton Notch; Katlyn scanning East Baldpate. Bottom: In the col between E & W Baldpate.

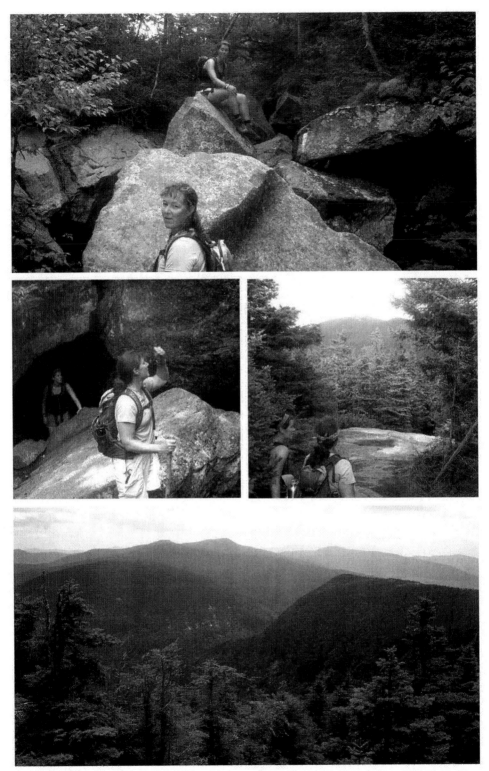

Top: Boulder scrambling in Mahoosuc Notch. Middle: Caving in Mahoosuc Notch; Katlyn and Marie scanning the Baldpates from Old Spec. Bottom: The Notch from Mahoosuc Arm.

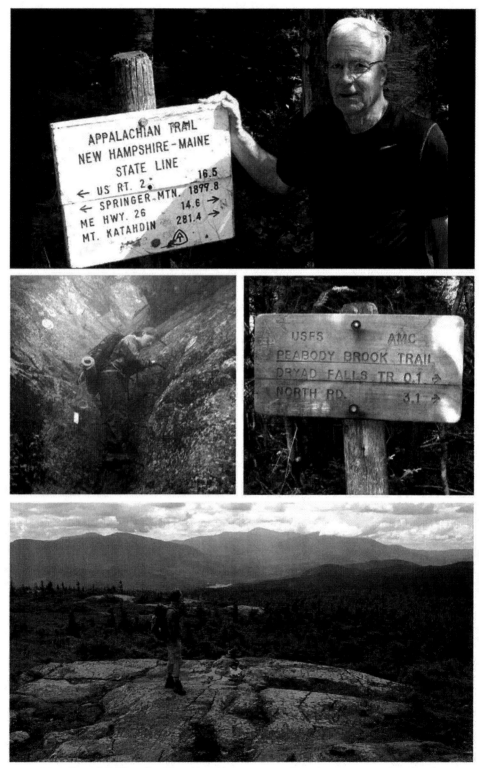

Top: State line. **Middle:** Ladder climbing up Goose Eye; 3.1 more tough miles to complete the Mahoosuc Range. **Bottom:** Steve scanning The Whites from Mt Success.

2012 – South - Tennessee and North Carolina

During President's Day weekend in February, Bethany and Kevin's condominium building in Hoboken, New Jersey caught fire, and within a few weeks, was totally demolished. They lost most everything they owned, including their two beloved cats, and Bethany's grand piano that she had purchased when she started at Steinway. They were not home at the time, and there were no human injuries in any of the 8 residential or 2 commercial units. Bethany and Kevin's insurance would help them with a new apartment a few blocks away, however, it is hard to insure for what you have accumulated in a lifetime. Kevin, as president of the small owner's association, would be involved in the possible rebuilding. The planning is ongoing.

With a great year of hiking in 2011, finishing the trail over the next few years had clearly become a goal. I figured if I could do over 250 miles a year, I could finish in 2014. *Oops.* Over the winter, I was able to drop about half of the weight that I'd put on since the beginning of the previous hiking season, but was still carrying about eight pounds more on my first hike of 2012. I was not the disciplined person I created in 2011. I fell off the wagon a few times, did not do as much yoga, but did take some spin classes. I was drinking coffee again. After tax season, my ego got the best of me, and I bought a road bike to try to improve my triathlon times. I was jumping to another age group, and was trying to be competitive. Not so much. People that are doing triathlons at my age are serious, and have those thin runner's bodies.

Since I was over 500 miles away from the trail both north and south, I decided I had to hike a full week at a time to make the drives worthwhile. I planned to do weeks in May and October in the south, and weeks in June and August in the north. I could take that much time off, since my work load in the summer did not take much time. I was giving up some of my work, as our partnership agreement expected. Four full weeks of hiking should get me well over 250 miles again. *Oops.*

My best friend from high school lived in Raleigh, North Carolina, and had always been saying that when I got down there, he had an interest in hiking with me. I was down there. John was the smartest guy in our Boyertown, Pennsylvania High School class of 350 students. He was the center on the football team, and he and I were doubles partners on the tennis team. John went to Yale as a math and economics major on an Army scholarship, and then was in the Army Corps of Engineers in Europe for his military commitment. After the service, he went to Harvard Business School. Like I say, smart.

John started his business career in New York City with airlines, and then banking, and then to a large public natural resource company, where he earned high-level positions in corporate finance. He met and married his wife Kim in New York City. He moved with his company to New Orleans and then Texas, where his two kids grew up. Later, he became part of a small group of executives based in Raleigh who would get investor capital to buy, improve and sell companies all over the world. Like I say, smart. I felt honored that he would want to keep in touch with me. John was retired now, so had the time to hike in between his frequent travels, ski and bike trips, and the time he spent at his summer home on Bald Head Island. He quickly picked up the trail name Old Baldy, for a lighthouse Kim was heavily involved with. He was not bald.

For my first trip, I would start down in Tennessee, and then John would join me for a few days as I finished up Virginia. I drove halfway down on Friday, May 4, and got up early on Saturday to continue. I had two miles near Pearisburg, Virginia to fill in. I drove 80 miles out of my way to do it. I took my bike along to shuttle myself along the road. The 2.1 trail miles paralleled Virginia 635 on the north side of Stony Creek, out in a remote area

15 miles east of Pearisburg. There was no cell reception. I left my car at the Cherokee Flats trailhead. While I was getting ready, a man who was fishing in Stony Creek came out of the woods and we spoke briefly. It was an easy 2-mile bike ride back to a small lot near the start of the section. There was a 100-foot access trail crossing Stony Creek to get to the AT.

The hike was easy, and I took my time. Michael from Woods Hole had mentioned that "The Captain" was along this section. Near the end of the two miles, I began to see his signs. The Captain lived on the road side of Stony Creek, but invited hikers to his home. He rigged a rope swing across the creek that you could sit on to pull yourself to the other side. He was sitting at a picnic table with his buddy, the fisherman whom I had met an hour before. The Captain had long, gray hair with a pony tail. He offered food and drink, but I declined. "Save it for the thru-hikers," I said.

Two thru-hikers had spent the night on the Captain's porch. They had just come through the Grayson Highlands a week before, where they said there was still snow. They were Catnap from West Virginia, and Danu, (a Greek Goddess, she explained) from Florida. Three dogs livened up the place. The Captain obliged, and took my picture on the swing. I left, and was soon crossing Stony Creek again on a beauty of a bridge. I picked up my bike and was off to Hampton, Tennessee, another 150 miles. On the way I passed the Bristol Motor Speedway and took some pictures.

I had arranged to meet Sutton Brown in Hampton at his store, Brown's Hardware and Grocery. Conversations with Sutton reminded me of the old Abbot and Costello routine, "Who's on first". I was never quite sure if he was poking fun of the northerner, or it was just his nature. I think we arranged to meet the next morning, but I was not really sure. I stayed at the Super 8 in Johnson City for the next few days.

The next morning, I arrived at Sutton's large home and hostel (Braemar Castle) in town. His family home was the former HQ of a logging company in the early 1900s. Sutton was nowhere to be found. I waited about half an hour past our scheduled meet time, and called his cell. He popped out of a neighbor's house with his dog, and we headed out. Sutton could not have been more friendly and accommodating. Sutton gave me the history of the Hampton area (which he loved) and his father and family, who were integral to it. A nearby bridge on Route 19E was named for his dad. Sutton went to college on a tennis scholarship, and was an accounting major. He met his wife when they were both whitewater rafting guides. His two sons were late high school and college. We had a long time to talk. We had a long drive around to Watauga Dam Road, and then back to the trailhead near Hampton on Dennis Cove Road. He told me he might ask someone else to do my shuttle for the next day, so we bid farewell.

My guidebook said about this section in part, "with its sheer cliffs and wooded slopes, waterfalls and rapids, the rugged gorge of Laurel Fork possesses a natural beauty that is one of the highlights of the entire AT." It did not disappoint. It would be 13 miles up to Watauga Dam Road.

I left the pretty trailhead area for an easy mile on an old railroad bed until a rocky climb down to Laurel Fork Falls. The scenery was spectacular, and the easy trail belied the ruggedness of the area. Laurel Fork Falls were some of the nicest that I had seen on the trail. I read later in the *2013 Thru-hiker's Companion* that a father and son drowned under the falls this year. Ducky, with a long ponytail, was sitting there with his back to me, mesmerized by the falls. I called out as I approached so as not to startle him. Ducky was from Ohio and seemed sad, as he said he was quitting his thru-hike because he was out of money. Most people say it costs about $1,000 a month to hike the trail. That includes supplies, gear and occasional hostel and motel rooms. A father-son team came to the falls from the north. They had hiked in a side trail from US 321. Ducky headed out and I followed, after the dad took my picture at the falls.

The hike continued to be gorgeous along the stream, and directly under the cliffs of the gorge. In another mile, I passed the Laurel Fork Shelter, and came to the junction with the Hampton Blueline Trail. Ducky was sitting at the junction, along with Dr. Slow and Forager. Dr. Slow was a 60-ish actual PhD from Hot Springs, North Carolina. She said she was "mostly done" with the trail, but I was not sure in what way. She reminded me of a neighbor of mine, with big gray hair that fell out of her Tilley hat when she took it off. Forager said he was a member of ATF (Addicted to Freedom). He said he had thru-hiked in 2009 on no money and going ultra-light. He had lived everywhere, but could not stay away from the trail. Both were headed to Damascus for Trail Days. None of the three of them seemed to want any part of the upcoming climb of Pond Mountain. I suspect they took the side trail to US 321 to avoid it. I saw Dr. Slow and Forager a few days later in Damascus. They looked comfortable sitting in chairs in front of the outfitter there. I'm sure they had not hiked to get there.

I was still in good shape, even though my weight was off my low. I was not in hiking shape though, and the climb up Pond Mountain was a tough two miles and 1,700 feet to Pond Flats. The trail was nice, and switchbacks mitigated the grade. From Pond Flats it was a long, easy three miles down to US 321 and Watauga Lake. Just before the road, I overtook a thru-hiking couple from California. She was struggling with a bad foot, and just trying to get to Damascus to rest it. She had 40 miles to go.

I ate lunch at the lake, which was enjoyable. It was a beautiful Sunday, and warm for early May. There were many swimmers and boaters out, which surprised me. I forgot I was in the south now. The hike around the lake was on rocky and rooty trail, and seemed like a long three miles until a few-hundred-foot climb up to Watauga Dam. AT hikers may cross the dam even though it is closed to the public. It was a steep walk on the dam access road, and then into the woods along a rocky crest. There were some nice, limited views back to the lake. I was glad to reach my car. It had become a long 7 ½-hour hiking day. I headed back to Johnson City and a sports bar.

The next morning, I met Bob Peoples at Watauga Dam Road. Bob would take me to the Cross Mountain trailhead on Tennessee 91. It would be a long 16-mile day along Iron Mountain Ridge through the Cherokee National Forest and the Big Laurel Branch Wilderness. Hiking south, I figured I would see many northbound thru-hikers. I did.

Bob Peoples is a legend in the area and beyond, and I was honored for him to shuttle me, once I learned more about him over the coming months. Bob owned and ran the Kincora Hostel on Dennis Cove Road. It held 26, and 19 had been there the night before. He does not charge anyone directly, but people make a donation (suggested $4) as they see fit. He keeps his pantry stocked, and hikers pay for things voluntarily. He relies on the hikers themselves to keep the place clean, and they do. I would not want to be an exception to this. Bob would have a way of taking care of it. He is a long-time trail angel and volunteer maintainer. He shuttles hikers to town twice a day for free, and gives free slack pack shuttles.

Bob was 69, and sadly his wife had passed away a few years earlier. He was clearly in great shape. In 2009, he hiked the Camino Real Trail in Spain with a friend. Each year, the week following Trail Days in Damascus, he runs Kincora Hard Core. It is a week of tough trail maintenance. Volunteers stay at his place and camp nearby for free. One hundred people show up, he is so respected.

There was graffiti about Bob at the Vandeventer Shelter. "When Bob Peoples stays in a shelter, the mice bring him food." "Bob Peoples sleeps with a pillow under his pistol." "Bob Peoples once got bitten by a snake. After three days of pain and anguish, the snake died."

From the trailhead at Cross Mountain, it was easy trail across the ridge for four miles to the Iron Mountain Shelter. I was making very good time. There were no views along the ridge. Surprisingly, I did not meet anyone until a tentsite past Turkeypen Gap at my halfway point. Four guys, Buddy Holly, Spam, Budda, and Mattress Pad, from different Florida cities, were just packing up, even though it was after 11:00 A.M. They had night-hiked until the middle of the night. Sometimes thru-hikers hike at night to avoid the heat of the day. It was only May and not hot, so I found this curious. The guys were a riot, so I stopped to have lunch as they gathered their things. Since only one in four make it to Katahdin, I tried to size up which one of them it would be.

I continued along the easy ridge and met Union Jill from England. I love British accents, especially watching golf on TV, which I do a lot.

There were 10 or more hikers at the Vandeventer Shelter. Most of them stayed at Kincora two nights before. One guy was a riot, and had the strangest accent I had ever heard. He was from Ohio, but it sounded like a combination of Boston/Pittsburgh/Atlanta. He said he got that a lot, and he was the only one that talked like he did. He said his batteries in his headlamp had given up as he was coming down Pond Mountain overnight, so had to stop. I gave him mine. Mudbug was there, who must have been my age, but looked younger.

As I hiked down the switchbacks (Bob Peoples' work) to the road, the thru-hikers came fast and furiously, including Philly Steve, a Philadelphia sports fanatic with a Phillies hat, and the Noodleheads, a married couple from Colorado. I again met the couple that I'd met approaching Watauga Lake the day before. She was visibly limping. I offered my car a mile away, but she was a gamer. Tree Trunk and Manula, a late-50s married couple from upstate New York came by.

From the shelter and along the way, there were some limited views down to Watauga Lake. After 29 miles in 2 long days, I was very glad to get to my car.

The next morning I did not need a shuttle, since John was going to meet me at Cross Mountain at about the time I expected to finish. I was planning to hike the 10 miles from McQueen Gap south back to Cross Mountain. Bob Peoples discouraged me from leaving my car at McQueen Gap because of vandalism. I was tired, and the weather had gotten bad with some rain expected. I no longer had the luxury of being a fair-weather-only hiker. I decided I could cut my hike down to 6.5 miles by starting at Low Gap on US 421. That would leave the other 3.7 miles south of McQueen Gap for another time. I could sleep in a little, and take my time before starting my hike, and still meet John when he expected me.

At the Low Gap trailhead, I met the funny-accent guy who I had given the batteries to. He thanked me profusely, since he would have had some dark nights without a headlamp until he got to Damascus. From the small parking area, I crossed the road and headed south. Shortly, I ran into the Noodleheads from Colorado again. I would see many of the same thru-hikers that I had seen the day before. It was clear for the moment, and the Noodleheads were trying to dry themselves out. I didn't think it would work, because it started to rain again soon after I left them. It had rained hard overnight, and would shower off and on for the next two days.

The easy trail and grade over the four miles to Double Springs Shelter did not take long. My camera stayed in my pack because of the rain. At the shelter, some of the thru-hikers I'd met the day before were there, trying to dry out. It stopped raining long enough for me to eat my lunch. A few more thru-hikers came in. As I was leaving, Philly Steve came by. He already knew about how the Sixers were doing in the basketball playoffs. It started to rain heavily. Mudbug came by holding an umbrella. He was the only hiker I could remember who used one. Tree Trunk and Manula came by.

From the shelter, it was an easy downhill. The last mile was through cow pastures in the rain. The cows barely acknowledged me. It stopped raining when I got to the Cross Mountain trailhead. The couple from California was there. She was limping more than ever. She still had over 20 miles to get to Damascus. I again offered help, but they declined. I was early and figured I would have to wait for John, but in a few minutes, he pulled in. His cooler was well stocked. We retrieved my car, and headed to our Abingdon motel, through Damascus. We made arrangements at the outfitter there for a shuttle in the morning. We said we would be there at 9:00 A.M.

It was great to catch up with John over the next few days. He was a lineman on the high school football team, but weighed less now than high school. He keeps himself in good shape by biking. He and his wife Kim biked a lot, and had just gotten back from a New York City ride that included all five boroughs and went over the Verrazano Narrows Bridge. They had done some B&B rides in several places, and even did a century ride (100 miles). He had never hiked much at all since the Army (Ranger School; he had some stories), and was a little worried about it. He did not need to be, and I believe we were pretty equal, ability wise. It worked out well.

For John's first day out, he decided to oversleep. We were about 10 minutes late getting to our shuttle in Damascus, which seemed to annoy the driver. He had a schedule. He took us out to McQueen Gap. The dirt road up the mountain was poor, which is why we decided to get a shuttle rather than use our two cars. I'm glad we did. As the driver dropped us off, it started to pour. We scurried to put on our rain gear, paid the driver, and he was down the road. I think John wanted to call after him, having second thoughts. The rain let up, but we kept our rain jackets on all day, mostly because of the fog and mist. There really were not any viewpoints on this section. It would be 11 miles to the center of Damascus.

The trail could not have been easier along the ridge of Holston Mountain. Other than a rise or two of a hundred feet, it was level until the last four miles downhill to Damascus, and then a street walk through town. We overtook Tree Trunk and Manula. When we broke for lunch, Mudbug came by, still with his umbrella. Since John lived in New Orleans when working, he seemed to know of mudbugs in the south, which was where Mudbug was from. We took some pictures at the Tennessee/Virginia line. Crossing it seemed like a big deal, as was arriving in Damascus.

Damascus, Virginia, may be the best-known and most popular trail town on the entire AT. The town caters to the hiking community, and is the home of "Trail Days". Trail Days is a five-day event, and a big deal. Tens of thousands of current and former AT hikers descend on the town. Daily showers are set up behind the Baptist Church. Free shuttles are provided into and out of town. Gear representatives are there, repairing and selling equipment. There is free food and medical screenings. The event culminates with the hiker parade, which tends to get a little crazy. Town officials have to caution that everyone must wear clothes. This year, Trail Days would be held the following week, beginning Wednesday, May 16. I had planned around it. The hard-core trail people were arriving in town early. Like I said, Trail Days is a big deal to some.

John and I hiked along the main street and took pictures of each other in front of Town Hall, the end of the section. We headed over to the ice cream place to get a bite to eat. Tree Trunk and Manula were there with a friend who was supporting their hike. They planned a zero (miles) day the next day.

John and I headed back to Abingdon. John knew Abingdon well. He and Kim stayed at a B&B in town the previous year when they did some biking on the Virginia Creeper Trail. We went to one of the restaurants that he and Kim had been to. John was a disciplined eater, and never had more than one drink at dinner. Smart. That is how he kept the pounds off. I could learn from him.

I had a section to fill in up in the Grayson Highlands, so the next morning John and I headed up the interstate to Marion and Virginia 16. We stopped at Mount Rodgers HQ so I could show him the facility and the nearby Partnership Shelter. We continued on to the Fox Creek Trailhead along Virginia 603. We dropped my car and drove around to the Grayson Highlands State Park. There were few cars in the lots, unlike July of the year before when I was there. It was a quiet Friday in May. We headed up the access trail from the parking lot to Massie Gap. It was still a little damp, and out in the open terrain, there was a cool chill. The weather would break, and eventually the sun would come out.

From Massie Gap we headed north along Wilburn Ridge. There were spectacular views, even with the gray sky. We both loved it. We met two trail crews from Konnarock, working the ridge. John kept saying he wanted to bring Kim back there some time. He did the next spring. After a break at the Wise Shelter, we hiked in the woods of the Little Wilson Creek Wilderness, but were soon on the open ridge again. Later, I spotted what I thought might be wild ponies ahead, and pointed them out. As we approached, we confirmed the sighting. They were very near the trail, and we could get them to eat the apples I had cut up in the morning. The animals were shyer than the ones I had seen at the conference the year before. It was neat to see, and John was enjoying himself. I'm not sure John had a bad day in his life.

We continued on to the "The Scales," once the site of scales to weigh cattle before being shipped to market. The cattle had grazed in the highlands. The area was now used by horses and riders, as several horse trails intersect here. We were only half-done our hike, and still had five miles in the woods. At the intersection of the Pine Mountain Trail we met Wren and Robin. They were inspired, new hikers, out for the day. Their husbands would pick them up at their finish. We decided to stop and eat lunch. Robin talked about hiking in the Whites this summer, going hut to hut. I did not say anything, but she must have noticed my big eyes. I told her a little about it, but did not discourage her.

As we hiked on, the trail had some roots and rocks, but no big deal to me. John did not care for it as much. He preferred the highlands. At the Old Orchard Shelter we met a guy and a girl thru-hiker. The girl had a crazy get up, with a loud skirt, shirt and bandana. She was fast, and soon passed us, flying by. The guy came out of the woods when we were at my car. We offered him a beer, but he preferred a soda, which we did not have. He did take the granola bars we offered, just trying to keep up his calorie intake.

We drove around to get John's car, and then headed out the Crooked Road to Damascus. It was a long hike, and a lot of driving today. The people at the ice cream store were getting to know us. We had a late dinner.

On Saturday we planned a short hike before our drive home. It was only

5.6 miles from Straight Branch back to Damascus. This was my last day to finish Virginia, which I had started eight years earlier in 2004. We left John's car in town and headed back out US 58, the Crooked Road again. It was only four miles. We actually had a little trouble finding the trail from the small parking area along the road, but were soon ascending up to Feathercamp Ridge. There were some nice views along the way on the easy, moderately graded trail. On the way down to the car, here came Tree Trunk and Manula again. I think I saw them five times. They were headed to Marion, Virginia this time, 80 miles up the trail, where they would meet their support person again for another zero day. Their picture was in the March 2013 AT magazine at the Katahdin signboard. They were 2,000-milers.

A flight of steps took us down to Main Street and along the Creeper Trail into town. I had completed the AT in Virginia. It seemed like a big deal. John recognized it. We retrieved my car, had an ice cream, and we both headed home. I heard from John over the next few days. He said he was a little stiff, but enjoyed himself and thought he might do it again sometime.

I was home in time for Bethany's graduation from NYU's Stern School of Business, getting her MBA. Graduation was at Radio City Music Hall. She had left Steinway after 10 years to work for a large financial institution. She would have 10 national accounts that she was responsible for in the credit card division. She wanted to diversify her experience, but did not rule out the possibility of getting back into the music industry, and did not burn any bridges. Steinway helped her buy a new piano in the fall to replace the one she lost in the fire, giving her a discount as if she still worked there. Kevin got a new job as well.

Ben's son John was six months old now, and getting interesting. Ben had been doing some business traveling to Europe and China, but now that he was a dad, did not like being away. He and Michelle are great, loving, attentive parents.

I would spend the summer hiking in New Hampshire and Maine. It was tough up there. I completed my 9th and 10th Triathlons. I was down another minute on my time at the New Jersey State event in July. LeBron James and the Miami Heat won the NBA title, and the London Olympic Games had come and gone. Lance Armstrong was stripped of his Tour De France titles.

I heard from John in September after his summer season at his place on Bald Head Island. He had joined the ATC. I think he thought I gave them his name. He was bitten by the AT bug. We planned a week in October. John would hike with me three days before leaving on a 2-week trip to Yosemite and the Northwest. We would hike in the Roan Mountain area.

I left home on Tuesday, October 10. I had planned to make up a tiny missed section near Humpback Rocks, but got a late start due to a funeral. A long-retired partner of the firm passed away after a long illness. His wife was a hero, caring for him at home as long as she could. I rolled into Salem, Virginia after 10:00 P.M., but was still up early the next morning and on the road.

For Wednesday, I planned to make up the 3.7 miles just south of Damascus from Low Gap to McQueen's Gap. I arrived in Shady Valley, Tennessee, and put my boots on in the parking lot of the closed general store. Shady Valley was the home of The Cranberry Festival, lettering on the water tower said right next to the blinking light on Tennessee 91. It was a cloudy but pleasant day. It was a 4-mile drive up to the ridge on US 421 to Low Gap. It looked like an easy hike, and it was. I would have to hike it round trip, a first for me. From the valley, I could see fog covering the mountain. It was like soup at the trailhead. The leaves were heavy on the small parking lot.

From Low Gap, I headed north. There were no views on the section, which was a good thing, since I could not have seen anything through the low clouds. I did not see a soul this day. It was eerie. There was a stone wall next to the trail for 100 yards. The McQueen Gap Shelter was the most dilapidated structure I had seen on the trail. It was built in 1934. I reached McQueen's Gap road and decided to eat a sandwich. No cars came by. I turned around and headed back to my car. I was finished in three hours.

I continued on to Roan Mountain, Tennessee. John and I arrived there within minutes of each other, and we drove over to the Visitor's Center of Roan Mountain State Park to look at the maps of the area. The displayed map was the ATC map for this section, so I already had it. There was not much to see at the visitor's center, so we headed to our motel in Erwin, Tennessee, which would be our home for four nights. It was great to see John again, and we got caught up at dinner.

Our hike on Thursday would be nine miles, from Iron Mountain Gap to Hughes Gap. We headed out Tennessee 107 from Erwin to the top of the ridge at Iron Mountain Gap. The trail in this area runs right along the Tennessee/North Carolina border. Once you cross the state line, all the state route numbers change. We continued with two cars to Buladean, North Carolina, and then across to Hughes Gap. We dropped my car (and the cooler) at Hughes Gap, and headed back to Iron Mountain Gap, where we would start our hike. The hike looked easy on the elevation profile. It was. The trail was nice. It was cool on top of the mountain, and we had long pants and heavy shirts. In two hours we were at Greasy Creek Gap. A hand-written sign indicated the way to a nearby hostel. One said to not go to the southeast, but to go the other way. It did not matter to us, since we were sticking to the trail. There was a mildly tough climb up to Little Rock Knob. It was 500 feet in half a mile. It was the toughest climbing John had seen on the trail so far. Our hike of the next day would be very much like it, but 2,000 feet over two miles up to Roan Mountain. At cliffs along Little Rock Knob, we enjoyed our only view of the day, to the north and west.

From Little Rock Knob it was an easy down to Hughes Gap. We met Hans Solo from Ohio. It was his fifth year of section-hiking the trail. While we were enjoying a beer at Hughes Gap, a large pickup came roaring into the small trailhead lot. Two women acting frantically jumped out of the truck and each took off on the AT in different directions. One of the women was the owner of the Greasy Creek hostel.

Their story was that they had a neighbor who was always creating problems for them. He had posted signs near the trailhead telling hikers that the hostel was closed due to a family death, which was not true. He was apparently a mean old fart, and was a constant problem for them. There was nothing the police could do for the hostel owner. The women retrieved the signs, but it seemed like the guy would go to great lengths to hurt the hostel business, like mowing his lawn at 6:00 A.M. After the women left to go back to their bottle of wine, John and I realized that the sign we had seen at Greasy Creek Gap was another of his pranks. He was trying to direct hikers in the wrong direction. We did not think of it in time to tell them.

As we were still there, two hikers came out of the woods from the north.

One was a former thru-hiker from Asheville, who was out for a long week-end with a neighbor kid. The kid had just been expelled from school, and the hiker was trying to get him out in the woods to get his head straight. We talked to them a while, and we offered the man a beer and the kid a Gato-rade. The kid seemed nice, and it was hard to imagine what he had done.

Our Super 8 Motel in Erwin was quite nice, with pleasant, accommo-dating owners. The price was right. I have found motels in Virginia and Tennessee to be very low-priced compared to the northeast. There were slim pickings for dinner in Erwin, so John and I drove up the interstate to John-son City, and ended up in the hotel sports bar where I ate back in May.

The next day we had a very short (5-mile) hike, climbing Roan Moun-tain from the south. We did not need to rush in the morning, so agreed to meet an hour later than normal. We had an hour drive back over to the burg of Roan Mountain, and then the 10 miles up the mountain to Carver's Gap. Carver's Gap has large, paved parking lots in this beautiful area. We left John's car and headed back down to the mountain to a cutoff road to get to Hughes Gap.

It was a cloudy day, and there would be some fog on top of the moun-tain. The elevation profile on my map looked fierce. It would be 2.6 miles, climbing 2,200 feet. It never seemed that difficult. A lot of work was being done on the trail in this area. I suspect that Bob Peoples had his fingerprints all over it. My book and maps were dated 2005. A new set was in the works. The old closed trail was visible, with a direct route. Beautiful new trail had been built using switchbacks, mitigating the formerly tough grade. Some of the new trail was cobblestone-like. Stone steps were plentiful. I understand that over ninety percent of the AT has been relocated since the original was built. This is not easy work.

We climbed leisurely up the grade on easy trail. On the climb, we met a group from Indiana, and another from Ohio. Both groups were section-hik-ers of the trail, and backpacking this beautiful section along the North Carolina/Tennessee border in the Roan Mountain area. We reached the site of the former Cloudland Hotel. I was really surprised about how easy the climb had been. On a rock face at a high point we met Larry from Tennes-see. Larry, a late-60s but weathered old guy, was section-hiking this year, but planning a thru-hike for the following year. He had stayed at Bob Peoples' hostel in Hampton, and talked about a run-in Bob had with the old fart neighbor of the Greasy Creek hostel owner. Bob apparently started up his chain saw when the man confronted him. Larry had not officially taken his trail name of Blizzard yet. He picked the name from his favorite DQ ice cream dessert.

As Larry walked away to the south, a dad and his two teenage girls that we had passed earlier were coming back up the mountain to head over to Carver's Gap. The area around the former Cloudland Hotel was an open and grassy field. The sign said "the hotel reflected the grand style of the late 1800s." The hotel was built on the North Carolina/Tennessee border. A stripe was painted down the middle of the floor. Alcohol was only allowed on one side. Unlike many of these old wooden hotels on mountain tops that had burned down, this one was actually dismantled after it closed in 1910.

It was another half-mile to the short side trail to the shelter at Roan High Knob. There was a damp chill in the air. It looked like the shelter would be busy tonight. A family from western Canada was huddled around a fire near the high point on a rock which was at elevation 6,285 feet, only 3 feet less than the summit of Mount Washington. After John took my picture on the rock, we spoke to the Canadians for a while. The young couple were southbound thru-hikers, who started at Katahdin on June 18. The wife's parents had joined them for a week of hiking. A few days earlier they had stayed at Mountain Harbor B&B, where I planned to stay a few days later. They were shivering around the smoky fire.

From the shelter, it was an easy descent on nice trail to the parking lot at Carver's Gap. We lingered over a beer at the car. The parking lot was full now. Many must have come in to hike the area over the weekend. We retrieved my car at Hughes Gap and after a shower, had dinner at a nice steakhouse in Johnson City.

The next day would be John's last, and a 14-mile day. My guide book described it well. "The traverse of the high balds of Hump Mountain, Yellow Mountain and the eastern portion of Roan Mountain is one of the most spectacular parts of the entire trail, with superb views from treeless meadows above 5,000 feet. Several of the finest remaining southern Appalachian balds are found here." It was all of that and more. Since it was mid-October, few of the wild flowers that dominate the open meadows in the spring and summer remained. I made a note to myself to visit Carver's Gap at that time of year.

John and I left my car down in the town of Roan Mountain at the AT trailhead on US 19E. We drove by it a few times until we found the small 2-car lot. Then we drove up the mountain again to Carver's Gap. Even though it was early on this Saturday, the parking lot was full, and we had to park along the road. It was breezy on the summits of the balds, but the weather was breaking, and some sun was peeking through the clouds. John wore gloves, being the southerner he had become. I was glad for my wind shirt. The change in the weather was a major break for us, and we would have spectacular views all day.

The hike to the first summit, Round Bald, was on easy, well-maintained trail. It was less than a mile. This would be a great hike for even a young family to enjoy a nice easy outing. Extensive work was done on the trail to protect the fragile humus of the area. From Round Bald we could pick out each of our successive peaks; Jane Bald, Grassy Ridge, Little Hump Mountain and the massive Hump Mountain almost eight miles away. It looked far, and the visual distance was intimidating to both of us.

Walking along the ridge was great, with unbelievable views both east to North Carolina and west into Tennessee. The fall colors across to adjacent mountains were past peak at this higher elevation. They were still beautiful. Everyone should experience this and can, even from Carver's Gap. It was very interesting to arrive at each summit and look back or forward at the well-defined trail. Many weekend hikers along the route looked tiny in the cols between the peaks.

From Grassy Bald, the trail descended into a scrub forest of small trees. All the leaves were down at elevation, so you did not have a sense if the trees were living or dead. Larger and more mature living trees were in the area of the Stan Murray Shelter. Two couples were breaking camp. They had hiked in from Carver's Gap the day before, and were headed down to Route 19E over the next two days. That was our destination of tonight.

The next mile and a half was in the woods, until a brief climb to a summit that had more great views of where we had been and where we were going.

We descended into Yellow Mountain Gap. We heard some gunshots. A few miles later we encountered a local father-son hunting team. They had not discharged their guns, but they were aware of a friend who was also hunting in the area. A sign at the junction with the Overmountain Victory National Historic Trail told the story of 1,000 area militia who crossed the Gap in the bitter cold of September of 1780 to walk 170 miles to engage the British at Kings Mountain. The snow in the gap was "shoe mouth deep." We began the steep ascent of Little Hump Mountain. The trail emerged from the woods on the way. I had to stop a few times to catch my breath. John did not seem to be having any trouble. A young day-hiker from Carver's Gap sped by us. We looked back into the gap and could spot the Overmountain Shelter, which looked like a nice red barn.

We had lunch at the summit of Little Hump Mountain. We were just halfway on our day. John could spot the condo buildings along the ridge near Banner Elk, North Carolina where he had been skiing with his family years earlier. From Little Hump, the trail circled around the east side, rather than a more direct route to Hump Mountain. We were hearing chain saws for a while. Was it Bob Peoples working on new trail? The sun was out, and we could shed our wind shirts. I got down to short sleeves.

It was spectacular on the way to Hump Mountain. We were soon in the col between Little Hump and Hump. There were several false summits on the way up Hump. Just as we thought we were arriving at the top, another apparent peak appeared in front of us. Then again. Finally we were there, on top of the massive, open summit mountain. We were meeting several people now who had hiked in from US 19E for the day. An older guy warned us about the difficult trail on the north side of Hump Mountain on our way down. The hike down would be 2,700 feet over the next five miles. It did not appear that steep on the elevation profile. The first mile was still in open balds down the east side of Hump. After entering the woods, the descent started out somewhat tough, but not nearly what I had become used to in the Mahoosucs. Difficult is relative. The trail was filled with rocks and roots in spots. We passed a group of five mixed-age women. Some seemed to be having difficulty, and they were headed south and up the mountain. It was getting later, and I'm not sure where they were planning to stay for the evening. There would be no place to camp out on the balds. They had a way to go to get to the tentsite at Bradley Gap.

It was well over an hour after entering the woods until we arrived at Doll Flats. At this point, the AT leaves North Carolina and enters Tennessee for good. There were four young guys completing setup of their solo tents. They were from Asheville, and were out for the weekend. They were hiking our hike but over three days, and staying out two nights. We ate our final snack of the day as we swapped stories of hiking and camping. As John and I were leaving, three young girls were arriving at the tent site. One had a pack, the other two did not. They all seemed out of place. We wondered if they were "surprising" the guys.

The grade continued down and was getting easier, but was becoming long. A viewpoint across the valley showed a perfectly rowed Christmas tree farm. I took the lead for a while and picked up the pace. John was on my heels. We both were looking forward to seeing what was in our cooler at John's car. When we got to the Apple House Shelter we went on by, barely acknowledging the occupants. We crossed the bridge over Buck Creek and were at the car. It was a long but very rewarding day of hiking. The beer tasted good. We still had to drive up the mountain to get the car and then back to Erwin. After a quick shower, we drove over to Johnson City for a late dinner.

John was driving home the next morning, but agreed to shuttle me before leaving. After an early breakfast, we checked out and dropped my car at Iron Mountain Gap, where we started our hiking earlier in the week. He drove me back to town and back up the ridge to Indian Grave Gap so I could begin my 11-mile day. John was then off to Raleigh.

From Indian Grave Gap I was climbing immediately, and it would be two miles up to Beauty Spot, on an old woods road for the first mile. It was easy. It appeared there had been a fire on the mountain. New scrub trees were starting to grow. After a gravel road crossing, the trail emerged from the woods and climbed in an open grassy area. You could see the trail pick its way to the summit of Beauty Spot. At the summit there were great views south toward Erwin. It was a sunny morning. We were in Pisgah National Forest, so I was surprised to see what appeared to be a cul-de-sac with a truck parked there. It almost seemed like the beginning of a development at the top of the mountain. My map said there were some roads and a parking lot in the area. I guess it was just access to other trails in the Unaka Mountain Wilderness which I would be skirting, but not entering.

I headed down and left the bald and was soon at Beauty Spot Gap. From there, I began the long ascent of Unaka Mountain. The summit of Unaka was a dense, dark hemlock forest, with a clean dirt floor. On the way down and out to the road, I passed several groups, all of whom John and I had seen a few days earlier. It was Larry (Blizzard) from Tennessee, the groups from Ohio and Indiana, and three single guys. They were continuing on their section hike. Some were planning to stay in the hostel in Erwin. They would be there the next day.

I stopped and ate my sandwich at Low Gap. An Asian southbound thru-hiker came by. It became cloudy and windy. I continued on a short distance to the Cherry Gap Shelter, which was deserted. The forest was beginning to claim Piney Bald and Little Bald Knob, but there still were limited views down into the valleys and Roan Mountain stood in the distance. It was an easy last mile to my car at Iron Mountain Gap.

I had made good time, so lingered at the trailhead a while to see who might pop out of the woods. Two southbound thru-hikers came along, but did not stay. They were in a hurry to get to the hostel in Erwin. Two old guys from Atlanta came down the mountain. They were 69 and 70, and were hiking the section from US 19E in Roan Mountain to Erwin this trip. One seemed to be struggling and was out of water. I gave him all I had. They were planning to stay at the Cherry Gap Shelter for the evening. I judged it would take two hours for them to get there with their big packs. Once they left, I packed up the cooler and drove over to the B&B and hostel where I planned to be the next two nights.

Mountain Harbor Bed and Breakfast and Hiker's Hostel is a beautiful spot within half a mile of the AT in the town of Roan Mountain. It was run by Mary and Terry, 60-somethings who had lived in California all their lives. Moving from California to the hills of Tennessee had to be quite the culture shock. Terry and Mary purchased it in 2003, a few years after it was opened.

The main home had three B&B rooms on the second floor. There was a large, welcoming, nicely decorated country kitchen/great room with a huge big screen TV, a separate dining room, and Terry and Mary's living quarters all on the main level. Mary's breakfasts (served at 9:00 A.M.) were to die for. There was a separate hostel cabin on the property that seemed way above traditional hostels from what I could tell from the pictures, although I never actually saw the inside.

A creek ran through the property, and two goats grazed the banks of the creek. Horses out back were harassed by one of their dogs. I checked into one of the B&B rooms for two nights. Cody was staying in the hiker hostel, and came out to greet me until she realized I was not the friend she was waiting for. Cody had thru-hiked the trail in 2011 and planned a reunion hike with a buddy and some other friends over the balds of the Roan Mountain area.

I drove into North Carolina to try to find dinner, but ended up at Mickey D's.

Breakfast on Monday morning was very busy. Cody and her crew were there. Three guys from New Jersey had arrived late Sunday night and were planning a 3-day hike over the balds. Janet and her son Ron were staying in one of the B&B rooms. They were from Florida, and were section hiking from Erwin to Damascus (over 100 miles) prior to Ron's upcoming wedding. Janet was game, but I think it was a little tough for her and she was having issues with her feet, not to mention her big pack. They would take a zero day on Monday, and I would see them the next morning at breakfast.

For my hike on Monday, Terry would shuttle me up to Walnut Mountain Road and I would hike the 10 trail miles south back to Mountain Harbor. Soon after Terry dropped me and I started down the trail, I heard Terry talking to someone who was parked at the trailhead. In five minutes, three guys hiking north came by. They saw my Philadelphia Eagles hat and wanted to know about all the Sunday games, including the Atlanta Falcons. They were from Atlanta. They said they were only going to the road and that Bob Peoples was picking them up. That was who Terry must have been talking to. Bob Peoples is everywhere.

The first four miles was a very easy gradual downhill to Elk River. After the three guys from Atlanta in the first five minutes, I would not see a soul the rest of the day. The leaves were heavy on the trail. Heavy rains overnight prevented the normal *whoosh* of leaf walking. There was a pretty small water-fall about an hour in. There was some rhododendron tunnel walking. The trail then followed along Elk River on a very easy footpath until beginning the long gradual climb up to Buck Mountain Road. I thought I heard voices and I was expecting to bump into Janet and Ron, not knowing at that point they had taken a day off. No one ever appeared.

Half a mile up the hill, I came to the junction for a side trail to Jones Falls. It was early, and only one-tenth of a mile, so I walked over. It was well worth the effort to see the nice, full-flowing falls from the overnight rains. It was a good spot for lunch. At the trail junction someone wrote a note on a 3x5 card to not miss this one (the falls). They were right. After lunch, I con-tinued climbing and entered an abandoned Christmas tree farm. The thick, perfectly rowed forest made for a dark hike for five minutes. It was eerie. I crossed Buck Mountain Road next to a cute as a button little church and continued up, circling around Isaacs Cemetery before reaching the summit. The views from the summit were great of all the surrounding mountains to the south and west and down into the valley as well. The visibility was very good this day, despite the somewhat gray sky.

I began the 900-foot descent to the Town of Roan Mountain, through open pasture at first, before entering Bishop Hollow. The half-mile hike directly down the hollow in overgrown fields was interesting, as you could see the valley below all the way down. I don't remember such an experience before. At these lower elevations, the leaves were still in nice color. I crossed a bridge and a road and a few more tenths and I was at US 19E. A car stopped to ask me where the trailhead was. They decided to park their car at Moun-tain Harbor, where many do who section hike in the area.

It was early and quiet when I arrived back at Mountain Harbor. I decided to drive over to Banner Elk, North Carolina for dinner. It was a quaint little ski town and quiet this time of year. I found a good place at a local sports bar for dinner.

I decided I needed to get home for some personal business and aban-doned my last day's hike. I packed up early and waited for Mary's breakfast before beginning my drive home. It was only me and Janet and her son for breakfast. Those in the hostel often did not wait (or want to pay) for breakfast at the later hour.

On the way home, I planned to fill in some missed blazes up at Reed's Gap and Humpback Rocks in Virginia. I arrived at Reed's Gap. A few cars were there. I hiked north on the AT for only half a mile to reach the parking area where I had cheated and walked down the road. I'm not sure why I would have done that. The half-mile could not have been easier. I turned around and walked back. I think I was away from my car for 30 minutes.

Driving up the Blue Ridge Parkway, I stopped at the lookout again and met a local section hiker out with his dog. He told me the shelter where he was planning to go. It was only another few miles. He needed water, so I gave him all I had. I continued up the Blue Ridge Parkway to Humpback Rocks. I did not have my Virginia map and book, so was not exactly sure which trail to take, so I went over to the visitor's center to get a map. Once I figured out where to go, it was past 4PM, so I decided to skip it and do it another time. There would still be many more days driving down Interstate 81.

That was it for the year. I had logged only 41 miles in the north and 117 in the south for a total of 158. My mileage was disappointing to me, but progress none the less. I did have a great time and was looking forward to some more "good" parts of the trail. For 2013, I had the challenges of Maine, the beautiful balds of the southern Appalachians, and the Cullowhee AT trail conference to look forward to. I couldn't wait.

By the end of 2012, I had gained back all of the weight I had lost at the beginning of 2011. I had to find that discipline again. My cumulative hiking now had carried me 1,534 miles in 162 days. I was now over 70% of the trail and had only about 650 miles to go, 300 in the north and 350 in the south. I was not making predictions any more about when I might finish. I'm hoping my body holds up. Before the end of the year, I had my Medicare card.

In October, Hurricane Sandy made landfall in New Jersey and New York, resulting in 110 deaths and billions in property damage. Power outages throughout the northeast of up to a week or longer were common. Some communities may never recover. In December, a 20-year-old man stole his mother's guns, killed her and 26 people at a school where she volunteered, including 20 first-graders. It hit us all like a ton of bricks as we wept for the families. The Mayan "end of the world" came and went.

For Christmas, Virginia gave me the newly ATC published book, *The Appalachian Trail-Celebrating America's Hiking Trail.* The history of how the trail happened was very interesting, the pictures were fantastic and brought back many memories, and together with the AT *Journeys* magazines and the ATC website, it is apparent that use of the trail, particularly by thru-hikers, is increasing.

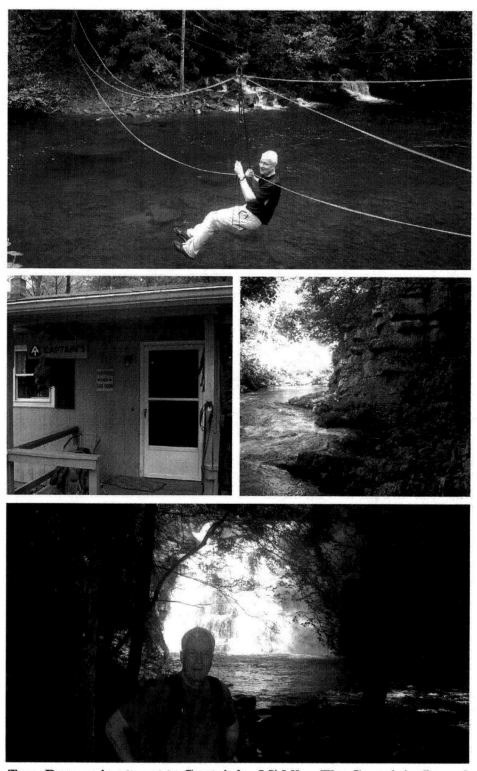

Top: Rope swing to get to Captain's. Middle: The Captain's; Laurel Fork Gorge. Bottom: Laurel Fork Falls.

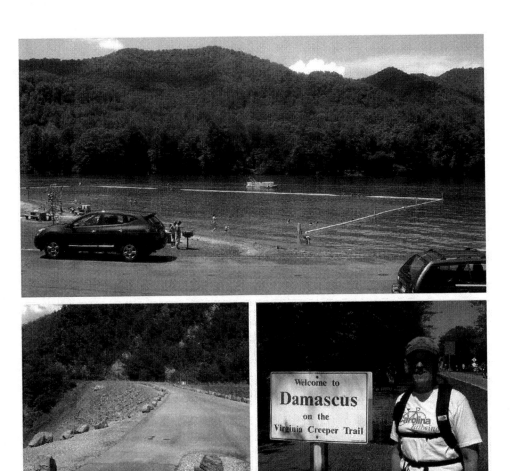

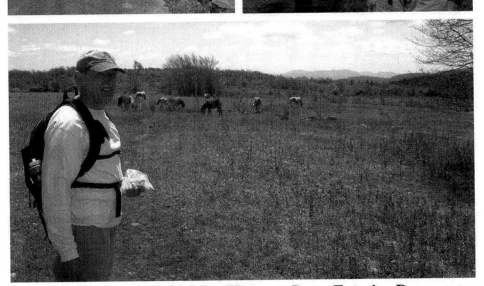

Top: Watauga Lake. Middle: Watauga Dam; Entering Damascus.
Bottom: John in the Grayson Highlands.

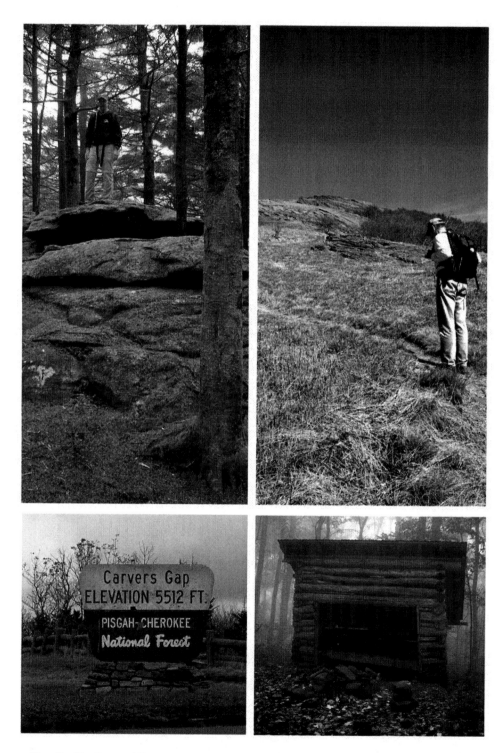

Top Left: Roan Mountain High Point. Top Right: Hump Mountain.
Bottom Left: Carvers Gap. Bottom Right: The McQueen Gap Shelter.

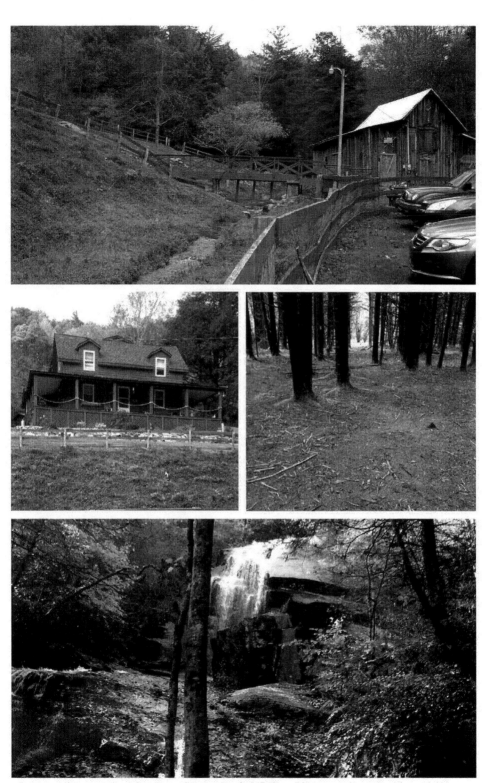

Top: Mountain Harbor Hostel. Middle: Mountain Harbor B&B; Unaka Mountain summit. Bottom: Jones Falls.

Epilogue

As I think about my 11 years (and counting) of hiking the AT, many things have changed in the world and my business and personal life. I consider myself to be very fortunate.

When I started hiking, I was 54. Now I'm eligible for Medicare.

My work life is still very important, but is no longer all consuming. I have no plan to retire, but am fortunate that I can gradually phase down my responsibilities at the firm as I choose. I still work hard during tax season, but can take time in the summer to continue my AT quest. I have five trips, including the Cullowhee conference, planned for 2013.

Ben and Bethany have grown from early 20-something new college graduates to their mid-30s with good careers, marriages and now a grandson for Virginia and me.

Virginia has her own interests, but makes my home life very easy in our new condo.

I have become a gym rat and even though I yo-yo with the weight, I have permanently lost 40 pounds. The health benefits are there. I take no meds and feel great, except for the stress (I don't know what I have to be stressed about) that creeps in now and then. I expect to be around a long time. Both my parents are in their 90s and doing fine.

I did not start hiking the trail because I needed something to do, but now it is a part of what I do, who I am, and what I think and talk about. The trail grabs you and won't let go.

When I started hiking, I knew almost nothing about it. I don't claim to be an expert on the trail, but have learned quite a bit by going to the AT conferences, visiting communities and hostels along the way, but mostly talking to all the hikers in the Appalachian Trail community. Most people in the east seem to know someone who has hiked the trail. The AT hiking numbers are growing by leaps and bounds.

Thru-hikers are probably the most recognized and thought of as the way to hike the AT. Northbounders (NOBO) and Southbounders (SOBO) hike with full packs. A few do fully supported slack packs. I have learned however, that there are also many who section hike the trail over periods of up to 20 years. All can report their completion to the ATC for recognition in the annual report. Many use a combination of backpacking and slack packing. I have just chosen to try to hike the entire trail by not sleeping on the ground. I hope to finish it that way. There is more than one way to hike the Appalachian Trail.

When I started the AT, I had no thoughts about ever actually finishing it. Now it is in sight. Not in my wildest thoughts did I think I would write a book about it. Finishing the trail will be my book two.

This book was rattling around in my head and had to come out. It did not seem hard. I look forward to hearing from those who might recognize themselves as they read along. I hope I did not offend. The people of the trail are really what it is all about. Not just getting from point A to point B.

See you on the trail.

Acknowledgements

Most every day I hiked, there was a shuttle driver who met me in the morning and then drove me to my starting point. I mentioned all of them in the book and I thank them all. Thank goodness for those willing to do this for us day hikers.

Although I did not stay in many hostels, my experiences at the Dutch House, Woods Hole, and Mountain Harbor were terrific. The warm environments that they offered were very appreciated by this day hiker.

The ongoing assistance of the Keane family in Maine is much appreciated. Maine is tough.

Thanks to Lee Ann at First Editing and Josh for his photo shop expertise on the collages.

Mostly thanks to my wife Virginia who could not have been more supportive of this venture for the last eleven years. She was my first shuttle driver and then became the supreme lunch packer and checklist verifier. As my travels grow more distant, she works hard to make sure I have the food and supplies that I need for the time I am away. She always knew where I was hiking and who to call if she did not hear from me. Virginia was a big help with the editing also, but she would not have needed to read the book. She lived it.